Risk Management in Transfusion Medicine

Risk Management in Transfusion Medicine

J. MILLS BARBEAU, MD, JD
Alpert Medical School of Brown University
Director of Laboratory Medicine
Department of Pathology and Laboratory Medicine
Lifespan Academic Medical Center
Providence, RI, United States

ELSEVIER

ELSEVIER

3251 Riverport Lane
St. Louis, Missouri 63043

RISK MANAGEMENT IN TRANSFUSION MEDICINE   ISBN: 978-0-323-54837-3

Publisher: Dolores Melani
Acquisition Editor: Robin Carter
Editorial Project Manager: Karen R. Miller
Production Project Manager: Poulouse Joseph
Cover Designer: Alan Studholme

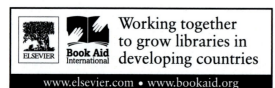

Working together to grow libraries in developing countries

www.elsevier.com • www.bookaid.org

Acknowledgment:
For Debbie

List of Contributors

Caroline R. Alquist, MD, PhD, D(ABHI)
Section of Transfusion Medicine and
    Histocompatibility
Department of Pathology and Laboratory Medicine
Ochsner Health System, and Assistant Professor
Ochsner Clinical School, University of Queensland
    School of Medicine
New Orleans, LA, United States

J. Mills Barbeau, MD, JD
Alpert Medical School of Brown University
Director of Laboratory Medicine
Department of Pathology and Laboratory Medicine
Lifespan Academic Medical Center
Providence, RI, United States

John R. Hess, MD, MPH, FACP, FAAAS
Professor of Laboratory Medicine and Hematology
University of Washington School of Medicine
Medical Director
Transfusion Service
Harborview Medical Center
Seattle, WA, United States

Joseph D. Sweeney, MD, FACP, FRCPath
Director
Coagulation and Transfusion Medicine
Professor of Pathology and Laboratory Medicine
Alpert Medical School of Brown University
Providence, RI, United States

Sarah Vossoughi, MD
Fellow of Transfusion Medicine
Columbia University/New York Blood Center
    Columbia University
Irving Medical Center
New York, NY, United States

Stuart P. Weisberg, MD, PhD
Assistant Professor of Pathology and Cell Biology
Department of Pathology and Cell Biology
Columbia University
New York, NY, United States

Preface

Welcome, reader. It is a pleasure to introduce the book *Risk Management in Transfusion Medicine*. The timing of this book is auspicious—there is currently an increasing awareness of the importance of risk management in healthcare. Blood transfusions are high-risk, potentially fatal, and among the most common procedures performed in medical practice. The complexity involved in the safe delivery of such a vast amount of blood from vein to vein every day is staggering. Transfusion Medicine is therefore an ideal vehicle for illustrating risk management concepts.

The ultimate goal of this book is to give the reader a profound understanding of risk management, not just in the context of transfusion medicine, but in healthcare generally. Readers who happen to find themselves sitting on hospital Boards of Directors should feel quite comfortable with their risk management responsibilities. Of course, one will inevitably learn a great deal about blood safety by reading this book, and readers who are involved in blood safety, quality, and clinical best practices will find this resource to be particularly valuable.

Please note that the term "transfusion medicine" is used in the text as an umbrella term that includes transfusion medicine, blood banking, and cellular therapy. More specific terms are used as appropriate.

—JMB

Contents

CHAPTER 1

Enterprise Risk Management—What It Is and Why It Matters

J. MILLS BARBEAU, MD, JD

INTRODUCTION

"Risk" can mean many things. Risk connotes an absence of safety, and the possibility of suffering a loss. In healthcare, patient safety efforts concentrate on risks such as the risk of falling or the performance of "risky" procedures. We use timeouts to minimize the risk of wrong-side surgery. Risk is associated with potential financial loss, legal liability, or both. Yet, we also talk about risk being related to opportunity, as when we decide that something is "worth the risk." In decision making, we frequently "weigh the risks," including the risk of doing nothing, before choosing a course of action. The corporate world defines risk as any factor that can jeopardize the organization's ability to achieve its business objectives.[1] Could this definition of risk apply to healthcare organizations?

What, then, is risk management? In practice, risk management typically involves identifying risks and minimizing them—by eliminating the risks, implementing procedures to reduce the risks, educating personnel on how to avoid the risks, or buying insurance to outsource the financial impact of the risks. Risk management is typically performed within a given service's span of responsibility, at the level of a department, unit, or division. A threshold issue is whether such a balkanized approach to risk management is maximally effective, or whether it might be preferable to address risks at the organizational level, taking advantage of economies of scale. One may counter that a local approach to risk management effectively brings risks to the attention of those with the most expertise and experience regarding risks in their spheres of activity. In addition, human nature being what it is, managing risk across departmental domains may give rise to feelings that one group is criticizing another or otherwise overstepping its bounds.

The term "enterprise risk management" (ERM) may not be familiar to most healthcare professionals. This is largely because enterprise risk management did not originate in healthcare, but rather in the corporate world. Although ERM may not have become part of healthcare culture or consciousness at the provider level, the impact of ERM is nevertheless felt at all levels of any large healthcare organization. To appreciate why enterprise risk management is important, it is helpful to understand some interesting historic background.

SARBANES-OXLEY ACT OF 2002

Some readers may recall the Enron and WorldCom corporate fraud scandals of 2001. Both Enron and WorldCom were successful, respected companies that had thrived throughout the 1990s. Enron was a large energy company, named "America's Most Innovative Company" by Fortune Magazine for six consecutive years up to 2001.[2] In 1999, Enron started an electronic commodities-trading website, and soon thereafter, it invested heavily in high-speed broadband networks. Unfortunately for Enron's employees and investors, the "dot com" bubble burst, and the arrival of economic recession in 2000 led to multibillion dollar losses for many web-based companies.[3] In an attempt to hide its losses, Enron's executives—with the support of its accounting firm, Arthur Anderson—engaged in fraudulent accounting practices.[4,5] By the time the fraud was discovered, shareholders and employee pensions had lost billions of dollars. Enron and Arthur Anderson collapsed and Enron's CEO, Jeffrey Skilling, was convicted of fraud, insider trading, and conspiracy.

WorldCom was also a progressive telecommunications company that prospered during the 1990s. In 1997, WorldCom announced a merger with MCI Communications Corporation, which would be the largest corporate merger in the US history. Two years later, WorldCom announced a merger with Sprint. The proposed new company would be larger than AT&T. However, the Justice Department balked at the Sprint-WorldCom merger on anticompetitive grounds and the merger failed. By then, the telecommunications industry

Risk Management in Transfusion Medicine. https://doi.org/10.1016/B978-0-323-54837-3.00001-8

was in decline. When the merger failed, WorldCom share prices dropped precipitously. The company was no longer the darling of investors. Financial weakness in WorldCom's organization began to become apparent. Similar to the CEO at Enron, WorldCom's CEO, Bernard Ebbers, began to doctor the books with the assistance of the same accounting firm, Arthur Anderson.[6,7] Whistle blowers within the company sounded an alert,[8] and WorldCom plunged into a downward spiral. The company filed for bankruptcy in 2002.[9] Similar to Skilling, Ebbers' career ended in federal prison.[10]

In the wake of the Enron/WorldCom scandals and Arthur Anderson's collapse, Congress passed the Sarbanes-Oxley Act of 2002.[11] It had become clear that many corporations made a practice of hiring a single accounting firm to act as both external auditors and internal consultants, as was the case with Arthur Anderson. As external, "independent" auditors, the accountants would perform the corporation's annual external audit on behalf of investors and shareholders. During the rest of the year the same accountants were paid handsomely by the corporation to act as consultants. Thus, the accountants were in essence working for the corporation, and the external audits were a sham. Sarbanes-Oxley mandates that external auditors of publically traded corporations shall not have such conflicts of interest. Furthermore, CEOs are personally responsible for the accuracy of the company's financial reports. The CEO and senior executives must all personally verify the company's internal controls. "Internal controls" is an auditing term for risk management.[12]

The mandate to implement comprehensive internal controls (i.e., risk management practices) requires company leadership and the external auditor to perform a "top-down risk assessment" of the entire organization.[13,14] Specifically, the company must identify *all* factors that could jeopardize the company's ability to achieve its business objectives. Leadership must establish a "systems culture" in which control consciousness permeates the entire organization and systems are in place to identify and share information about risk. Comprehensive control activities, embodied in clear policies and procedures, must harmonize risk management across the enterprise, and the risk management process must be continuously monitored and improved.

The Sarbanes-Oxley Act has had a far-reaching impact, which extends into the realm of healthcare. Although compliance is mandatory only for publically traded corporations, the enterprise risk management paradigm has become the standard for all significant business enterprises. This makes good business sense. Not only do such practices protect against losses, but a comprehensive, fully integrated risk management program also favorably impacts a company's credit rating. After all, a company that has effectively minimized its risks is a less "risky" investment for shareholders and lenders. Healthcare organizations, similar to other large companies, avail themselves of bonds, loans, and capital markets. A good credit rating improves access to capital, which in turn enables organizations to seize business opportunities when they arise. Effective risk management can be a competitive advantage in competitive markets, healthcare[15] or otherwise.[16]

Enterprise risk management also allows the company to weather disruptive events. Market volatility and uncertainty, economic shocks, and new competition or technology can rapidly upset the competitive terrain (Fig. 1.1). An organization that has thoroughly

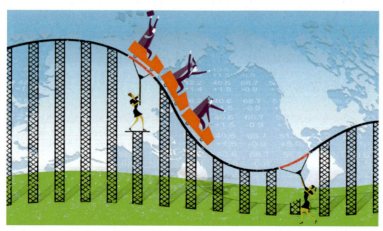

FIG. 1.1 An organization that has thoroughly assessed its vulnerabilities and prepared accordingly is better able to weather disruptive events, thus gaining a competitive advantage.

assessed its vulnerabilities and prepared accordingly will be better able to weather such events.[17] As a result, disruptive events disproportionately impact companies that are less prepared. The more resilient organizations find themselves emerging in a competitively advantageous position, demonstrating that a conscientiously applied risk management program can be a competitive business strategy.

It is no wonder that healthcare CEOs have taken notice of enterprise risk management. Similar to traditional, for-profit corporations, healthcare organizations also answer to boards of directors whose members are well versed in contemporary best business practices. In the present competitive healthcare environment, hospital leadership would be foolhardy not to have a robust ERM program in place. In 1980, the American Hospital Association established the American Society for Healthcare Risk Management (ASHRM), which is generally regarded as the leading professional membership group for practitioners in healthcare risk management. ASHRM publishes a textbook entitled "Risk Management Handbook for Healthcare Organizations," now in its sixth edition. The very first chapter of this 3-volume text is "Basics of Enterprise Risk Management in Healthcare."[18]

PERFORMING A RISK AUDIT

As we have seen, enterprise risk management involves identifying all risks across the enterprise, then managing those risks by controlling, eliminating, or outsourcing them. The process begins with an enterprise-wide risk audit organized around risk domains.

To envision the concept of risk domains, consider a stylized manufacturing facility, shown in Fig. 1.2:

Imagine that the company produces running shoes. The physical plant consists of land, buildings, and manufacturing equipment. Raw materials are purchased and brought to the factory to be turned into product. Investors have contributed capital to build the plant and purchase the raw materials, and the investors interests are represented by a board of directors. Employees operate the machines, and consumers pay money for the shoes. Tracking the cash flow, order processing, billing, and accounting are essential functions. Significantly, all of the company's business operations occur in a milieu of laws and regulations, including Occupational Safety and Health Administration (OSHA) and Environmental Protection Agency (EPA) regulations, labor laws, tax laws, corporate laws, and others.

The company's activities are carried out in a context of uncertainty and risk: Foreign and domestic competition, disruptive technology, consumer preferences, the global and domestic economy, and accessibility of money markets are all dynamic variables that can jeopardize the company's ability to achieve its business objectives.

The elements that go into manufacturing a product like running shoes are remarkably analogous to those of a healthcare organization. Place a siren and a red cross on the truck pictured in Fig. 1.2, and substitute consumer health in place of running shoes as the product being provided, and most of the elements of production remain unchanged. If one doubts the conveyor belt analogy, consider Fig. 1.3, taken from the author's office door, showing a contemporary, automated hospital laboratory:

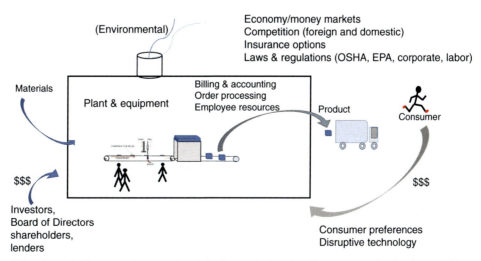

FIG. 1.2 This schematic illustrates the operational challenges facing virtually every organization that provides a product.

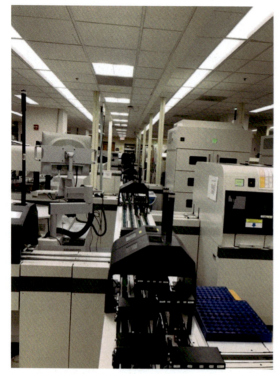

FIG. 1.3 Contemporary high-throughput clinical laboratories demonstrate many of the features seen in highly automated assembly lines.

TABLE 1.1
The ERM Process
• Catalog all risks in the organization using risk domains
• Identify the relationships among risks (break down "silos")
• This reveals the actual scope of each risk and reveals potential efficiencies in risk management
• Score the risks in terms of the likelihood of each potential harm (PROB) and severity should the harm occur (SEV)
• Assign a risk priority number (RPN) to each risk: (PROB) × (SEV) = (RPN).
• Assess each risk in light of the organization's strategic goals
• Given the enterprise's strategic goals, manage each risk by the following:
• Controlling the risk (policies/procedures to minimize risk);
• Outsourcing the risk (e.g., purchasing insurance); or
• Eliminating the risk (cease the activity)

In ERM, risk is defined as anything that can jeopardize the organization's ability to achieve its business objectives. Viewed in this light, the operational elements of the organization illustrated in Fig. 1.2 can be considered as "risk domains." The key functions that are carried out within the organization can be guideposts for a comprehensive risk audit of the entire organization. For a medical center, a comprehensive list of risk domains might consist of the following:

- Strategic plan (executive management)
- Operations and clinical activities
- Physical plant
- Financial and economic environment
- Regulatory and legal environment
- Technology and scientific innovation
- Human resources
- Hazards/disasters (natural, environmental, infectious, and terrorist)

Once the risk domains are defined, the comprehensive risk audit can begin.

ERM is based upon an organized set of activities, as shown in Table 1.1. The first step is to catalog all of the risks identified in each risk domain. Once that is accomplished, the next step is to identify the relationships among those risks, across all risk domains. This is an important precept of enterprise risk management: Once the risks are identified, tracing their interrelatedness across domains is crucial. One cannot prioritize a risk without knowing the true magnitude of that risk. It is therefore important to tally the extent of each risk across all risk domains.

Institutions tend to form silos, and as discussed earlier, there is often an unspoken assumption that risks should be assessed and managed within each service's span of responsibility. Each silo is familiar with its own risk profile, and is typically comfortable managing its own risks. However, a global risk may manifest differently throughout the organization.

Imagine an example involving patient identification in a large hospital. On admission, each patient is issued an armband that displays the patient's name, date of birth, medical record number, and CSN number (CSN stands for contact serial number, more commonly known as an "encounter" number). Several carefully crafted procedures instruct staff how to properly identify patients in the various settings in which patient identification is necessary, such as phlebotomy, radiology, laboratory specimen intake, and blood transfusion.

An enterprise-wide risk audit might discover that the blood bank's bar code reader sometimes captures the CSN number instead of the patient's medical record number. Meanwhile, Radiology has its own

Agency for Healthcare Research and Quality (AHRQ)

Statistical Brief #149, Feb 2013.

Blood transfusion is the most common procedure in hospitals

Transfusion risk management impacts all services in the organization

Table 1. Number of stays, stays per 10,000 population, and percentage change in rate of the most frequent all-listed procedures for hospital stays, 1997 and 2010

All-listed CCS procedures	Number of stays with the procedure in thousands		Stays with the procedure per 10,000 population (rate)		Percentage change in rate
	1997	2010	1997	2010	1997–2010
All stays (with and without procedures)	34,681	39,008	1,272	1,261	−1%
All stays with any procedure	21,257	24,740	780	800	3%
Percentage of all stays with a procedure	61%	63%			
Blood transfusion	1,098	2,815	40	91	126%
Prophylactic vaccinations and inoculations	567	1,837	21	59	185%
Respiratory intubation and mechanical ventilation	919	1,638	34	53	57%
Repair of current obstetric laceration	1,137	1,292	42	42	0%
Diagnostic cardiac catheterization; coronary arteriography	1,461	1,283	54	41	−23%
Cesarean section	800	1,278	29	41	41%
Upper gastrointestinal endoscopy; biopsy	1,105	1,206	41	39	−4%
Circumcision	1,164	1,150	43	37	−13%
Artificial rupture of membranes to assist delivery	853*	917	31	30	−5%
Fetal monitoring	1,002	875	37	28	−23%
Diagnostic ultrasound of heart (echocardiogram)	632	858	23	28	20%
Hemodialysis	473	850	17	27	58%
Arthroplasty knee	329	730	12	24	96%
Enteral and parenteral nutrition	277	613	10	20	95%
Percutaneous transluminal coronary angioplasty (PTCA)	581	562	21	18	−15%
Laminectomy; excision intervertebral disc	425	532	16	17	10%
Colonoscopy and biopsy	531	528	19	17	−12%

FIG. 1.4 This extract from a table by the Agency for Healthcare Research and Quality (AHRQ) shows that among all medical procedures performed in U.S. hospitals in the year 2010, blood transfusion was the most common.

billing system. When a patient is sent for X-rays or a CT scan, the radiology department routinely generates its own armband, labeled with the patient's name and the radiology billing number. During an admission, edema or other factors may lead to the repositioning of armbands. When patients have surgery, armbands are often repositioned in the operating room. The radiology armband may end up being the only one on the patient's wrist, or the only one attached to the patient at all. Variations on the theme might include transfers between hospitals within the same medical center or same-day "passes" for medical procedures, with the original armband remaining on the patient while new bands and encounter numbers are issued.

The scenarios discussed earlier, while exaggerated for emphasis (one hopes), are intended to emphasize that patient identification errors may be occurring throughout a hospital without any single service comprehending the extent of the problem or its many causes. Meanwhile, blood requests and laboratory orders are placed on radiology billing numbers or CSN numbers. Therefore, orders for blood may not be fulfilled and laboratory results may not be reported, having been diverted into LIS error files. Billing and accounting may be impacted. Patient care may be

delayed, or worse. Patient identification is the Joint Commission's highest 2018 National Patient Safety Goal.[19] By failing to systematically identify and assess the risks posed by the institution's patient identification practices, the organization may be at much greater risk than it appreciates.

Focusing on blood transfusions and transfusion-related procedures, we observe that like patient identification, transfusions occur on virtually every service in a healthcare institution, including surgery, trauma, hematology-oncology, internal medicine, obstetrics, and the emergency department. According to the Agency for Healthcare Research and Quality (AHRQ),[20] in the year 2010 blood transfusion was the most common procedure performed in hospitals (see Fig. 1.4). Add therapeutic apheresis, sickle cell exchanges, peripheral blood stem cell transplants, and other aspects of cellular therapy, and it becomes clear how extensively transfusion-related activities transcend clinical silos.

RISK RESPONSE

Once the enterprise's risks have been cataloged and their relationships identified, ensuring that the true scope of each risk is assessed, the next step is to score the risks and rank them. Each risk is scored according to its likelihood of occurrence (PROB) and the severity of harm if the risk does occur (SEV). Likelihood and severity are then combined to assign each risk a risk priority number (RPN). At this point, all significant risks have been identified and ranked. They may then be mapped or otherwise displayed graphically for consideration by executive management.

Upon completion of the ERM risk audit, all risks that can impact the organization's strategic goals are ranked according to the risk priority number of each risk. The final step is to assess each risk in light of the organization's strategic goals. An enterprise's strategic goals are set by executive management. Given those goals, leadership can manage each risk by controlling it, outsourcing it, or eliminating it. *Controlling* a risk involves training, education, and implementation of procedures designed to avoid or at least minimize the risk. *Outsourcing* a risk may involve strategic partnerships, or more often, buying insurance to outsource the financial impact of the risk. *Eliminating* a risk is achieved simply by choosing not to participate in the activity.

Consider the risks inherent in providing an obstetrics service. Labor and delivery services are far from risk-free. An institution's strategic goals relative to providing obstetric services will depend on variables such as the degree of market saturation, demographic needs, the comprehensiveness of care the organization wishes to provide, and state and local political support. Clearly, the decision whether to control, outsource, or eliminate the risk of delivering babies will depend on the institution's strategic goals.

The breadth of transfusion-related activities in healthcare is vast, transcending silos and touching virtually all clinical practices. The primary goal of this book is to help transfusion medicine specialists comprehend and articulate the full scope of risk management activities undertaken by their services. There is a secondary goal as well. It is also important for the enterprise to fully understand the risk management contribution made by its BB/TM services. Enterprise risk management is a context in which the adage "if you don't measure it, it doesn't count" rings true. Given the number of transfusions and transfusion-related procedures, and the risk inherent in each, an institution with a comprehensive program to control transfusion risks is a decidedly safer institution. Investors, directors, insurers, third-party payers, lenders, employees, and the public all care about patient safety. It is imperative to educate one's institution and other stakeholders about

the effective, interdisciplinary transfusion risk management program that exists at the institution. Every chapter of this book is designed to help facilitate that conversation.

REFERENCES

1. Fraser JRS. How to prepare a risk profile. In: Fraser J, Simkins BJ, eds. *Enterprise Risk Management (Kolb Series in Finance)*. Hoboken: John Wiley & Sons, Inc; 2010:171–188.
2. Tran M, Khow S. *Enron: The Man Who Founded Enron, Kenneth Lay, has Died Just Weeks Before his Jail Sentence was to be Announced*. The Guardian; July 6, 2006. www.theguardian.com/business/2006/jul/06/corporatefraud.enron. Accessed Oct. 1, 2018.
3. CNN Library. *Enron Fast Facts*; April 27, 2017. www.cnn.com/2013/07/02/us/enron-fast-facts/index.html.
4. Brown K, Dugan IJ. Arthur Andersen's fall from grace is a sad tale of greed and miscues. *Wall St J*. June 7, 2002. www.wsj.com/articles/SB1023409436545200. Accessed October 1, 2018.
5. Weil J, Emshwiller J, Paltrow SJ. Arthur Anderson admits it destroyed documents related to Enron account. *Wall St J*. Jan. 11, 2002. www.wsj.com/articles/SB1010695966620300040. Accessed October 1, 2018.
6. Druker J, Sender H. WorldCom accounting debacle shows how easy fraud can be. *Wall St J*. June 27, 2002. www.wsj.com/articles/SB102513134054041480. Accessed October 1, 2018.
7. Van J, Alexander D. *Andersen was WorldCom Auditor*. Chicago Tribune; June 26, 2002.
8. Pulliam S, Soloman D. How three unlikely sleuths exposed fraud at WorldCom. *Wall St J*. Oct. 30, 2002. www.wsj.com/articles/SB1035929943494003751. Accessed October 1, 2018.
9. Romero S, Atlas RD. *WorldCom's Collapse: The Overview; WorldCom Files for Bankruptcy; Largest U.S. Case*. New York Times; July 22, 2002.
10. Searcy D, Young S, Scannell K. Ebbers is sentenced to 25 years for $11 billion WorldCom fraud. *Wall St J*. July 14, 2005. https://www.wsj.com/articles/SB112126001526184427. Accessed October 1, 2018.
11. Sarbanes-Oxley Act of 2002, Pub. L. No. 107-204, 116 Stat. Vol. 745 (codified in sections 11, 15, 18, 28, and 29 U.S.C.S. [2005]).
12. Everson MEA, Soske SE, Martens FJ, et al. *Committee of Sponsoring Organizations of the Treadway Commission: "Internal Control – Integrated Framework*. Available at: May 2013. www.coso.org.
13. Sarbanes-Oxley, supra at 11, Sec. 404 (internal controls).
14. Everson MEA, Chesley DL, Martens FJ, et al. *Committee of Sponsoring Organizations of the Treadway Commission: "Enterprise Risk Management – Integrating with Strategy and Performance*. Available at: June 2017. www.coso.org.

15. Celona J, Driver J, Hall E, Value-driven ERM. *Making ERM an engine for simultaneous value creation and value protection. Monograph by American Society for Healthcare Risk Management.* Available at: 2010. www.ashrm.org/pubs/files/white _papers/Monograph_ERM2010.pdf.

16. Walker R. Benefits of competing on risk. In: *Winning with Risk Management. Hackensack.* World Scientific Publishing Co; 2013:197–209.

17. Walker R. Operations pose embedded risks to the enterprise. In: *Winning with Risk Management. Hackensack.* World Scientific Publishing Co; 2013:37–62.

18. Carroll RL, Norris GA, Zuckerman M. Basics of enterprise risk management in healthcare. In: Carroll R, Nakamura PLB, eds. 6th ed. Risk Management Handbook for Healthcare Organizations; Vol. 1. San Francisco: John Wiley & Sons; 2011:1–18.

19. The Joint Commission on Accreditation of Healthcare Organizations, National Patient Safety Goal, NPSG.01.01.01 (eff. January 2018).

20. *Agency for Healthcare Research and Quality (AHRQ), Statistical Brief #149.* February 2013.

CHAPTER 2

Quality Systems in Transfusion Medicine

J. MILLS BARBEAU, MD, JD

It is not an exaggeration to say that contemporary healthcare quality management was pioneered in the clinical laboratories. One needs to look no further than the efforts of Oswald Hope Robertson during World War I, when he instituted the world's first blood bank. During the Battle of Cambrai in 1917, Robertson provided transfusions using bottles that combined "sterile fluid handling, citrate anticoagulation, ABO blood typing using hemagglutination not hemolysis, heterophile syphilis testing, and ice storage made with gas refrigeration."[1] Robertson documented his standard operating procedure (SOP) in the British Medical Journal[2] so that the process could be faithfully reproduced–which it was. By the end of the war, approximately 30,000 soldiers had received transfusions by Robertson's technique.

Of course, blood banks and clinical laboratories did not invent every quality management technique currently used in healthcare. Nevertheless, risk management and quality management have been part of laboratory practice throughout the era of modern medicine. An informal listing of representative laboratory quality and risk management techniques is shown in Table 2.1.

A more formal list of key quality improvement (QI) techniques routinely practiced by laboratory, blood banking, and transfusion medicine services is shown in Table 2.2.

THE RELATIONSHIP BETWEEN RISK AND QUALITY

It is useful at the outset to consider the relationship between risk and quality. On its face, risk management seems self-explanatory: Risk management is the process of controlling risks to prevent harm. However, as mentioned in the first chapter, risk (and harm) can take many forms. A healthcare organization's failure to capture a long-sought business opportunity can be a source of harm, not just to the enterprise, but also to patients. For example, if a healthcare organization is unable to obtain the capital necessary to open a labor and delivery ward in an underserved community, the community is harmed, as is the healthcare organization that missed an important strategic opportunity.

Quality is similarly multifaceted. Quality healthcare delivery includes avoidance of harm, but the concept of quality is much more nuanced. Quality involves not only safety, but cost-effectiveness, while providing the right care at the right time, in a patient-focused manner. Quality involves achieving *maximum effectiveness* without spending unnecessary resources. The notion of quality thus includes efficiency and stewardship of healthcare resources, so the greatest number can benefit at the least cost. The Institute of Medicine's "Crossing the Quality Chasm" emphasizes precisely those features when it describes quality care as safe, effective, patient centered, timely, efficient, and equitable.[3]

From this vantage, we can see that risk management and quality improvement can meet in a paradigm in which safety, efficiency, patient-centered care, and equitable distribution of healthcare resources come together. For example, Lean Management and Six Sigma, referred to Table 2.2, are fundamental quality improvement strategies. They are also risk management strategies. Lean Management refines processes to accomplish them in the minimum number of steps, eliminating redundancy and the opportunity for errors. Six sigma reduces variability in processes, reducing the number of different ways a task is performed, which also reduces errors. Reducing the risk of errors by reducing process inefficiencies is highly cost-effective: Output increases while laboratory error (risk of patient harm) is reduced. This is the essence of quality and safety. A closer examination of the quality improvement techniques listed in Table 2.2 is thus worthwhile.

Risk Management in Transfusion Medicine. https://doi.org/10.1016/B978-0-323-54837-3.00002-X

TABLE 2.1
An Informal Listing of Commonly Used Laboratory Quality and Risk Management Techniques

LABORATORY RISK MANAGEMENT TECHNIQUES INCLUDE:

• Proficiency testing	• *Standards for Blood Banks and Transfusion Services (etc.)*
• Automation	• Six Sigma, Lean
• LIS	• Quality system essentials (QSE)
• Infectious disease testing, quarantine, lookback	• RFID specimen tracking
• Patient blood management/stewardship	• Armbands
• Unique identifiers	• Human factors/ergonomics
• Adverse event reporting/root cause analysis	• Massive Transfusion Protocols (MTP)
• Transfusion review committee	• Remote blood releasing systems
• AABB, FDA, CLIA, TJC, CMS, etc.	• And more

TABLE 2.2
Formal Quality Improvement Techniques Routinely Practiced by Laboratory, Blood Banking, and Transfusion Services

QUALITY IMPROVEMENT TECHNIQUES

- Failure mode and effects analysis (FMEA)
  - *Prospective* risk assessment: Identify potential failures and score them using RPN
  - A "mini" ERM audit
- Root cause analysis (RCA)
  - Deep-dive *retrospective* review of an event to identify causal factors; focus on the system
- Six Sigma
  - Reduces variability in laboratory processes
  - Six sigma: Processes must be 99.9996% perfect
  - Errors below 3.4 defects per million opportunities
  - DMAIC: Define, Measure, Analyze, Improve, Control (and repeat)
- Lean
  - Minimize steps/eliminate redundancy
- Quality System Essentials
  - Designed specifically for Blood Banking/ Transfusion Medicine

ERM, enterprise risk management; *RPN*, risk priority number.

FAILURE MODE AND EFFECTS ANALYSIS

In healthcare, failure mode and effects analysis (FMEA) is sometimes overlooked in favor of its better-known sibling, root cause analysis (RCA). RCA involves a retrospective review of an event to identify causal factors. FMEA, on the other hand, is a *prospective* risk assessment. Failure mode and effects analysis is similar to the enterprise risk management process discussed in the first chapter. FMEA can be considered as a "mini" ERM audit. The key difference between enterprise risk management and FMEA is the difference in breadth. FMEA is seldom, if ever, applied on an enterprise-wide scale. It is instead used to assess the risk of failure of a specific, discrete process.

Failure mode and effects analysis was developed by the US space program in the 1960s. The analysis requires the identification of all possible failures that might occur in a given process, and for each failure, an assessment of the likelihood of its occurrence (OCC), the severity of its impact on the system if it does occur (SEV), and the probability that the failure will go undetected prior to the failure (DET). As with enterprise risk management, a risk priority number is assigned to each risk. In the case of FMEA, the formula is RPN = (OCC) (SEV) (DET). It is interesting that DET, the probability that the failure will go undetected, is included in the formula. If the likelihood that the failure will *not* be detected is 100%, then the risk priority number is the same as it would be using the enterprise risk management formula, since DET simply multiplies by 1. If the likelihood that the failure will go undetected is only 50%, then the RPN is reduced by half. As one can see, the enterprise risk management RPN in essence assumes that the risk will not be detected, so the enterprise risk management formula is somewhat less flexible than NASA's formula. For that reason, some healthcare practitioners use the NASA formula.

Process step	Potential failure mode	Potential failure effects	sev	Potential causes	occ	current process controls	Det	RPN
Order Generated	Wrong test is ordered by LS Staff/ Provider	Correct test is not done	8	Wrong language used to describe the test	2	Order error is put into red folder	3	48
			8	Informatics: Synonyms are not present in EPIC/Tests are misspelled/ order name is wrong	6	Request that a new test be built (via email, with synonyms added), Requestor Complaints	8	384
			8	Lab guide is incorrect/ incomplete	4	Steve is/ is not notified of a new process	5	160
		Charging for the wrong test	7	Send Outs ordered incorrect test	2	Lab guide	6	84
		Paying for the incorrect test	6	Provider ordered incorrect/ ambiguous test	3	Human intervention by Lab Specialist	5	90
		Financial impact in Lifespan	6	Provider ordered incorrect/ ambiguous test	3	None	10	180
		Delay in care	7	Provider ordered incorrect/ ambiguous test	3	None	10	210
		Provider dissatisfaction	7	Wrong test ordered and Provider does not get the results of the test	3	None	10	210
	Test not ordered in the system: Soft and EPIC (hard copy requisition)	Re-work by the Send Out department (staff needs to order)	4	Staff/ physician lack of knowledge/ experience/ effort	5	None (Potential future process state control- feedback to physician and staff)	10	200
		Specimen gets lost or misdirected	6	lack of tracking	5	Staff/Provider may call back and notify of problem	4	120
			6	lack of tracking	5	RSENDs get in-lab status that notifies provider/ orderer	2	60
		Incorrect test is ordered	7	Provider ordered incorrect/ ambiguous test on manual requisition	6	Red folder	3	126
			7	Not all tests built into EPIC or Soft	3	Workbook	2	42
			6	Not all tests built into EPIC or Soft	3	Workbook	2	36

FIG. 2.1 A representative excerpt from a failure mode and effects analysis (FMEA) performed at the author's institution. OCC = likelihood that the failure will occur; SEV = severity of impact; DET = probability that the risk will be undetected prior to the failure; RPN = risk priority number.

A small excerpt from an FMEA performed at the author's institution is presented in Fig. 2.1.

The failures with the highest RPNs are often presented graphically in a Pareto chart, which provides a succinct summary of the greatest of risks in the process being studied (see Fig. 2.2):

ROOT CAUSE ANALYSIS

To fully understand root cause analysis, one must understand that event reporting is the most important element of the process. Success lies in having a robust, nonpunitive system for identifying adverse events and near misses ("close calls"),[4] without fear of reprisal. The mindset with which one should approach adverse events and near misses is that the system is more likely to have failed the employee than the other way around. There are two good reasons to make this assumption. First, the vast majority of individuals who enter healthcare professions want to do a good job and help patients. Second, searching for system failures rather than focusing on employee mistakes is likely to reveal global solutions that will positively impact the entire organization.

A near miss should be considered a gift to a healthcare organization. Why? Because no actual harm occurred, but a risk was revealed. The healthcare entity has thus been granted an opportunity to prevent actual harm in advance. Of course, an actual adverse event should be treated with an even higher degree of respect, since a patient—and by implication her caregivers–suffered actual harm. In all cases, whether adverse events or near misses, a learning healthcare organization that is committed to patient safety will extract all information that can be gleaned from every such incident.

A useful and intuitive way to characterize RCA is to describe it as a process of asking "Why?" repeatedly until every step leading to the error has been thoroughly explored. When all contributing factors are exhaustively examined, the fundamental cause or causes, that is, the "root" cause, is established. One of the keys to a successful root cause analysis is to assemble a team whose members have, in aggregate, an excellent understanding of the circumstances in which the event occurred. For example, a transfusion event might involve experienced individuals from the blood bank, the emergency department, the trauma team, and hospital IT, along with the individuals specifically involved in the actual

Pareto Chart:
RPN rank order

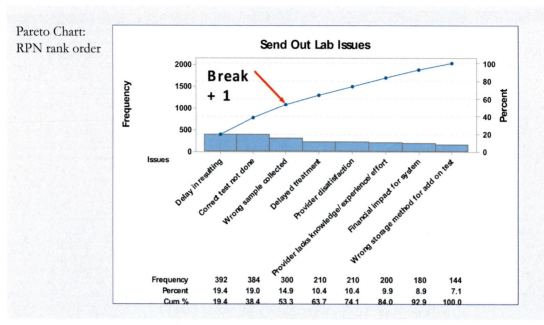

FIG. 2.2 A Pareto chart provides a graphic visualization of the highest concerns in terms of their risk priority numbers.

incident. Several meetings may be necessary before the root causes are identified to everyone's satisfaction.

Once the cause or causes have been identified, the next step is to formulate a "corrective action," that is, an improvement designed to prevent the problem from happening in the future. The change or changes must then be audited to confirm that the solution is adhered to and it is working effectively. Depending on the nature of the problem, long-term watchful monitoring may be the most effective strategy, particularly for rare events.

LEAN AND SIX SIGMA

Lean Management and Six Sigma[5] are important quality improvement techniques that are typically employed in conjunction with each other, often under the general term Lean-Six Sigma. As previously noted, Lean is focused on avoiding redundancy in processes and eliminating steps that do not add value. Six Sigma eliminates variability in processes. If the same task is performed in different ways each time it is undertaken, the likelihood of errors increases. If a single robust and efficient process can be identified, the individuals performing the task will do so with more confidence, while expending less energy in ad hoc decision making. The

goal of Six Sigma is to make each process 99.9996% perfect, reducing the error rate to below 3.4 defects per million opportunities. Together, Lean and Six Sigma are a powerful combination. There is one caveat: implementing a Lean-Six Sigma quality improvement project can be a significant undertaking. Projects should be selected carefully.

A Lean-Six Sigma project begins by mapping process flows. The earliest efforts to clearly define and delineate all of the elements of an established laboratory process can be messy–which is, in fact, a clear sign that Lean-Six Sigma is needed. As an illustration, a preliminary flow map of a send-out laboratory's various workflows is presented in Fig. 2.4.

The reader is not expected to examine the details of Fig. 2.4. The image is a first draft of an effort to define a send-out laboratory's workflows, illustrating how difficult it can be to parse, clarify, and define all of the workflows involved in sending patient samples to a reference laboratory. The team has begun the laborious process of identifying all of the subroutines within each workflow. Eventually, the process steps begin to clarify, as shown in Fig. 2.5, which illustrates the placement of a send-out order.

Once all of the steps in each process are identified, such as processing barcoded samples, for example, the

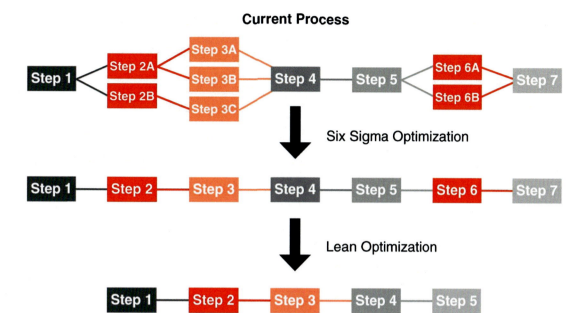

FIG. 2.3 Lean-Six Sigma achieves process improvement by (1) eliminating steps that do not add value, (2) reducing variability, and (3) reducing errors. Bishop, Clin Chemistry, seventh Ed., Wolters Kluwer/Lippincott Williams & Wilkins, Phil. 2013.

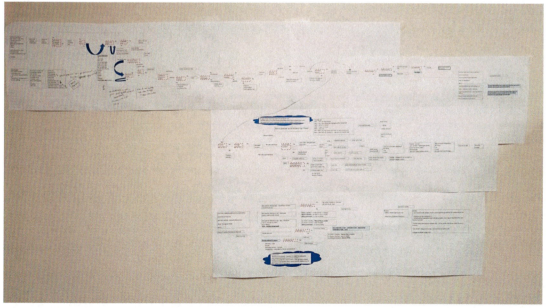

FIG. 2.4 The first step of a Lean-Six Sigma project is to map out laboratory workflows. This image shows a bird's-eye view of the first draft of a send-out laboratory's workflows. The process of defining workflows inevitably undergoes considerable refinement during the first stage of a project.

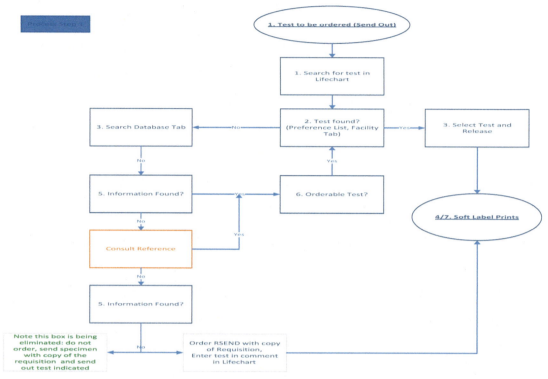

FIG. 2.5 Eventually, even subroutines are identified in detail; in this case the workflows for ordering a send-out test are revealed.

use of "spaghetti diagrams" can be very helpful in mapping each task (Fig. 2.6A):

Now that the workflows for processing barcoded patient samples are understood and mapped out, we can employ Lean-Six Sigma techniques. Eliminating unnecessary steps (Lean management) can greatly simplify the process, reducing opportunities for error. Eliminating variability in how each task is performed (Six Sigma) brings the process further under control. Changes are made in the laboratory to accommodate the improved workflows, as revealed by the new spaghetti diagram (Fig. 2.6B).

QUALITY SYSTEM ESSENTIALS

We have arrived at this chapter's destination, the Quality System Essentials (QSEs). The QSEs are uniquely associated with the American Association of Blood Banks (now officially named AABB), and they have had a far-reaching impact on laboratory quality management worldwide.

Many readers are familiar with the AABB's Standards for Blood Banks and Transfusion Services ("Standards"), now in its 30th edition. The original Standards were published by AABB in 1958, under the title "Standards for a Blood Transfusion Service". The 1958 Standards was only 19 pages long, compared to the present 119 pages. The focus of the early standards was technical rather than clinical, addressing labeling requirements, ABO and Rh typing, storage requirements, simple sterility testing, the 21-day expiration for whole blood collected in acid citrate dextrose anticoagulant, basic record keeping, and an abbreviated set of donor eligibility requirements.

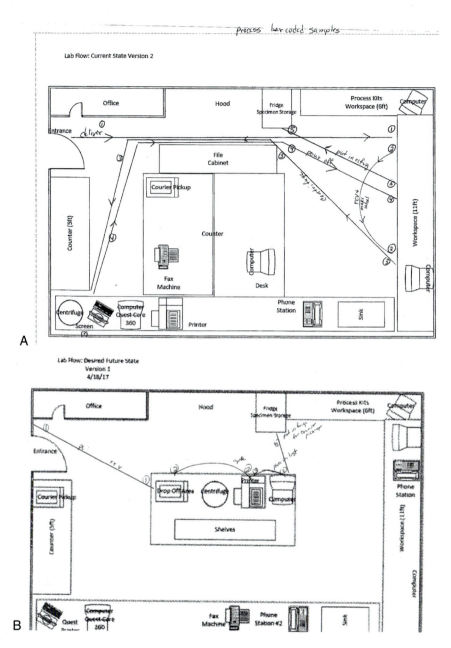

FIG. 2.6 Spaghetti diagrams are very helpful for identifying variability in workflows as well as unnecessary steps in a process (A), thus revealing changes that will optimize workflows (B).

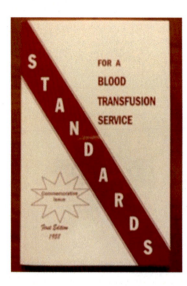

laboratory quality management principles with laboratory technical requirements.

Coming out of the workshop, FDA published a nonbinding guidance document[7] and AABB published "The Quality Program," a blueprint for unifying technical operations with quality practices in blood banking. Finally, in 1997, AABB incorporated "10 Quality System Essentials" into the Standards.[6] The QSEs were innovative, because they added a quality management component to the technical specifications. For the first time, technical laboratory activities began to be guided and supported by a comprehensive framework of quality and safety practices, including the development of standard operating procedures, ongoing process improvement, and external proficiency assessments.

A now iconic image summarized the new relationship between a transfusion service's technical workflow and the quality system that sustains and supports that workflow:

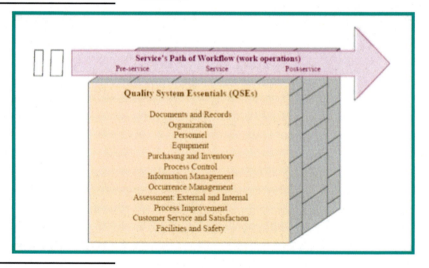

In the mid-1970s, FDA announced that it would regulate blood as a drug. By the early-1980s, HIV had entered the blood supply. When the threat of transfusion-transmitted HIV had not been eliminated by the 1990s, the Institute of Medicine, Centers for Disease Control, Congress, and the FDA exerted increasing pressure on blood banks to be more proactive. FDA was determined to move blood safety "from a program of detection to a program of prevention".[6] In 1992, FDA convened a workshop to explore how to unite medical

The image reveals how the laboratory's technical operations (workflow) are to be supported by a comprehensive quality management system—a "supervisory" overlay that ensures quality and safety. Today, the QSEs are literally the chapters of the Standards.

The QSE relationship between a clinical laboratory's technical workflow and the quality system that supports it was revolutionary. It has become the FDA's working paradigm for all laboratory quality management systems. The QSEs have been adopted by NCCLS/CLSI

(1999), ISO 15189 (2003), and numerous countries around the world. The importance of the QSE system is illustrated by the "Laboratory Quality Management System Training Toolkit" jointly presented in Lyon, France, by WHO, CDC, and CLSI. The presentation specifically stated that the Quality System Essentials are the "building blocks" of the Quality Management System model for laboratories. To emphasize that point, the presentation included a crosswalk between the 12 QSEs, ISO 15,189, and CLSI GP26-A3.

AABB Quality System Essentials were a watershed: they were the first comprehensive quality management system developed specifically for clinical laboratories. They were jointly developed by AABB and the FDA, and AABB's standard-setting relationship with FDA remains strong to this day. Furthermore, the QSEs have been adopted worldwide.

It is clear that Blood Banking and Transfusion Medicine services have a great deal to offer their institutions and their patients in terms of best practices in quality and safety. In the next chapter, we will examine the regulatory environment in which transfusion medicine operates. In Chapter 4, we will explore how the QSEs are structured, and how each of the Essentials supports a crucial pillar of comprehensive quality assurance and risk management. Then, in Chapter 5, we will see how those principles play out in the context of protecting blood recipients from transfusion-transmitted infectious diseases.

REFERENCES

1. Stansbury LG, Hess JR. The 100th anniversary of the first blood bank. *Transfusion.* 2017;57:2562–2563.
2. Robertson OH. Transfusion with preserved red blood cells. *Br Med J.* 1918;1:691–695.
3. Institute of Medicine. *Committee on the Quality of Health Care in America. Crossing the Quality Chasm: A New Health System for the 21st Century.* Washington, DC: National Academy Press; 2001.
4. Adverse events, near misses, and errors. In: *U.S. Department of Health and Human Services Patient Safety Network.* ; 2017. Available at: https://psnet.ahrq.gov/primers/primer/34/adverse-events-near-misses-and-errors.
5. *S3: Simple Six Sigma for Blood Banking, Transfusion, and Cellular Therapy. Walters and Carpenter Badley.* AABB Press; 2007.
6. Lipton S. *Transfusion.* 2010;50:1643–1646. Berte, *Clin Lab Med* 2007;27:771–790.
7. *FDA Guideline for Quality Assurance in Blood Establishments.* ; July 11, 1995. https://www.fda.gov/downloads/BiologicsBloodVaccines/GuidanceComplianceRegulatoryInformation/Guidances/Blood/ucm164981.pdf.

CHAPTER 3

Regulatory Oversight of Transfusion Medicine

J. MILLS BARBEAU, MD, JD

A comprehensive discussion of risk management would be incomplete if it did not consider the regulatory environment in which transfusion services operate. Yet, the regulatory environment can sometimes be so pervasive that we almost forget its presence, like the air we breathe. A very large proportion of healthcare regulations are aimed at managing risk, and we would be missing an elephant in the room if we did not acknowledge the presence of regulations in our risk management activities.

We should try to guard against thinking of regulations as monolithic commandments that must be continuously mollified with compliance documentation. As mentioned in Chapter 2, there is often a great deal of give and take between the government and its regulated industries. This is particularly true in healthcare, where the government depends heavily upon the medical expertise of those who are subject to its regulations. Frequently, when the government appears unresponsive to the needs of the healthcare industry, the problem is often more a result of the sheer size of the healthcare industry than governmental callousness. Simply put, the government moves slowly.

This chapter provides an overview of the regulatory environment, as it impacts risk management practices in transfusion medicine and blood banking. We will see that our professional best practices often interdigitate with regulatory requirements, so that professional standards and regulatory mandates are sometimes one in the same. It must also be observed that statutes and regulations sometimes empower, rather than limit, the regulated industry, as might be seen in aspects of the Clinical Laboratory Improvement Amendments of 1988 (CLIA).[1] It must be noted that, although individual states, such as states like Washington and New York, may have extensive regulatory schemes, this chapter does not delve into those regulations as they vary considerably from state to state.

FDA REGULATION

To understand the relationship between the transfusion medicine community and the Food and Drug Administration (FDA), it will be helpful to start with some history. The United States Congress made efforts to pass comprehensive legislation regarding drugs and adulterated food as early as the 1870s, but such efforts failed due to industry opposition and Congressional concerns about legislative overreach.[2] Regulatory efforts eventually bore fruit with the passage of the Food and Drugs Act of 1906,[3] which President Theodore Roosevelt signed with great fanfare on June 30, 1906. The history leading up to that event may not be familiar to all readers. In 1905–06, Collier's magazine published a series of articles on "The Great American Fraud,"[4] which decried the fraudulent practices of the patent medicines industry. Hucksterism reigned, with medicines being advertised to cure tuberculosis, cancer, arthritis, and baldness, often by the same product. These potions often contained little more than alcohol and sugar water. Worse still, the elixir, often sold through the mail, might contain cocaine or morphine, leading to addictions that would keep the customer coming back for more.

Immediately upon the heels of Collier's expose on fraudulent drug marketing practices, Upton Sinclair published The Jungle,[5] which revealed employee abuses and unhygienic practices in the food industry, specifically, Chicago's meat packing industry. The public was outraged–and revolted, in both senses of the word. The sale of meat fell precipitously. Roosevelt leveraged the momentum of public awareness to push through legislation on meat inspection as well as the 1906 pure food and drug law.

What may not be as well known to readers is the fact that the Food and Drugs Act of 1906 was preceded historically by legislation governing biologics, specifically the Biologics Control Act of 1902.[6] It was the Biologics Control Act, not the Food and Drugs Act of 1906, that was the first federal law to regulate the interstate sale of

Risk Management in Transfusion Medicine. https://doi.org/10.1016/B978-0-323-54837-3.00003-1

a specific class of drugs. The Biologics Control Act was "An Act to regulate the sale of viruses, serums, toxins, and analogous products in the District of Columbia, to regulate interstate traffic in said articles, and for other purposes." It was signed into law, rather quietly, by President Roosevelt on July 1, 1902.

To place the Biologics Control Act in perspective, it is important to recognize that the late 19th century was the golden age of microbiology and immunology.[7] The development of vaccination against smallpox, quinine for malaria, and mercury compounds for treating syphilis (salvarsan and neosalvarsan) ushered in a new era of empowerment against infectious diseases.

The first Nobel Prizes were awarded in 1901, and the first prize ever awarded for Medicine and Physiology was to Emil von Behring for "his work on serum therapy, especially its application against diphtheria."[8] In 1890, while working in Robert Koch's laboratory in Berlin, Behring and Kitasato[9] had injected laboratory animals with diphtheria and tetanus toxins, and succeeded in stimulating antibodies ("antitoxins") against those organisms. The sensitized animal's serum could then be injected into patients, often young children who had contracted those life-threatening diseases. The ability to prevent the death of children with diphtheria was nothing short of miraculous.

A chemicals and pharmaceuticals company named Hoechst worked with von Behring to produce antitoxin commercially. Soon thereafter, in 1894, Emil Roux of the Pasteur Institute in Paris reported that large quantities of antitoxins could be produced by horses, leading the way to large-scale production of diphtheria antitoxin. As a result of antitoxin production, the mortality rate from diphtheria in Paris quickly decreased from 52% to 25%. Joseph Kinyoun, the founder and first director of the United States' Laboratory of Hygiene, traveled to Europe to visit Roux's and Koch's laboratories (Kenyoun had studied under Koch). In the spirit of the times, the Pasteur Institute provided a supply of diphtheria toxin for Kinyoun to send back to the Hygienic Laboratory in Washington, DC, for immunizing horses to produce antitoxin. Before long, the Hygienic Laboratory was one of the major producers of diphtheria antitoxin in the United States. Fig. 3.1.

The importance of city and state public health laboratories during this time period cannot be overlooked. In the final decades of the 19th century, the United States' centralized federal bureaucracy had not yet come into existence. The Bacteriological Laboratory of the New York City Health Department was instrumental in production and implementation of diphtheria antitoxin in the United States, as well as the standardization

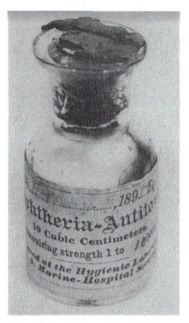

A bottle of diphtheria antitoxin produced by the Hygienic Laboratory in 1895. (Courtesy of the Smithsonian Institution.)

FIG. 3.1

of procedures for producing safe, sterile, and effective products. Indeed, state labs continued to play a major role in addressing the public health threats posed by all of the infectious diseases of the day, such as cholera, smallpox, and typhoid.

Unfortunately, not all laboratories producing antitoxins had sufficient expertise in laboratory techniques for assuring the sterility of their products, such as temperature controls, aseptic syringes, and sterility checks. There was a growing awareness that not all products were safe. Fig. 3.2 Unfortunately, it required a tragedy to galvanize a public demand for action. In 1901, a 5-year old girl in St. Louis died in a hospital from tetanus.[10] The girl's working diagnosis was meningitis, but she was injected with diphtheria antitoxin prophylactically–just in case. Inspectors quickly discovered that the horse that produced the diphtheria antitoxin, whose name was Jim, had been destroyed after contracting tetanus. Inexplicably, Jim's serum had not been recalled after he was destroyed. Soon, 12 more children died of tetanus after receiving Jim's contaminated serum. Recognizing the urgent need for regulatory action, medical professionals and local officials in Washington, DC quietly proposed legislation. It was immediately passed by both houses of Congress, thus becoming the Biologics Control Act of 1902.

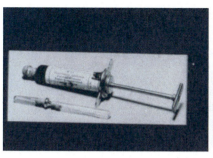
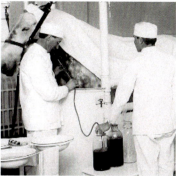

Production of diphtheria antitoxin by inoculating horses required great care to maintain purity and avoid contamination. Courtesy of National Archives and Records Administration.

FIG. 3.2

Dr. Kinyoun had established the Laboratory of Hygiene of the Marine Health Service in 1887. Originally located on Staten Island, the Laboratory of Hygiene was responsible for quarantining and inspecting ships arriving in the United States, and also for testing incoming immigrants for infectious diseases. The Laboratory of Hygiene thus had expertise in microbiology as well as performing on-site inspections.

In 1891, the Laboratory of Hygiene was moved from Staten Island to Washington, DC, but the laboratory remained within the Marine Health Service. When the Biologics Control Act was passed in 1902, the Marine Health Service was renamed the Public Health and Marine Hospital Service. The Biologics Act granted the Public Health and Marine Hospital Service authority to inspect the premises of biologics manufacturers. The Act changed the name of the Laboratory of Hygiene, renaming it the Hygienic Laboratory of the Public Health and Marine Hospital Service, and the laboratory was charged with administering the Biologics Act. Inspections and bacterial testing of biologics were conducted by the Hygienic Laboratory's Division of Pathology and Bacteriology.

In 1930, the Ransdell Act changed the name of the Hygienic Laboratory to the National Institute of Health (NIH). The NIH's responsibilities were expanded beyond inspections and oversight, with more emphasis placed on research. The Division of Pathology and Bacteriology remained within the NIH and continued to oversee the Biologics Control Act, but in 1937, organizational changes led to the reassignment of biologics from the Division of Pathology and Bacteriology to a newly established Division of Biologics Control. From 1937 to 1972, minor name changes and division reassignments continued, but on July 1, 1972, NIH's Division of Biologics Standards was transferred to FDA, where it became FDA's Bureau of Biologics.[11,12]

The transfer of biologics oversight from NIH to FDA was due to the increasingly divergent expertise of the agencies: NIH focused on research and FDA focused on inspections and regulation. NIH finally lost authority over biologics manufacture when a 1972 General Accounting Office report demonstrated that NIH was improperly licensing biologic products under the Biologics Control Act, the products having failed to meet requirements for proof of effectiveness.[13]

In terms of regulatory authority specifically over blood products, the original language of the Biologics Control Act of 1902 had indeed addressed blood–clearly, but not in much detail. The 1902 Act had defined biologics to include vaccines, antitoxins, serums, and "blood for transfusion and other medical purposes." Given that Karl Landsteiner had not discovered the ABO blood groups until 1900, the lack of specificity could be forgiven. Fig. 3.3.

In 1970, Congress amended the Biologics Control Act specifically to include *blood products*. Thus, when the Bureau of Biologics came within FDA's scope 2 years later, the agency's authority over the full scope of blood and blood products was already established. Upon the Bureau of Biologics' arrival at FDA, the agency promptly issued detailed procedures for overseeing the safety, effectiveness, and labeling of licensed biologics, specifically including blood banks, which were now required to be federally registered.[14] Regulations governing good manufacturing practices for collecting, processing, and storing blood components were published in 1974.[15]

ABO System

- Karl Landsteiner (1900): Serum from one person sometimes **agglutinated** red cells from another

People fell into groups:

- Serum from people in **group A** agglutinated red cells from people in **group B**, and vice versa.

- Group A and group B serum could not agglutinate RBCs from a third group, called **group O**

- Serum from **group O** people agglutinated RBCs of both group A and group B

- 1902: Discovery of the **"AB" blood group**
  - Serum from the AB group did not agglutinate anyone's red cells
  - Serum from group O people agglutinated RBCs of group A, group B, and group AB

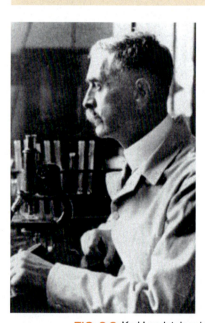

FIG. 3.3 Karl Landsteiner in his laboratory.

Today, the majority of regulations pertaining to blood testing, blood products, and blood collection can be found in the Code of Federal Regulations, Title 21 (Food and Drugs), Chapter 1 (Food and Drug Administration Department of Health and Human Services), Subchapter F (Biologics), Part 640 (Additional Standards for Human Blood and Blood Products). In addition, as we will see in Chapter 4, several important draft and final guidance documents governing blood and blood products are located in the Federal Register.

THE CLINICAL LABORATORY IMPROVEMENT ACT OF 1967 AND THE CLINICAL LABORATORY IMPROVEMENT AMENDMENTS OF 1988 (CLIA '88)

One tends to associate regulation of blood banks with the FDA. However, blood banks and transfusion services are clinical laboratories, so they are also governed by CLIA. The first US federal law ever to regulate the practice of clinical laboratory medicine was the Clinical Laboratory Improvement Act of 1967.[16] Only about

10% of laboratories fell within the scope of CLIA '67, as only large, independent clinical laboratories that were engaged in interstate commerce and participated in the Medicare program fell within the reach of the Act. The great majority of clinical laboratories in 1967 were small physician office laboratories or local hospital labs, which tended not to be within the statute's reach. Therefore, the legislation had relatively minor impact, although it should be noted that CLIA '67 did begin, albeit on a small scale, to introduce some federal involvement into quality control, proficiency testing, and personnel standards in the laboratories that were covered by the Act.

CLIA '88[17] had a far greater impact. CLIA '88 defines a clinical laboratory as follows:

A facility for the examination of materials derived from humans for providing information for the diagnosis, prevention, or treatment of any disease or impairment of, or the assessment of health of, human beings.[18]

In other words, virtually every clinical laboratory in the United States falls under the jurisdiction of CLIA '88.

Much of the impetus for the passage of CLIA '88 was a perceived lapse in cytology testing practices leading to missed Pap smear diagnoses. Congress and the public concluded that quality standards in contemporary laboratory testing were not sufficiently rigorous, and greater government oversight was essential.[19] It may well have been the case that the 1967 statute was fine, except it did not reach enough labs to make a difference. Be that as it may, the resulting federal oversight ushered in by CLIA '88 was considerably broader than its 1967 predecessor,[20] and the new Act brought in a new approach to laboratory oversight. Instead of the historic practice of stratifying oversight according to the type of clinical laboratory involved, CLIA '88 based its oversight on the complexity of each test, as well as the harm that might be caused by erroneous results. The Department of Health and Human Services (DHHS) characterized this approach as regulating according to "technical complexity" of the test, rather than the "location" of the testing – in other words, according to a risk-based paradigm.

A clinical laboratory must have a valid CLIA certificate before it may legally test human specimens and be eligible to receive payments from Centers for Medicare and Medicaid Services (CMS).[21] CLIA '88 originally categorized laboratory tests into three levels of complexity: *waived* tests, *moderate-complexity* tests, and *high-complexity* tests.[22] Any given laboratory, no matter its size or test volume, might perform tests of any level of complexity. Both moderate-complexity tests

and high-complexity tests required a heightened level of quality control and risk management. If a laboratory performed moderate- or high-complexity testing (or both), then the lab was required to adhere to a program of proficiency testing, patient test management, quality control, quality assurance, and personnel standards. By contrast, tests in the "waved" category did not require adherence to the requirements that applied to moderate- and high-complexity testing. If the laboratory performs only waived testing, then things are simple: the laboratory merely applies for a *certificate of waiver*. Once the certificate of waiver arrives with the laboratory's assigned CLIA number, the lab may perform its waived testing and it may bill CMS.

The criteria for assigning a given test to a complexity level were specified in the statute. Waived tests must (1) employ methodologies that are so simple and accurate that the likelihood of erroneous results was negligible; (2) incorrectly performed tests posed no reasonable risk of harm; and (3) the test was cleared by FDA for home use. Moderate- or high-complexity tests were categorized according to the degree of knowledge needed to perform the test; the training and experience required; the complexity of reagent and materials preparation; the complexity of operational steps; the characteristics of calibration; the nature of the quality control and proficiency testing materials; the amount of troubleshooting and maintenance required; and degree of interpreting and judgment required.

CMS was charged with implementing CLIA '88, but the US FDA was tasked with categorizing laboratory tests according to their complexity as waived, moderate complexity, or high complexity.[23,24] Transfusion medicine tests were categorized according to complexity, just like any other laboratory test that is performed for examination of materials derived from humans. Examples of blood banking and transfusion medicine-related tests categorized as high-complexity under CLIA '88 include compatibility testing to determine donor/recipient compatibility; recipient and donor ABO group/D(Rho) typing; special antigen typing; direct antiglobulin test; unexpected antibody detection and identification; and crossmatch procedures. There are also many high-complexity tests involved in donor testing.

It is necessary to understand the three-tiered CLIA '88 regulatory structure of waived, moderate-complexity, and high-complexity testing to understand the statute. However, the reader will no doubt have noticed that, in practice, it might be difficult to distinguish why some tests are placed in the moderate-complexity category while others are in the high-complexity category. Presently, FDA continues to assign test methods into the three complexity levels as envisioned by the statute. However, the 2003 update of CLIA regulations combines the moderate- and high-complexity tests into a single "nonwaived" category.[25] As a result, tests are presently referred to as being waived or nonwaived, with the "nonwaived" category comprising both moderate- and high-complexity tests.

The CLIA certification process is more complicated for laboratories that perform nonwaived testing. To obtain a CLIA certificate, a doctoral-level individual who is qualified under CLIA to direct the proposed laboratory must first apply for a *"certificate of registration,"* which allows the laboratory to test samples for 11 months. The laboratory operates under the certificate of registration until an on-site "survey" (i.e., an inspection) confirms that the laboratory is in compliance with CLIA requirements. The survey is performed either by CMS itself, by a CMS agent such as a state agency, or by a CMS-approved accreditation organization such as The Joint Commission or the College of American Pathologists. Upon completion of a successful survey by CMS or a CMS agent, the laboratory is issued a *"certificate of compliance."* If the laboratory chose to be inspected by an accreditation organization such as The Joint Commission (TJC) or the College of American Pathologists (CAP), the laboratory instead receives a *"certificate of accreditation."* In either case, the laboratory receives its CLIA number and it is placed on a 2-year inspection and recertification cycle for the life of the laboratory.

Currently, seven accreditation organizations have been approved by CMS. These organizations are said to have "deemed" status from CMS, as in "judged, or deemed, worthy" to represent CMS in the inspection and certification process. The organizations with deemed status from CMS are as follows:

- The Joint Commission (TJC) –focused on hospitals, including hospital laboratories
- College of American Pathologists (CAP)—comprehensive coverage of clinical laboratories
- AABB (formerly the American Association of Blood Banks)—accredits organizations collecting, processing, distributing, or transfusing blood and blood components
- COLA (formerly the Commission on Office Laboratory Accreditation)—focused on office and community hospital testing
- American Society for Histocompatibility and Immunogenetics (ASHI)
- American Osteopathic Association (AOA)—for AOA-accredited hospitals
- American Association for Laboratory Accreditation (A2LA)—comprehensive coverage of clinical laboratories

The vast majority of laboratories are accredited by COLA (office labs), CAP (all lab types), and TJC (hospital laboratories), in that order.[26]

A notable aspect of the 2003 update of the CLIA regulations is its adoption of Control procedures (quality control) in 42 CFR §493.1256 subpart K.[27] These very specific control requirements follow the specimen through the preanalytic, analytic, and postanalytic phases of sample analysis. They apply to all clinical laboratories, so it is important to be familiar with their content. The following table has selected key aspects of §493.1256 Subpart K and summarized them for ease of review. The reader is referred to the Code of Federal Regulations for details.[27]

§493.1256	Standard: Control Procedures
§493.1256(a)	For each test system, the laboratory is responsible for having control procedures that monitor the accuracy and precision of the complete analytical process.
§493.1256(b)	The laboratory must establish the number, type, and frequency of testing control materials using, if applicable, the performance specifications verified or established by the laboratory as specified in §493.1253(b) (3), verification of performance specifications.
§493.1256(c)	The control procedures must: 1. Detect immediate errors that occur due to test system failure, adverse environmental conditions, and operator performance. 2. Monitor over time the accuracy and precision of test performance that may be influenced by changes in test system performance and environmental conditions, and variance in operator performance.
§493.1256(d)	The laboratory must: 1. Perform control procedures as defined, unless otherwise specified in the additional specialty and subspecialty requirements at §§493.1261–.1278 (which includes immunohematology). 2. For each test system, perform control procedures using the number and frequency specified by the manufacturer or established by the laboratory when they meet or exceed the requirements in paragraph (d) (3) of this section.
§493.1256(d) (7)	Over time, rotate control material testing among all operators who perform the test.
§493.1256(d) (8)	Test control materials in the same manner as patient specimens.

§493.1256	Standard: Control Procedures
§493.1256(d) (9)	When using calibration material as a control material, use calibration material from a different lot number than that used to establish a cut-off value or to calibrate the test system.
§493.1256(d) (10)	Establish or verify the criteria for acceptability of all control materials.
	1. When control materials providing quantitative results are used, statistical parameters (for example, mean and standard deviation) for each batch and considerable number of control materials must be defined and available.
	2. The laboratory may use the stated value of a commercially assayed control material provided the stated value is for the methodology and instrumentation employed by the laboratory and is verified by the laboratory.
	3. Statistical parameters for unassayed control materials must be established over time by the laboratory through concurrent testing of control materials having previously determined statistical parameters.
§493.1256(f)	Results of control materials must meet the laboratory's results and, as applicable, the manufacturer's test system criteria for acceptability before reporting patient test results.
§493.1256(g)	The laboratory must document all control procedures performed.
§493.1256(h)	If control materials are not available, the laboratory must have an alternative mechanism to detect immediate errors and monitor test system performance over time. The performance of alternative control procedures must be documented.

The universally applicable quality control requirements set forth in §493.1256 are very important, but perhaps even more important for transfusion specialists is §493.1271,[28] which provides specific quality control procedures for immunohematology, that is, blood banking and transfusion medicine. Highlights of §493.1271 are extracted:

§493.1271	Standard: Immunohematology
§493.1271(a) (1)	Patient testing. The laboratory must perform ABO grouping, D(Rho) typing, unexpected antibody detection, antibody identification, and compatibility testing, by following the manufacturer's instructions.

§493.1271	Standard: Immunohematology
§493.1271(a) (2)	The laboratory must determine ABO group by concurrently testing unknown red cells with, at a minimum, anti-A and anti-B grouping reagents. For confirmation of ABO group, the unknown serum must be tested with known A1 and B red cells.
§493.1271(a) (3)	The laboratory must determine the D(Rho) type by testing unknown red cells with anti-D (anti-Rho) blood typing reagent.
§493.1271(c)	Blood and blood products must be stored under appropriate conditions that include an adequate temperature alarm system that is regularly inspected.
§493.1271(c) (1)	An audible alarm system must monitor proper blood and blood product storage temperature over a 24-h period.
§493.1271(c) (2)	Inspections of the alarm system must be documented.
§493.1271(d)	Retention of samples of transfused blood. According to the laboratory's established procedures, samples of each unit of transfused blood must be retained for further testing in the event of transfusion reactions.
§493.1271(e) (1)	Investigation of transfusion reactions. The laboratory that performs compatibility testing, or issues blood or blood products, must promptly investigate all transfusion reactions occurring in facilities for which it has investigational responsibility and make recommendations to the medical staff regarding improvements in transfusion procedures.
§493.1271(e) (2)	The laboratory must document, as applicable, that all necessary remedial actions are taken to prevent occurrences of transfusion reactions, and that all policies and procedures are reviewed to assure that they are adequate to ensure the safety of individuals being transfused.
§493.1271(f)	The laboratory must document all control procedures performed, as specified in this section.

OTHER REGULATIONS THAT IMPACT TRANSFUSION RISK MANAGEMENT

It is not difficult to identify other federal regulations that impact aspects of transfusion risk management. In fact, given the regulatory environment in the 21st century, and particularly in healthcare, the problem is knowing where to stop. Many regulations and guidance documents that flow freely from the font of FDA and CLIA often aim to take blood bank technologists and transfusion medicine practitioners by the hand to lead them through the minutia of how the government wishes blood banks to deliver safe blood products to patients. Conversely, many other federal statutes, such as HIPAA,[29] regulate patient risk as well. Improper disclosure of a patient's protected health information (PHI) is potentially very damaging to patients, so that the HHS Office of Human Rights is charged with enforcing HIPAA. HIPAA can certainly be considered a federal regulation to improve patient safety, and it certainly applies to blood banks and transfusion services.

In 2013, HIPAA was expanded to include the HITECH Act.[30] HITECH established a program to incentivize adoption of electronic health records. Successful achievement of "meaningful use" milestones in the implementation of certified electronic health record (EHR) systems allowed users to qualify for financial incentives from the Center for Medicare and Medicaid Services. HITECH is certainly directed toward improving patient safety and the quality of patient care. EHR systems have the potential to reduce errors and enhance communication. Continuity of care can be much better assured if a patient's health care record can be transmitted to other caregivers electronically, wherever the patient and the caregiver might be located. Electronic health records can bring best practice alerts to a physician's fingertips, improving care, and potentially reducing health disparities and enhancing care delivery in remote areas.

These are all laudable goals, and they are actively and intentionally driven by regulations, specifically by healthcare quality and patient safety regulations. Here, however, regulatory goals and current healthcare best practices may not harmonize, at least not in the near term. EHR features, such as drop-down lists, templates, multiple open charts on a single screen, and the ability to copy–paste have the potential to create novel sources of patient risk.[31] If a healthcare institution responds to the federal HIPAA/HITECH meaningful use incentives by installing a new electronic health record, the transfusion medicine service will certainly be effected– whether the service's LIS is updated with the rest of the hospital or the service retains the legacy LIS while the rest of the institution adopts another EHR. Enormous time and resources will be spent either way.

Many other regulations specifically designed to minimize healthcare risks have an impact on transfusion risk management. These regulations would certainly include regulations governing workplace environment, health, and safety. These regulations are largely designed to protect employees, but here, synergy typically applies: a safe workplace translates directly into improved patient care. Furthermore, a safe workplace also minimizes the institution's overall risk profile, which improves the institution's financial stability, as discussed in Chapter 1.

The Occupational Safety and Health Administration (OSHA) promulgates "Occupational Exposure to Hazardous Chemicals in Laboratories" (also known as the "OSHA Laboratory Standard")[32] and "Hazard Communication" (also known as "HazCom").[33] The OSHA Laboratory Standard protects workers from chemical, physical, and biological safety standards, and it is the source of the Chemical Hygiene Plan (CHP). The CHP addresses the specific chemical hazards in the laboratory for which the CHP is designed. The laboratory must develop standard operating procedures for those hazards, implement exposure control and monitoring measures, implement appropriate protective equipment, and provide information and training to the laboratory workers. The OSHA Laboratory Standard regulation is written to address risks that are specifically related to laboratories, rather than more general industrial risks. HazCom requires a written Hazard Communication Plan that includes an inventory of hazardous chemicals, properly labeled containers, safety data sheets (SDSs), and worker training.

Finally, it is important to recognize another very important source of regulatory authority: ourselves. Recall, for example, the discussion regarding private, nonprofit organizations that have been granted deemed status by CMS to represent CMS as an accrediting organization for clinical laboratories under the CLIA program. The standard to qualify for deemed status is that the organization must apply standards and criteria that are equal to, or more stringent than, the applicable CLIA requirements set forth in 42 CFR §493. Organizations such as AABB and CAP have for many years established professional standards that exceed CLIA requirements. As a result, today many laboratory best practices exceed the minimum regulatory requirements. As a byproduct of these efforts, professional organizations that consistently strive to *improve* patient care, reduce risk, and shepherd healthcare resources, gain a great deal of credibility over many decades of working with regulatory agencies. Very often, this literally translates into a seat at the table when new regulations are being contemplated.

REFERENCES

1. Clinical Laboratory Improvement Amendments (CLIA) of 1988; 42 CFR 493.
2. Young JH, ed. *The Early Years of Federal Food and Drug Control.* Madison: American Institute of the History of Pharmacy; 1982.
3. Pure Food and Drug Act of 1906 (P.L. 59-384; 34 Stat. 768).
4. Adams SH. *The Great American Fraud, the Patent Evil.* Collier's Weekly; 1905–06.
5. Sinclair U. *The Jungle.* New York: Doubleday, Page & Company; 1906.
6. The Biologics Control Act of 1902. P.L. 57-244; 32 Stat. 728, Chapter 1378.
7. Parascandola J. The public health service and the control of biologics. *Pub Health Rep.* 1995;110:774–775.
8. *Nobelprize.org, the Official Website of the Nobel Prize.* 2018. https://www.nobelprize.org/nobel_prizes/medicine/laureates/index.html.
9. Junod SW. *Biologics Centennial: 100 Years of Biologics Regulation. FDA Update*; November–December, 2002. https://www.fda.gov/downloads/AboutFDA/WhatWeDo/History/ProductRegulation/UCM593491.pdf.
10. Milstien JB. Regulation of vaccines: strengthening the science base. *J Pub Health Policy.* 2004;25(2):173–189.
11. 37 Federal Register. Vol. 12. 1972:865.
12. *Blood Policy and Technology.* Washington, DC: U.S. Congress, Office of Technology Assessment; 1985. TA-H-260.
13. Leveton LB, Sox HC, Stoto MA, eds. *HIV and the Blood Supply: An Analysis of Crisis Decisionmaking.* Washington, DC: National Academies Press; 1995.
14. 37 Federal Register. Vol. 17. 1972:419.
15. 39 Federal Register. Vol. 18. 1974:614. 40 Federal Register 53, 532, 1975.
16. Dept. of Health and Human Services Health Care Financing Administration. Medicare. Medicaid and CLIA programs; revision of the laboratory regulations for the Medicare, Medicaid, and clinical laboratories improvement Act of 1967 programs. *Fed Reg.* 1990;55:9538–9610.
17. *Public Law 100-578. Clinical Laboratory Improvement Amendments of 1988. Stat 42 USC 201. H.R. 5471.* October 31, 1988.
18. U.S. Department of Health and Human Service, Center for Medicare and Medicaid Services. *Laboratory Requirements, Code of Federal Regulations, Title 42 – Public Health, Chapter IV, Part 493* (rev.). Washington, DC: U.S. Government Printing Office; 2000.
19. Boodman SG. *How Accurate Are Medical Lab Tests? Washington Post*; September 1, 1992. https://www.washingtonpost.com/archive/lifestyle/wellness/1992/09/01/how-accurate-are-medical-lab-tests/3ce37a3b-bbac-4304-bbca-8cfa73f155f7/?noredirect=on&utm_term=.a335cfc0367a.
20. Centers for Disease Control. Regulations for Implementing the Clinical Laboratory Improvement Amendments of 1988: A Summary. Vol. 41. MMWR; 1992:001(RR-2).
21. Presently, There Are Two Exceptions. The States of New York and Washington Are Exempt from CLIA Certification Because CMS Has Approved Those States' Laboratory Program as Being Equivalent to CLIA Certification.
22. U.S. Department of Health and Human Services. Medicare, Medicaid, and CLIA programs: regulations implementing the clinical laboratory improvement Amendments of 1988 (CLIA). Final rule. *Fed Regist.* 1992;57: 7002–7186.
23. Available at: *CMS Initiatives to Improve Quality of Laboratory Testing under the CLIA Program.* 2018. https://www.cms.gov/Regulations-and-Guidance/Legislation/CLIA/Downloads/060630BackgrounderrlEG.pdf.
24. Rivers PA, Dobalian A, Germinario FA. A review and analysis of the clinical laboratory improvement amendment of 1988: compliance plans and enforcement policy. *Health Care Manage Rev.* 2005;30(2):93–102.
25. U.S. Centers for Medicare. Medicaid Services (CMS). Medicare, Medicaid, and CLIA programs: laboratory requirements relating to quality systems and certain personnel qualifications. Final rule. *Fed Regist.* 2003;16: 3640–3714.
26. Rauch CA, Nichols JH. Laboratory accreditation and inspection. *Clin Lab Med.* 2007;27:845–858.
27. *42 CFR §493.1256. CFR, Title 42, Chapter IV, Subchapter G, Part 493, Subpart K, Section 493.1256.* 2003.
28. 42 CFR §493.1271.
29. *Health Insurance Portability and Accountability Act of 1996 (HIPAA; Pub.L. 104–191, 110 Stat. 1936, Enacted.* August 21, 1996.
30. *Health Information Technology for Economic and Clinical Health (HITECH) Act, Pub. L. No. 111-5, 123 Stat. 226.* 2009.
31. Hoffman S. *Electronic Health Records and Medical Big Data.* New York: Cambridge University Press; 2016.
32. 29 CFR 1910.1450.
33. 29 CFR 1910.1200.

CHAPTER 4

Procedures for Protection

J. MILLS BARBEAU, MD, JD

INTRODUCTION

In the second chapter, we saw how the Quality System Essentials (QSEs) were jointly developed by Food and Drug Administration (FDA) and AABB, and we noted the extent to which the QSEs have become the framework for clinical laboratory best practices worldwide. It will therefore come as no surprise that the QSEs are the infrastructure on which the AABB's Standards for Blood Banks and Transfusion Services (BB/TS Standards, or Standards) are built. At the time of this writing, the 31st edition of the BB/TS Standards is going into press.

In the United States, the FDA has regulatory authority over blood banking. In light of the fact that the quality system essentials were cooperatively developed by FDA and AABB, one might wonder whether adherence to the AABB Standards is mandatory for US blood banking and transfusion services. The answer is no. The BB/TS Standards do indeed incorporate all relevant federal statutes, regulations, and guidance documents. Therefore, adherence to the Standards is a reliable pathway to meeting or exceeding federal requirements, but the Standards are not mandatory per se.

In contrast, US Federal laws, FDA Final Guidance documents, and regulatory rule making published in the Code of Federal Regulations (CFR) do carry the force of law in the United States. It is true that lawmakers and regulatory bodies typically avail themselves of subject matter expertise provided by organizations such as AABB, the American Red Cross, America's Blood Centers, the American Society for Apheresis, and the American Society for Gene & Cell Therapy, to name a few. Nevertheless, in the United States, the federal government always has the final say.

Today, the science and practice of blood transfusion and blood safety is an increasingly international affair. In writing the BB/TS Standards, AABB did not simply follow federal guidelines. It also invited the participation of representatives from a range of allied organizations, including Canadian Blood Services, Hema-Quebec, the United States Department of Defense, the College of American Pathologists, British and EU colleagues, and

FDA. The BB/TS Standards were specifically developed with an eye toward international best practices.

This internationalism is significant, because AABB plays a unique role, domestically and internationally, in laboratory accreditation for transfusion medicine, blood banking, and cellular therapy. Cognizant of global efforts to harmonize quality practices in healthcare, the BB/TS Standards reflect international principles of quality management, including harmonization with International Society of Blood Transfusion (ISBT) standards, with the result being that the AABB Standards for Blood Banks and Transfusion Services are a reliable guide to best practices domestically and abroad. As a byproduct of incorporating international best practices into the BB/TM Standards, AABB accreditation is often accepted as a basis for earning accreditation in foreign countries.

UNDERSTANDING THE STANDARDS

The BB/TS Standards are organized, section by section, according to the Quality System Essentials discussed in Chapter 2. Some of the section titles have evolved over the years–for example, "Personnel" is now "Resources (Human Resources)"—but the concepts have remained the same, and the section headings for the BB/TS Standards remain recognizable. As always, the section headings of the BB/TS Standards continue to be the list of Quality System Essentials, as follows:

1. Organization
2. Resources (Human Resources)
3. Equipment
4. Supply and Customer Issues
5. Process Control
6. Documents and Records
7. Deviations, Nonconformances, and Adverse Events
8. Assessments: Internal and External
9. Process Improvement Through Corrective and Preventative Action
10. Facilities and Safety

Risk Management in Transfusion Medicine. https://doi.org/10.1016/B978-0-323-54837-3.00004-3

When considering each section of the Standards, it is useful to keep in mind that the goal is to provide an operational structure for delivering lifesaving blood to patients while protecting donors and recipients from harm. The Standards are the fundamental elements–the "nuts and bolts"—of risk management in transfusion medicine. Each QSE is a domain of activity that is necessary to assure product safety, quality, potency, and effectiveness. Structurally, each QSE is a supervisory function that combines managerial oversight with clear, written practices and procedures that ensure the ongoing reliability of the service. At the same time, it is important to note that there is a certain flexibility built into the BB/TS Standards' Quality System Essentials. Individual services are expected to craft policies and procedures adapted to their own practice settings.

Given the BB/TS Standards' central role in transfusion risk management, it is appropriate to spend time on each of the QSEs individually, to understand the scope of each and the operational function that each performs in managing risk.

QSE 1: Organization

Organizationally, laboratory leadership consists of a medical director and executive management. Leadership roles must be defined, and the leadership must have authority over, and responsibility for, the laboratory. A quality system must be established, and quality and operational policies and procedures must be developed and implemented. Emergency preparedness and an emergency management plan must also be established. Lab leadership is also responsible for establishing procedures to identify customers' needs and expectations, and creating a confidential process for personnel to communicate concerns they may have regarding quality or safety.

QSE 2: resources (human resources)

There must be a sufficient number of laboratory personnel to perform the functions of the service, and they must possess the proper qualifications and training to carry out all of the activities of the service. There are many ways to approach qualifications and training. Many institutions have established minimum educational and licensure requirements at the institutional level. If not, or if the requirements are not adequate in the judgment of the service, appropriate requirements must be set forth in a policy. Some states have set forth licensure requirements for technologists in clinical laboratories and transfusion services, but others have not. In fact, some states have discontinued mandatory qualifications for laboratory personnel as a bureaucratic cost-cutting measure, eliminating professional requirements to avoid administrative costs in the responsible

state agencies. Whatever the case may be, transfusion services must exercise independent responsibility for determining the qualifications and training (including ongoing education and training) needed to be able to carry out all of the activities of the service.

QSE 3: equipment

Laboratory equipment is critically important for providing safe and effective blood and blood products. Policies and procedures must be in place for selecting, qualifying, installing, and calibrating equipment; verifying, validating, monitoring, and maintaining the equipment; and investigating equipment malfunctions. Storage devices for blood and components, along with alarm systems to detect temperature perturbations, must be qualified and properly maintained. Information systems, including hardware, software, and backup systems, must be maintained and monitored.

In many health care institutions, responsibility for maintaining medical equipment is assigned to a division outside of the laboratory, often referred to as the biomedical department, or "biomed." There is nothing wrong with such an arrangement, as long as the outside department understands the laboratory's medical and regulatory responsibilities, and cooperates with the laboratory's need for continuous monitoring of the activities being carried out on the laboratory's behalf. The biomedical department must also be prepared to provide governmental and credentialing bodies access to its facilities and records during inspections.

QSE 4: supply and customer issues

Supplier qualification is another important element of quality system essentials. Many institutions have purchasing departments, and they may also participate in group purchasing organizations (GPOs) that permit the institution's access to economies of scale in purchasing. State-owned healthcare institutions must also adhere to statutory requirements relating to fair purchasing, avoiding conflicts of interest, and any other legal and regulatory mandates. Importantly, however, the laboratory must nevertheless participate in the selection of all suppliers that will provide critical materials, equipment, and services to the laboratory, prior to acceptance of an agreement. If a supplier fails to meet requirements, the laboratory is responsible for informing the institution's contracting authority of all nonconformances.

QSE 5: process control

Process control is the essence of risk management, not just for blood banking and transfusion medicine, but for all clinical laboratories. More than any other Quality System Essential, process control focuses directly on patient care. Not surprisingly, Process Control is the longest section of the BB/TS Standards. The rules are specific, detailed, and prescriptive. The word "shall" appears frequently, and indeed, many of the directives in the Process Control section of the BB/TM Standards are mandated by federal statutes and regulations.

As discussed, the BB/TS Standards are designed to deliver blood safely to those who need it, without harming the donor or the recipient. Donor protection is achieved by verifying that the donor is physically fit to donate blood, and by practicing safe blood collection procedures. Process controls in the manufacturing steps and adherence to strict product specifications are aimed at ensuring product safety, purity, potency, and effectiveness. Recipient safety practices focus on preventing transfusion-transmitted infectious diseases and other important harms such as immune-mediated transfusion reactions, circulatory overload, and inappropriate blood ordering.

The present discussion will focus on donor protection and quality control in the manufacture of blood products. Processes to protect recipients against infectious risks are discussed in Chapter 5 (Infectious Risks in Transfusion Medicine). Immunological concerns and risk-based blood ordering practices are addressed in Chapters 6 and 7.

Process controls for managing donor risk.

To be eligible to donate blood, one must be 16 years old or older, unless applicable state law specifies otherwise. Studies have shown that individuals who begin donating blood at a young age are more likely to become lifelong donors,[1] and some commentators have suggested that the age limit for donation should be lowered below age 16. There is no upper age limit for donating blood, as long as the donor is healthy.

The FDA has devoted considerable time and resources to developing donor eligibility rules regarding a prospective donor's minimum allowable predonation hemoglobin and hematocrit. Prior to May, 2015, all donors were required to have a predonation Hb ≥ 12.5 g/dL or Hct ≥ 38% to be eligible to donate blood. As females tend to have lower hemoglobin and hematocrit levels than males, many more females than males were "deferred" (i.e., rejected) from donating blood. Data reported by the American Red Cross in the year 2006 showed that, of all prospective donors that were determined to be ineligible to donate, 70% of those rejections were due to low hemoglobin or hematocrit.[2] This amounted to over 600,000 prospective donors lost that year. A study using the REDS II database[3] found that 9.9% of all blood donation attempts

failed due to low hemoglobin levels. Remarkably, only 1.6% of donation attempts by males were deferred due to low hemoglobin, whereas 17.7% of donation attempts by females were deferred for that reason.

The loss of so many healthy female blood donors was highly problematic, particularly in light of the fact that the World Health Organization (WHO) threshold for anemia in adult females is 12.0 g/dL, meaning that females are not anemic at hemoglobin levels as low as 12.0 g/dL. Thus, FDA was requiring female donors with hemoglobin in the 12.0–12.5 g/dL range to be deferred even though they were not anemic. Many commentators urged the FDA to relax the mandatory thresholds by permitting females to donate blood if their hemoglobin was ≥12.0 g/dL or hematocrit ≥36%.

After careful consideration, and upon the recommendation of FDA's Blood Products Advisory Committee, the agency made what was to many a startling announcement: FDA left the requirement for female blood donors unchanged and they raised the eligibility thresholds for male donors to Hb ≥ 13.0 g/dL or Hct ≥ 39%. The new rule went into effect on May 23, 2016. Why would FDA do such a thing? The simple answer is iron stores. FDA did not issue its final determination until the results of the REDS-II-RISE study,[4] which evaluated iron deficiency in blood donors, was published. The study revealed an unexpectedly high prevalence of iron depletion in frequent blood donors. Because of those findings, FDA's Blood Products Advisory Committee voted unanimously to *raise* the minimum Hb/Hct levels for male donors, but they found that the evidence did not support changing the minimum standards for female donors.[5] Thus, the current requirement for female donors remains Hb ≥ 12.5 g/dL or Hct ≥ 38%, and the requirement for male donors has been increased to Hb ≥ 13.0 g/dL or Hct ≥ 39%.

Donor safety also requires that there be strict limits on the amount of blood that one may donate. The maximum volume of blood that may be removed during a whole blood donation is 10.5 mL per kg of body weight. Blood donors must also weigh at least 110 lbs (50 kg) to be eligible to give blood. It may seem arbitrary to designate a minimum weight limit for donating blood. However, the basis for the requirement is largely due to a combination of donor safety and logistics. At 10.5 mL/kg of body weight, a person who weighs 110 lbs can donate a maximum of 525 mL of blood. A standard blood collection bag is designed to hold a total volume, including anticoagulant, preservatives and donor blood, of 450 mL ± 10%. Thus, at maximum, the bag can be filled to a slightly less than 500 mL. The bag itself therefore ensures that the blood draw will not exceed the maximum limit for donors weighing 110 pounds and above, and of equal importance, the unit contains the proper amount of anticoagulant and preservatives for about 450 mL of blood. Thus, a safe volume is drawn, proper anticoagulation and preservatives are ensured, and there is no need to measure volumes during the collection process.

A prospective donor's blood pressure must be 90–180 mmHg systolic and 50–100 mmHg diastolic pressure. The 180 mmHg upper limit reflects a lack of data regarding whether it is safe to donate at blood pressures above 180 mmHg, combined with concerns that such a high level of hypertension might make donors vulnerable to severe adverse events if a significant blood volume is removed quickly.[6] On the other end of the spectrum, diastolic pressures below 50 mmHg raise the concern that the blood donation might represent an unsafe percentage of an individual's blood volume.

In addition to blood pressure requirements, the donor's heart rate is required to be between 50 and 100 beats per minute, and the pulse must be regular. The rules regarding blood pressure and pulse rate are not absolute, however. The responsible physician who oversees donations may examine the donor, explore the donor's health history, and/or consult with the donor's physician, and determine that the health of the donor will not be adversely affected by donating.[7]

The most familiar image of a blood donation involves the insertion of a needle into the donor's antecubital vein and drawing blood into a clear plastic bag. This is the "whole blood" donation. To prevent iatrogenic iron depletion, whole blood donors are required to wait 8 weeks before making another blood donation. The same requirements also apply to red blood cell donations that are performed by apheresis. Some apheresis blood donors are large enough to give double red blood cell donations, in which case the donor must wait 16 weeks before the next donation of red blood cells or whole blood.

There are important donor safety rules relating to donations by apheresis. First, a brief overview of apheresis may be helpful. When one spins a tube of whole blood in a centrifuge, the components of the blood separate into layers according to their density. Centrifugal force moves the red blood cells out the farthest, traveling to the bottom of the tube. Platelets and white blood cells (WBCs) settle immediately above the red cells in a thin layer referred to as the buffy coat. White blood cells can be separated from platelets using centrifugation, but that requires removing the buffy coat and performing a second spin at higher rpm, often referred to as the "hard" spin. Above the buffy coat is

the straw-colored plasma layer. Plasma contains a variety of important blood elements, such as antibodies and coagulation factors.

Fig. 4.1 shows how centrifugation causes blood to separate into layers, including red blood cells, the buffy coat (which is comprised of platelets and white blood cells), and plasma.

Similarly, after a whole blood donation, centrifugation is used to separate whole blood into layers that can be collected as RBCs, platelets, or plasma (Fig. 4.2). Apheresis works on the same principle (Fig. 4.3 and 4.4). Apheresis machines draw the donor's blood into a bowl-like container that spins the blood into its component layers. An automated needle draws off the desired layer. White blood cells can also be collected using apheresis, but WBC collection is a specialized procedure, primarily used in stem cell collections for bone marrow transplantation and for removing blast cells in acute leukemic crises.

An important difference between whole blood donations and apheresis donations is that specific blood components such as platelets, plasma, and RBCs, can be collected in isolation by apheresis. As whole blood donations are drawn directly into a collection bag, they necessarily contain a mixture of all blood components as they exist in the donor's bloodstream. This difference is important because we can afford to donate a great deal more plasma or platelets than the volumes that happen to be contained in a 450 mL whole blood donation. The number of platelets produced by a whole blood donation is $\geq 5.5 \times 10^{10}$, whereas the number collected in an apheresis donation is $\geq 3.0 \times 10^{11}$. That means that apheresis instruments can collect 5–6 times as many platelets than whole blood derived ("random donor") platelets in a single donation.

Drawbacks of apheresis collection include the greater amount of time required to collect components by apheresis (Fig. 4.5), compared with an 8–12 min whole blood donation. Plasmapheresis and red cell apheresis donations take about 30–45 min. Platelet apheresis may take an hour or more. Apheresis needles also have a larger bore than the needles used to collect whole blood, and the donor's arm must be kept straight throughout the procedure. Apheresis collection is more expensive as whole blood donation, due to the cost of apheresis instruments and the need for specially trained personnel.

All of the requirements for whole blood donations also apply to apheresis donations. The donor must have hemoglobin/hematocrit levels of 12.5 g/dL or 38% for women; 13.0 g/dL or 39% for men. As with whole blood donations, apheresis donors must weigh more than 110 lb (unless approved by FDA). If a volume of

Spinning Down A Blood Sample

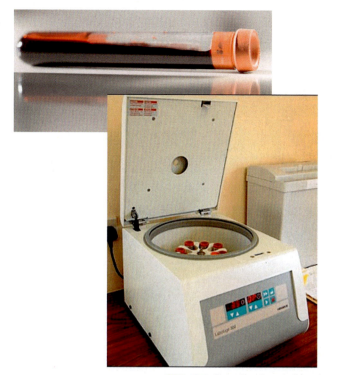

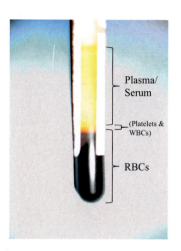

Plasma/
Serum

(Platelets &
WBCs)

RBCs

FIG. 4.1 Spinning down a blood sample.

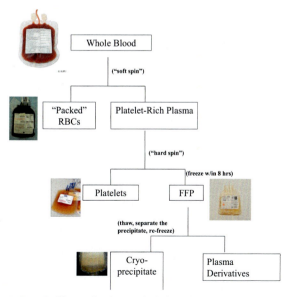

Whole Blood

("soft spin")

"Packed"
RBCs   Platelet-Rich Plasma

("hard spin")

(freeze w/in 8 hrs)

Platelets   FFP

(thaw, separate the
precipitate, re-freeze)

Cryo-
precipitate   Plasma
Derivatives

FIG. 4.2 After collecting a whole blood donation, the blood bank uses centrifugation to process the donor's blood into components.

APHERESIS TECHNOLOGY

- Centrifugal separation of the cellular blood elements and plasma.

- The ***cellular*** elements (RBCs, platelets, lymphocytes) layer out according to density.
  - A selected layer can then be drawn out.

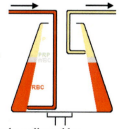

- ***Plasma*** goes to the top, and can be collected by filtration through a membrane.
  - Progress is being made toward selectively removing elements (e.g., immunoglobulins) from plasma by immuno-affinity techniques.

FIG. 4.3 Apheresis machines draw the donor's blood into a bowl-like container that spins the blood into its component layers. Specific blood components can be collected through a needle, and the remaining components are returned to the patient by the apheresis instrument.

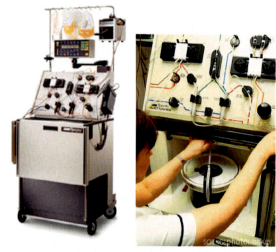

FIG. 4.4 Apheresis instruments appear complex, but fundamentally they function as shown in Fig. 4.3. Note the bowl shown on the right in Fig. 4.4.

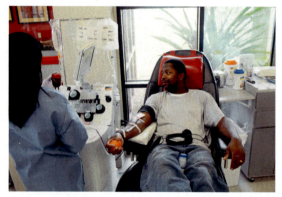

FIG. 4.5 A blood donation using an apheresis instrument. Copyright, Terumo BCT, Inc. 2017. Used with Permission.

whole blood greater than 200 mL cannot be returned from the apheresis instrument due to technical reasons, the patient is treated as having donated a unit of whole blood, with a mandatory 8-week deferral period until the next donation. As mentioned earlier, a "double" red blood cell donation by apheresis must be followed by a 16-week deferral period.

Several rules exist to minimize risks that are specific to apheresis donors. BB/TM Standards distinguish between "infrequent" and "frequent" plasmapheresis donors. *Infrequent* donors give plasma no more than once every 4 weeks. *Frequent* plasmapheresis donors are those who donate more often than every 4 weeks. Stricter rules are in place to protect frequent donors.

Apheresis Platelets

- Yield $\geq 3.0 \times 10^{11}$ plts/unit (in 90% of units sampled).
- Counts greater than 300K usually yield a double-dose ($\geq 6.0 \times 10^{11}$ platelets).
- Donation frequency limited to:
  - Once per two days;
  - No more than twice per week;
  - No more than 24 times per year;
  - Not within 48 hours of taking aspirin;
  - Plt count > 150K/µL (using a previous count is OK);
  - H/H $\geq$ 12.5/38% if female; 13.0/39% if male
  - BP 90-180/50-100; 50-100 bpm; temp $\leq$37.5C/99.5F
  - Exceptions with physician certification.

FIG. 4.6 Quality and safety regulations for platelet collections by apheresis.

Frequent plasma donors may undergo plasmapheresis once every 2 days (48 h) at a maximum of two procedures per 7 days. Red cell losses must be <200 mL per 8 weeks, and baseline serum protein electrophoresis or quantitative immunoglobulins must be performed at baseline and every 4 months thereafter.

Platelets collected by apheresis must yield $\geq 3.0 \times 10^{11}$ platelets/unit (a quality assurance requirement rather a donor safety requirement). The donor's predonation platelet count must be greater than 150,000/µL. Donors with platelet counts greater than 300,000/µL may yield a double-dose collection ($\geq 6.0 \times 10^{11}$ platelets). Platelet donation apheresis frequency is very similar to that of frequent plasma donors: Once every 2 days (48 h) and no more than twice per week. However, one additional limitation applies to platelet donors: one cannot donate platelets by apheresis more than 24 times per year (Fig. 4.6).

Protections for donors who provide RBCs by apheresis are primarily directed toward avoiding anemia or the depletion of iron stores. The same minimum hemoglobin and hematocrit qualifications for whole blood donations (12.5 g/dL or 38% for women; 13.0 g/dL or 39% for men) also apply to apheresis donations. As with whole blood donations, apheresis donors may donate one unit of red blood cells every 8 weeks. Apheresis technology makes it possible to collect a double dose (2 units) of RBCs if the donor is large enough not to exceed 10.5 mL per kg of body weight. However, after a double dose, the donor must wait 16 weeks before the next donation. Donors are given a saline infusion during RBC donations by apheresis to minimize volume depletion. A 2-unit collection must be calculated not to cause the donor's hematocrit to go below 30% or hemoglobin below 10 g/dL after volume replacement.

Blood product quality control (protecting recipients).
The FDA Center for Biologics Evaluation and Research (CBER) has regulatory oversight over blood and blood components. Within CBER, the Office of Blood Research and Review (OBRR) is charged with ensuring the safety, purity, potency, and effectiveness of blood and blood products. FDA's approach to blood safety incorporates the notion of redundancy. Five "layers" of protections keep the blood supply safe If one layer fails, protections are still in place. The first layer is donor selection, education, and risk factor screening. Donor deferral registries are next. The third layer is infectious diseases testing of the donated units. Fourth is the quarantining of units until infectious diseases testing is negative. Fifth is monitoring, investigating, and taking corrective action to address errors or accidents in the manufacturing process.

OBRR, working in cooperation with members of the regulated community, defines product standards for the manufacture of blood components in accordance with Current Good Manufacturing Practices (cGMP). The aim of these practices is to control quality throughout the entire manufacturing process to ensure the safety, purity, and potency of blood products. It is useful to think of blood as a drug: Not only are blood components regulated by FDA, but they must also meet safety, purity, and potency standards like drugs.

We have already seen a snapshot of how whole blood donations are processed into components, as shown in Fig. 4.2. We will now look at the process in more detail. To prepare red blood cells from a whole blood donation, the technologist begins by centrifuging the donor unit with a "soft spin." The RBCs migrate furthest, which is why they are frequently referred to as "packed RBCs." The technologist then draws off the 200–250 mL of straw-colored supernatant. This supernatant is referred to as "platelet-rich plasma" (PRP), as the platelets and plasma do not separate during the soft spin. The PRP then undergoes a "hard spin" that separates the platelets from the plasma.

Platelets cannot be frozen or refrigerated because they are very easily activated, causing them to clump. Instead, platelets are placed on a rotator that gently rocks them at 20–24°C (room temperature) to keep them from contact that will lead to platelet activation. Due to the risk of bacterial growth at room temperature, platelets have a shelf life of only 5 days, which explains why platelets are always in very short supply.

Plasma, on the other hand, can be frozen. If plasma is frozen within 8h of donation, it can be stored in the freezer at −18°C for 1 year. The short 8-h window gives rise to the term "fresh frozen plasma" or FFP. As a concession to the expanded use of "bloodmobiles," FDA has recently permitted plasma to be frozen within 24h of collection and still be eligible for the 1-year shelf life at −18°C. However, plasma that is frozen within 24h rather than 8h must be labeled as FP24, rather than FFP.

Cryoprecipitate is made by removing FFP from the freezer and thawing it in a refrigerator at 1–6°C. At that temperature, a slush precipitates out of the liquid. If the slush is separated and refrozen at −18°C within 1h, the aptly named cryoprecipitate can be stored for a year. Cryoprecipitate is a very compact source of fibrinogen. It also contains a significant amount of Factor VIII, but the use of cryoprecipitate to treat hemophilia A has waned due to the availability of recombinant Factor VIII.

The various blood components are governed by highly specific quality standards to ensure maximum purity, potency, and effectiveness. We will touch on some examples of important quality specifications to convey the rigorousness and complexity of the manufacturing process.

Red blood cells are most commonly derived from whole blood donations. The separation of red blood cells from whole blood by centrifugation does not yield a perfectly pure collection of RBCs. Red blood cells are metabolically active, so they require nutrients to remain viable during storage. In total, a unit of pRBCs consists of red blood cells ($\approx$260 mL), plasma ($\approx$50 mL), preservatives ($\approx$50 mL), WBCs ($\approx 10^8$), a trace amount of platelets, and iron (200 mg). FDA mandates, as a quality control requirement, that the hematocrit of a unit of RBCs must be <80% in all RBC units. Storage temperature requirements are also mandated by the FDA: RBCs must be stored at 1–6°C, and when they are shipped (across town or to the O.R.) their temperature must be maintained within the range of 1–10°C. RBCs can be frozen and stored for 10 years at −65°C, but once thawed, they must be stored at 1–6°C, and they expire 24h post-thaw. RBCs that have been irradiated expire 21 days post-irradiation or on the original expiration date, whichever is sooner.

FDA-approved RBC preservatives consist of the "primary" anticoagulant (primary because it is added to the bag prior to receiving the blood donation) and additive solutions. The shelf life of RBCs varies according to the anticoagulant and additive solutions that are used:

Primary anticoagulants
- Citrate phosphate dextrose (CPD): 21-day shelf life for RBCs.
- Citrate phosphate dextrose adenine-1 (CPDA-1): 35-day shelf life for RBCs.

Additive solution ("Addsol"): Extends shelf life of CPD-treated RBCs to 42 days.
- Addsol is added after the RBCs are spun and separated from the whole blood.
- Addsol can only be used with CPD, not with CPDA-1.

Platelets are traditionally derived from whole blood donations, in which case they are designated as "platelet concentrate" because the platelets are centrifuged with a "hard spin" and thus concentrated. One also hears the term "pooled" platelets, reflecting the fact that five to six platelet concentrates must be pooled together to constitute an appropriate dose for most adult patients. A third term for platelets that are derived from whole blood donations is "random donor" platelets, referring to the fact that multiple donors contribute to the unit, as opposed to so-called "single-donor" platelets collected from a single donor by apheresis.

Under FDA rules, platelet concentrate must contain at least 5.5×10^{10} platelets and the pH must be at least 6.2 in 90% of units sampled. There are typically about 10^7 white blood cells in each unit of random donor platelets, but one can reduce the number of WBCs being transfused by adding a leukoreduction filter. Leukoreduced platelets are required to contain fewer than 8.3×10^5 platelets in 90% of units sampled (Fig. 4.7).

Collecting platelets using apheresis is an efficient alternative to spinning whole blood and separating the platelets. The body produces considerably more platelets than are necessary for clotting, and apheresis machines can specifically draw platelets from the donor's blood without depleting other blood elements. A single plateletpheresis donor can supply as many platelets as five or more whole blood donors. FDA quality standards mandate that a single unit of apheresis platelets must contain at least 3.0×10^{11} platelets, which is approximately five times the 5.5×10^{10} minimum required for each unit of platelet concentrate derived from whole blood.

Another advantage of apheresis technology is that contemporary instruments are able to draw platelets without collecting an excessive number of leukocytes, despite platelets' tendency to run with WBCs in the buffy coat. Therefore, single donor platelet units are typically leukoreduced as a matter of course, satisfying the FDA minimum requirement of $<5.0 \times 10^6$ WBCs in 90% of units sampled.

QSE 6: documents and records
Document control is a very important but sometimes overlooked risk management practice. Perhaps the greatest risk from inadequate document control is the use of unofficial procedures such as "cheat sheets." For convenience, laboratory employees may sometimes jot down notes on how to perform a particular procedure rather than consulting the Procedure Manual each time they perform the test. Inspectors sometimes look

Platelets

PLATELET CONCENTRATE   ("pooled" or "random donor" plts):

Volume: 50 mL
Contents: Platelets ($\geq 5.5 \times 10^{10}$)
            Plasma
            Fibrinogen ($\approx$80 mg)
            WBC's (10^7)
            pH $\geq$ 6.2 (in 90%)

Leukoreduced platelets:
Same, except
$< 8.3 \times 10^5$ WBC (in 90%)

APHERESIS PLATELETS   ("single donor" platelets):

Volume: 100 mL
Contents: Platelets ($\geq 3.0 \times 10^{11}$)
            Plasma
            Fibrinogen ($\approx$150 mg)
            WBC's (10^6-10^8)
            pH $\geq$ 6.2 (in 90%)

Leukoreduced Pltpheresis:
Same, except
$< 5.0 \times 10^6$ WBC (in 90%)

FIG. 4.7 Primary constituents of random donor versus apheresis platelets. FDA-mandated quality control requirements are in red.

in the back of drawers to see if they find such notes, sometimes to the chagrin of surprised lab managers. A significant concern is that procedures, reagents, or instruments may have changed without the handwritten cheat sheets being updated. Anyone who follows the unofficial procedure may then perform the test incorrectly without knowing it.

A cardinal rule of good laboratory practice is that policies and procedures must be available at all times to the technologists performing the work. The corollary rule is that the documents must be up to date and accurate. Proper document control involves maintaining a master list of documents, and policies and procedures for tracking all documents, updating them, and informing employees of significant changes. When policies are amended, prior versions must be removed and replaced. Document management rules also require policies and procedures to be reviewed a minimum of every 2 years.

Facility records must enable the tracing of any blood or blood product from the source to the final disposition. In the event of a unit's recall, it must be possible to track the unit all the way from the donor to the recipient (if the unit has been transfused), and to perform a "look-back" to see whether blood from that donor was transfused to other recipients. In all cases, records of any significant activities performed by the laboratory must be maintained, and must indicate the performing technologist, the time and date of the activity, results obtained, equipment used, and the facility where the activity was performed.

An extensive set of document retention rules regarding both donation records and patient records is found in Reference Standard 6.2A (the appendix to Standard 6). The majority of donor and patient records, many related to donor and recipient testing (ABO, crossmatch, blood irradiation, adverse events in collection or transfusion, emergency release) must be kept for 10 years. A smaller number of rules related to minor matters such as transfusion consent forms, bedside patient identification, and personnel training records must be kept for only 5 years. The specific rules may be found in the Standard 6.2A.

QSE 7: deviations, nonconformances, and adverse events

Deviations are products that differ from specifications. A nonconformance is when blood or blood products do not meet the criteria for acceptability, that is, they do not conform to the specified requirements for release. Nonconforming products must be quarantined to prevent their being released unintentionally to a patient.

Procedures must be in place for identifying deviating and nonconforming components and capturing them for investigation, assessment, and disposition.

Adverse events are harms that befall a patient as a result of medical care. In transfusion medicine, adverse events include allergic reactions, acute and delayed hemolytic transfusion reactions, transfusion-related acute lung injury (TRALI), transfusion-associated circulatory overload (TACO), and the like. Fatalities must be reported to the FDA, pursuant to 21 CFR 606.170(b).[8] The Medical Director must provide notice to FDA within 24 h that a fatality appears to be related to transfusion or collection, and must submit a more comprehensive follow-up report within 3 days. There must also be a procedure for identifying, evaluating, and reporting nonfatal adverse events related to transfusion or donation, as well as processes for recognizing and responding to immediate (acute) transfusion reactions, including notification of the medical director and workup of potential acute hemolytic transfusion reactions. If a delayed transfusion reaction is suspected, a laboratory workup must be performed.

QSE 8: assessments–internal and external

The laboratory must participate in self-assessments and external assessments, which include proficiency testing ("challenges" involving the workup of specimens provided by outside entities) and external inspections (laboratory inspections by outside organizations). The results of the assessments must be reviewed, and when appropriate, the cause of failures must be identified and corrective action taken to prevent similar failures in the future. The results of assessments as well as corrective actions must be reviewed by executive management and the medical director.

Facilities performing transfusions must establish a program for monitoring the full breadth of transfusion-related activities, including blood ordering, blood transfusion, appropriateness of blood use, sample collection, labeling, patient identification, and adverse events. Quality indicator data must also be reviewed on a scheduled basis.

QSE 9: process improvement through corrective and preventative action

The laboratory must have a process for evaluating deviations, nonconformances, and complaints, and for performing corrective action to address all such events. Each event must be described, an investigation performed and documented, and the cause determined. A corrective action plan must be formulated and implemented, and the outcome monitored to be sure that the corrective action has been performed and that it has been effective. The reader is referred to Chapter 2 for more details about formal process improvement strategies.

QSE 10: facilities and safety

The laboratory must have policies, processes, and procedures to ensure that the work environment is safe and meets all applicable regulatory standards. This includes biological, chemical, and radiation safety, as well as the safe disposal of biological material such as blood and tissue.

REFERENCES

1. Satake M. Planning donor recruitment strategies with an eye on the future. *ISBT Sci Ser*. 2016;11(S2). https://doi.org/10.1111/voxs.12275.
2. Elder A, Bianco C, eds. *Screening Blood Donors: Science, Reason, and the Donor History Questionnaire*. Bethesda, MD: AABB Press; 2007.
3. Mast AE, Schlumpf KS, Wright DJ, et al. For the NHLBI retrovirus epidemiology donor study – II. *Transfusion*. 2010;50:1794–1802.
4. Cable RG, Glynn SA, Kiss JE, et al. Iron deficiency in blood donors: the REDS-II donor iron status evaluation (RISE) study," NHLBI retrovirus epidemiology donor study-II (REDS-II). *Transfusion*. 2012;52:702–711.
5. Federal Register. Vol. 80, No. 99. Friday; May 22, 2015: 29867–29868.
6. Federal Register. No. 99. *Rules and Regulations, at 29866*. Vol. 80. ; May 22, 2015:29842–29906.
7. Federal Register. No. 99. *Rules and Regulations, at 29868-29869*. Vol. 80. ; May 22, 2015:29842–29906.
8. 21 CFR 606.170(b). *"Guidance for Industry: Notifying FDA of Fatalities Related to Blood Collection or Transfusion"*; September 22, 2003.

CHAPTER 5

Transfusion-Transmitted Infectious Diseases

J. MILLS BARBEAU, MD, JD

In Chapter 4, we examined measures to minimize risk for the altruistic blood donors who save countless lives every year. This chapter turns to the protection of blood recipients. There are unfortunately many ways to harm patients receiving blood transfusions, but two categories of risk are particularly important: immunologic incompatibility and transfusion-transmitted infectious diseases. This chapter examines infectious risks.

Infectious organisms have found their way into human bloodstreams for as long as humans and microorganisms have coexisted. In fact, there is considerable evidence that humans and microbes have influenced each other quite profoundly, to the extent that infectious agents in blood are a study in coevolution. Cserti and Dzik have posited that "the origin, distribution, and relative proportion of ABO blood groups in humans may have been directly influenced by selective genetic pressure from *P. falciparum* infection."[1] Kwiatkowski has characterized malaria as "the strongest known force for evolutionary selection in the recent history of the human genome."[2]

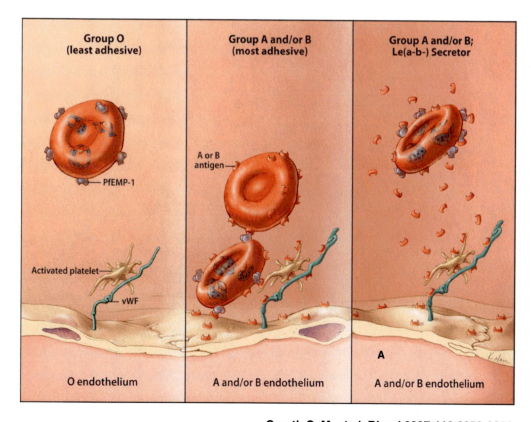

Cserti, C. M. et al. Blood 2007;110:2250-2258

Risk Management in Transfusion Medicine. https://doi.org/10.1016/B978-0-323-54837-3.00005-5

Delivering blood to patients is a complex endeavor. It is worthwhile to consider the various kinds of activities that must be performed flawlessly to deliver a safe, pure, and potent blood product to the patient. The practice of blood banking and transfusion medicine involves elements of:

- Public Health
- Manufacturing
- Transplantation and Immunological Science
- Infectious Diseases
- Direct patient care

All of these elements must fit seamlessly together or the product will fail. The public health function attends to the challenges of equitably and efficiently delivering a quality product that is in short supply. FDA, CDC, and CMS, as well as the professional societies that participate in both the rulemaking and the execution of the rules, carry out the public health function. The blood banking function performed by blood suppliers (and to a lesser extent, by transfusion-focused hospital services) is a high-stakes manufacturing process that must adhere to very strict tolerances of safety, purity, and potency. Clinically and scientifically, the field of transfusion medicine depends on a very high level of expertise in immunology and infectious diseases. Finally, transfusion medicine is direct patient care. When all is said and done, we bring our life-giving product literally to the patient's bedside.

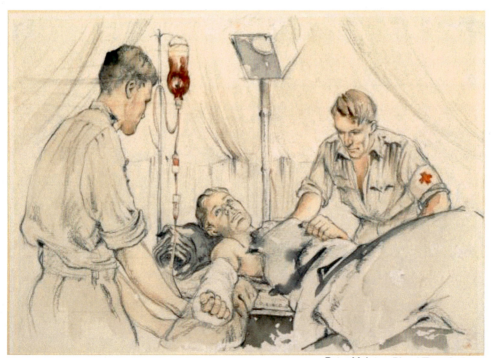

Peter McIntyr, *Blood Transfusion*

Ultimately, the safety of a blood product depends on two key elements: Immunologic compatibility with the patient and freedom from infectious diseases. This chapter focuses on the infectious diseases aspects of transfusion medicine, including the public health considerations in designing policies that minimize infectious risks in the blood supply.

The FDA adheres to a multilayered approach to keeping donor blood free of infectious agents.[3] The layers are overlapping safeguards that reinforce each other so that safety does not depend upon any single safeguard. The layers comprise the following:

- Donor screening
- Blood testing
- Donor deferral lists
- Quarantine
- Problems and deficiencies

DONOR SCREENING

The donor screening process is extraordinarily important for minimizing risk to blood recipients. The screening process begins with educational information provided to prospective donors. Next, potential donors are asked to answer a series of questions in a Donor History Questionnaire, designed to identify infectious risks.

Full-Length Donor History Questionnaire (DHQ)

	Yes	No
Are you		
1. Feeling healthy and well today?	❑	❑
2. Currently taking an antibiotic?	❑	❑
3. Currently taking any other medication for an infection?	❑	❑
4. Have you taken any medications on the Medication Deferral List in the time frames indicated? (Review the Medication Deferral List.)	❑	❑
5. Have you read the educational materials today?	❑	❑
In the past 48 hours,		
6. Have you taken aspirin or anything that has aspirin in it?	❑	❑
In the past 8 weeks, have you		
7. Donated blood, platelets or plasma?	❑	❑
8. Had any vaccinations or other shots?	❑	❑
9. Had contact with someone who was vaccinated for smallpox in the past 8 weeks?	❑	❑
In the past 16 weeks,		
10. Have you donated a double unit of red cells using an apheresis machine?	❑	❑
In the past 12 months, have you		
11. Had a blood transfusion?	❑	❑
12. Had a transplant such as organ, tissue, or bone marrow?	❑	❑
13. Had a graft such as bone or skin?	❑	❑
14. Come into contact with someone else's blood?	❑	❑
15. Had an accidental needle-stick?	❑	❑
16. Had sexual contact with anyone who has HIV/AIDS or has had a positive test for the HIV/AIDS virus?	❑	❑
17. Had sexual contact with a prostitute or anyone else who takes money or drugs or other payment for sex?	❑	❑
18. Had sexual contact with anyone who has ever used needles to take drugs or steroids, or anything not prescribed by their doctor?	❑	❑
19. Male donors: Had sexual contact with another male?	❑	❑
20. Female donors: Had sexual contact with a male who had sexual contact with another male in the past 12 months?	❑	❑
21. Had sexual contact with a person who has hepatitis?	❑	❑
22. Lived with a person who has hepatitis?	❑	❑
23. Had a tattoo?	❑	❑
24. Had ear or body piercing?	❑	❑
25. Had or been treated for syphilis or gonorrhea?	❑	❑
26. Been in juvenile detention, lockup, jail, or prison for more than 72 consecutive hours?	❑	❑

Full-Length Donor History Questionnaire (DHQ)

	Yes	No
In the past three years, have you		
27. Been outside the United States or Canada?	❑	❑
From 1980 through 1996,		
28. Did you spend time that adds up to 3 months or more in the United Kingdom? (Review list of countries in the UK)	❑	❑
29. Were you a member of the U.S. military, a civilian military employee, or a dependent of a member of the U.S. military?	❑	❑
From 1980 to the present, did you		
30. Spend time that adds up to 5 years or more in Europe? (Review list of countries in Europe.)	❑	❑
31. Receive a blood transfusion in the United Kingdom or France? (Review country lists.)	❑	❑
Have you EVER		
32. Female donors: Been pregnant or are you pregnant now?	❑	❑
33. Had a positive test for the HIV/AIDS virus?	❑	❑
34. Used needles to take drugs, steroids, or anything not prescribed by your doctor?	❑	❑
35. Received money, drugs, or other payment for sex?	❑	❑
36. Had malaria?	❑	❑
37. Had Chagas disease?	❑	❑
38. Had babesiosis?	❑	❑
39. Received a dura mater (or brain covering) graft or xenotransplantation product?	❑	❑
40. Had any type of cancer, including leukemia?	❑	❑
41. Had any problems with your heart or lungs?	❑	❑
42. Had a bleeding condition or a blood disease?	❑	❑
43. Have any of your relatives had Creutzfeldt-Jakob disease?	❑	❑

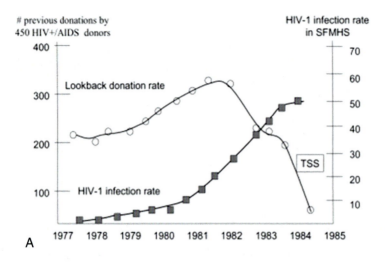

A

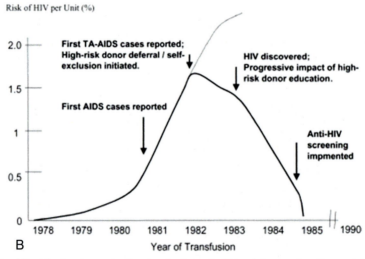

B

FIG. 5.1 Michael Bush's classic graph, showing the impact of blood donor education and donor history questionnaires in reducing the risk of HIV in the blood supply during the earliest years of the HIV epidemic.

The graphs produced by Michael Busch (Figure 5.1) illustrate the power of donor education and screening interviews. The top graph shows the accelerating human immunodeficiency virus (HIV) infection rate during the time period in which HIV was first recognized, along with the lookback blood donation rate of 400 HIV+ blood donors. The lower graph shows the risk of HIV per unit during the same period. The graphs demonstrate the steeply rising prevalence of HIV in the blood supply, which continued to rise until it was determined that HIV was causing transfusion-associated AIDS cases. Educational information and self-exclusion immediately reversed the trend, going from a steep increase to a rapid decline of HIV in donor blood.

Further understanding of HIV, along with impactful donor education, drove down HIV's prevalence in the blood supply even more steeply. Finally, on the far-right end of the curve, laboratory testing of donor blood drove the graph's tail almost to zero. Donor education and donor history questionnaires are highly impactful risk reduction tools.

The American Red Cross collected and published extensive data in 2006, which are summarized in Table 5.1. It is interesting to see how many prospective donors were deferred from donating blood because of the physical examination and donor history questionnaire.

It is interesting to note that, by far, the greatest number of deferrals was due to low hemoglobin or

TABLE 5.1
American Red Cross Blood Donor Deferrals, 2006

Reason for Deferral	Number of Donors Deferred	% of Total Donors (n = 7,788,748)			
PHYSICAL EXAMINATION			**HIV/Hep Total**	**41,898**	**0.54**
Hb/HCT (12.5/38%)	664,365	8.53	Hep after 11 yo	1,495	0.02
BP (≤180/100)	46,998	0.60	Live or sex w/ hepatitis+	6,493	0.08
Pulse (50-100)	26,875	0.35	HIV+/STDS/$ or drugs for sex	679	0.01
Other (tat, wt, arm, age, freq)	32,956	0.42	IV drug use	1,307	0.02
Total PE	**771,194**	**9.90**	MSM since '77	2,960	0.04
			Sex w/ at-risk	2,104	0.03
DONOR QUESTIONNAIRE			Txfn/txplt/tatoo	25,782	0.33
Currently ill	9,343	0.12	**Malaria (total)**	**49,243**	**0.63**
Infection/Abx	24,972	0.32	Had in past 3 y	138	<0.01
Ht/Lung Dz	7,965	0.10	Lived endemic	2,020	0.03
Bleeding Dz	5,054	0.06	Travel endemic	47,085	0.60
Cancer	14,666	0.19	**vCJD: In UK/Euro**	**10,589**	**0.14**
Other conditions	4,581	0.06	**vCJD: Dura/GH**	**413**	**<0.01**
Meds/vaccines	8,711	0.11	**Total Questionnaire**	**177,435**	**2.28**

hematocrit. The total number of blood donors was 7,788,748—a remarkable number. Fully 8.53% of all prospective donors were deferred due to low hemoglobin or hematocrit, which amounts to 664,365 donors total.

Malaria risks were the second most significant cause of deferrals after hemoglobin/HCT, with 49,243 deferrals for malaria risk. A total of 41,898 were deferred for STDs, hepatitis risk, IV drug use, money or sex for drugs, incarceration, and tattoos.

INFECTIOUS DISEASES TESTING
Mandatory Infectious Diseases Testing
Infectious diseases testing is the next safety layer, whereby laboratory assays detect specific infectious agents or classes of agents (such as bacteria) if they are present in the donor's blood. All infectious disease test kits used for donor blood testing must be FDA-approved. Currently, FDA requires all donor blood to be tested for the following:
- Hepatitis B virus
- Hepatitis C virus
- HIV-1 and -2
- Human T-lymphotropic virus (HTLV)-1 and -2

- *T. pallidum* (syphilis)
- West Nile virus
- Chagas
- Zika virus

Hepatitis B Virus
Hepatitis B is tested for anti-Hepatitis B core protein (anti-HBc) and Hepatitis B surface antigen (HBsAg). Ultra-sensitive HBsAg testing has been used since 2006. Hepatitis B are a very common cause of severe liver infection worldwide. Approximately 90% of healthy adults who are exposed to Hepatitis B recover spontaneously and produce anti-Hepatitis B surface antigen (anti-HBs) antibodies, conferring lifelong immunity. Ten percent of adults progress to chronic infection. Most significantly, 50% of children and 90% of infants who are infected with Hepatitis B progress to chronic infection, putting them at risk for cirrhosis and hepatic carcinoma. One might wonder whether it would be useful to add Hepatitis B nucleic acid testing (NAT) to the screen. Stramer et al.[4] revealed that the efficacy of the HBV vaccine for the prevention of clinical disease (even if not always prevention of infection), and the cost of interdicting donations that contain HBV DNA from

seronegative donors, are high in the face of unknown benefit. Thus, serologic testing remains the standard.

Hepatitis C virus
All blood donations must be tested for Hepatitis C virus using anti-Hepatitis C serology and Hepatitis C NAT.

Human Immunodeficiency virus
All blood donations must be tested for HIV-1 and -2 using FDA-approved NAT.

The issue of allowing men who have sex with men (MSM) to donate blood has been controversial for years. Until quite recently, any male-to-male sexual contact since 1977 (i.e., when HIV reached the United States) triggered an automatic lifetime prohibition against donating blood. Sexual contact with someone who is HIV positive triggers a 1-year deferral, but MSM sexual contact meant a lifetime deferral.

There are several 1-year deferral triggers, such as sexual contact with an HIV+ individual, paying money or drugs in exchange for sex, having sexual contact with someone who uses needles for illicit drugs, or being incarcerated for greater than 72 h. The logic behind a 1-year deferral after an HIV exposure is straightforward. HIV transmission will declare itself—one way or the other—within a year. The longest reported interval to HIV seroconversion was by a healthcare worker after a needlestick. Seroconversion reportedly took 213 days (average being 22–45 days). The data were not especially reliable, but a presumed 6–9-month maximum window for seroconversion to HIV+ status was a conservative basis for FDA's 1-year deferral rule for HIV exposures.

In 2006, AABB and the American Red Cross endorsed a proposal to reduce MSM deferrals to 12 months. The announcement caused significant press coverage. However, in 2007, FDA reaffirmed the permanent MSM deferral, observing that MSMs have an increased HIV prevalence, and they are the largest group who test positive in donor screening. FDA referred to data indicating that MSMs are more likely to unknowingly donate during the "window" period. FDA stated that MSM donations would increase the risk of inadvertently donating HIV+ blood, which in turn creates an increased risk of accidentally transfusing HIV+ blood (e.g., due to a failure to quarantine).

FDA also noted that MSMs have increased risk of infections such as HBV, HCV, and HHV-8. The document concluded by stating as follows: "No alternate set of donor eligibility criteria (even including practice of safe sex or a low number of lifetime partners) has yet been found to reliably identify MSM who are not at increased risk for HIV or certain other transfusion transmissible infections."[5]

In December 2015, FDA released its Guidance for Industry, Revised Recommendations for Reducing the Risk of Human Immunodeficiency Virus Transmission by Blood and Blood Products.[6] The Guidance announced FDA's revised donor deferral recommendations for individuals with increased risk for transmitting HIV infection. The document traced FDA's history of efforts to reduce HIV transmission by blood products, beginning in 1983. It then reviewed current evidence in the literature, Australia's experiences changing its MSM policy, and the recommendations of the Interagency Blood, Organ, & Tissue Safety Working Group (BOTS Working Group). The Guidance concluded with a recommendation to update the donor history questionnaire (DHQ), which now asks: "For male donors: a history in the past 12 months of sex with another man." Hence, healthy MSM donors are now excluded from donating for only one year after sexual contact with another man, instead of a lifetime deferral.

Human T-Lymphotropic virus
FDA regulations require testing donors for anti-HTLV-1 and -2 antibodies. Human T-cell lymphotropic virus was the first retrovirus to be discovered in humans. In fact, when HIV was discovered, it was originally named HTLV-3. These T-cell tropic viruses can lead to aggressive adult T-cell lymphoma. Moreover, 1%–5% of people infected by HTLV-1 develop cancer as a result. Modes of transmission of the HTLV-1 virus are very similar to that of HIV: through blood transfusion, sexual contact, sharing needles, and vertically during birth or through breast-feeding. HTLV-2 also affects T-cells, but there are usually no associated symptoms, although it appears to be a lifelong infection. The routes of transmission for HTLV-2 are also similar to those of HIV.

T. pallidum **(syphilis).** Syphilis was the first infectious disease to be tested in donor blood units, beginning in World War I—recall from Chapter 2, Oswald Hope Robertson, who instituted the world's first blood bank during the Battle of Cambrai. In 2015, FDA solicited comments and data on whether to discontinue the requirement for syphilis testing, but insufficient data was submitted to support discontinuation. Platforms cleared for syphilis testing are shown in Table 5.2. These assays remind us that all infectious disease testing of donor units must be performed using assays that have been cleared by FDA, a fact that has significant implications for the scope of testing available to the Agency. For example, as of this writing, no Creutzfeldt-Jakob disease (CJD) or variant Creutzfeldt-Jakob disease (vCJD) tests have been licensed for donor testing, preventing FDA from including such testing in mandatory screening, despite FDA's preference for such screening to be mandatory.[7]

West Nile virus

West Nile virus (WNV) is a mosquito-borne flavivirus that appeared in the United States in 1999. Donor blood has been screened for West Nile virus since 2003, using NAT. Eighty percent of people who are infected by WNV are asymptomatic. The virus is transmissible by transfusion. West Nile virus is seasonal, but the timing and severity of outbreaks are unpredictable. The 2012 season, for example, was quite serious, causing a total of 5674 cases, with 286 deaths. Half of the cases (2873 cases, or 51%) were neuroinvasive.[8]

Because of the unpredictability of outbreaks, a nuanced testing paradigm was necessary. The paradigm that has been developed relies on mini-pool NAT. A mini-pool (MP) comprises 6–16 donations per pool. A positive result from the mini-pool leads to testing each of the samples individually to determine which sample or samples were positive. A single positive mini-pool triggers reversion to individual-donation NAT (ID-NAT), a process that is referred to as "triggering." Data have shown that MP testing is not very sensitive (by some reports only about 50%),[8] so it is desirable to add a strategy of occasional targeted ID-NAT testing that supplements the MP testing during the quiet periods between triggering events.

TABLE 5.2
Cleared Donor Screening Tests for Treponema Pallidum (Syphilis)

Tradename(s)	Format	Specimen Collection	Donors	Manufacturer	Clearance Date
Olympus PKTP System	Treponemal	*Living:* Serum, Plasma	Living	Fujirebio Inc.	2/21/2003
ASI TPHA Teat	Treponemal	*Living:* Serum	Living	Arlington Scientific, Inc	1/30/2003
CAPTIA TM Syphilis(T. Pallidum)-G Package Insert (PDF - 355 KB)	Treponemal	*Living:* Serum, Plasma	Living	Trinity Biotech	4/2010
TPHA Screen	Treponemal	*Living:* Serum, Plasma	Living	Immucor	10/24/2012
ASiManager-AT	Non-treponemal	Living: Serum, Plasma Cadaveric: Serum, Plasma	Living, Cadaveric	Arlington Scientific, Inc	2/24/2014

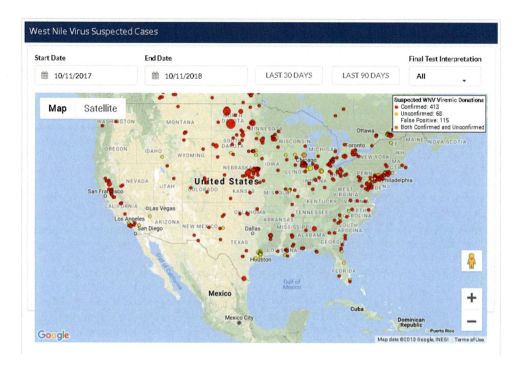

The map provided above by AABB is continually updated, showing West Nile virus suspected viremic donations, in this example between 04/28/2018 and 07/27/2018. Presumed viremic donations (PVDs) are defined as follows: (1) a WNV-reactive donation with a >17 signal-to-cutoff ratio; or (2) a WNV-reactive with a <17 signal-to-cutoff ratio that is repeatedly reactive. PVDs have a greater than 90% chance of being confirmed. Based on a decade of data, AABB recommends adopting *one* of the following criteria for conversion from MP-NAT to ID-NAT, that is, from minipool testing to individual donor testing:

1. One PVD with evidence of other WNV activity in the collection region.
2. Two PVDs in a 7-day rolling period if there is no other WNV activity in the collecting region.
3. One PVD if the collection facility elects not to consider regional activity.

Zika virus

Zika virus (sometimes referred to as ZIKV) is an enveloped, single-stranded RNA arbovirus in the *Flavivirus* genus. It is closely related to West Nile and Dengue viruses. Zika virus is transmitted by *Aedes* mosquitos,

usually *Aedes aegypti*, as is chikungunya. In recent years, Zika has demonstrated scattered but increasing activity in Micronesia, French Polynesia, Brazil, and Colombia. In December 2015, the United States was impacted as Puerto Rico reported mosquito-borne Zika transmissions. Within a year, an estimated 13% of the Puerto Rican population was infected with Zika virus. By that time, it was clear that routes of exposure included perinatal, intrauterine, sexual, laboratory-acquired, and blood-borne.[9]

Approximately 80% of individuals who become infected by Zika virus remain asymptomatic. When symptoms are present, they may consist of mild fever, rash, headache, and conjunctivitis. Unfortunately, Zika virus infection can sometimes lead to harm to developing fetuses, such as microcephaly, other congenital defects, and fetal or infant death.

By March 2016, Puerto Rico was receiving all of its blood products from the continental United States. In April 2016, individual donation NAT (ID NAT) for Zika virus was approved by FDA under an Investigational New Drug (IND) application. In August 2016, Zika virus was listed as a relevant TTI, and joined the list of organisms that are subject to individual donor testing. FDA issued a guidance requiring all blood suppliers to test all blood donations (universal ID NAT) for Zika virus. Louis Katz, CEO of America's Blood Centers, reported that blood suppliers screened more than 1 million units of blood during the first year, at a cost of $137 million. Because many regions of the United States are not geographically hospitable to Zika virus—for example, regions lacking an Aedes mosquito population—many blood centers considered the universal individual testing to be overanxious and, from a risk-based decision making perspective, flawed.[10]

In July 2018, a second test system was licensed for Zika NAT. FDA announced that blood suppliers could move from universal testing (ID NAT) to MP NAT, much as occurred in the case of West Nile virus. Regional blood suppliers can now use MP NAT testing for Zika virus, returning to individual testing only when their geographic region shows Zika activity.[9]

Chagas

Chagas disease is caused by *Trypanosoma crusi*, a parasite found predominantly in Central and South America.

The insect vector that carries *T. crusi* is a triatomine insect, also known as a reduviid, or "kissing" bug. The insect becomes infected with the *T. crusi* parasite while taking a blood meal. Later, when the triatomine insect feeds again on a sleeping human, typically on the victim's face, the bug defecates feces contaminated with *T. crusi*. The victim then rubs where the bug fed, inoculating the feces further. The triatomines are called kissing bugs because of their habit of landing on their sleeping target's face.

Chagas disease has an acute stage that lasts for 6–8 weeks after the bug bite. The acute phase is usually asymptomatic, or sometimes accompanied with fever, malaise, swelling at the site of inoculation, and possibly lymphadenopathy. The acute phase is followed by a chronic indeterminate phase, with potentially lifelong low-level, intermittent parasitemia. Decades after the initial infection, 30% of people will have onset of chronic, symptomatic disease with cardiomyopathy and arrhythmias, and/or gastrointestinal disease such as megaesophagus or megacolon.[11]

An AABB biovigilance map of 157 confirmed positive Chagas cases in the United States during the period 1/1/2017–7/27/2018 is shown:

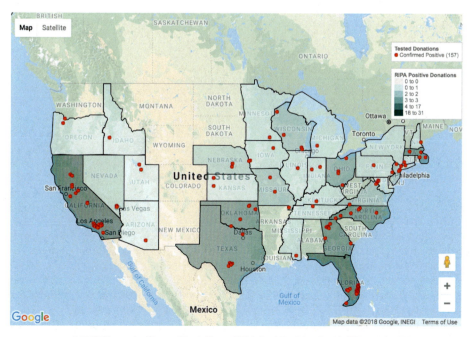

AABB Network: Chagas Biovigilance RIPA-Positive Map for 1/1/2017 – 7/27/2018

The tripomastigote (blood stage), amastigote (tissue stage), and epimastogote (triatomine insect stage) life stages of *T. crusi* are shown:

Trypanosoma crusi

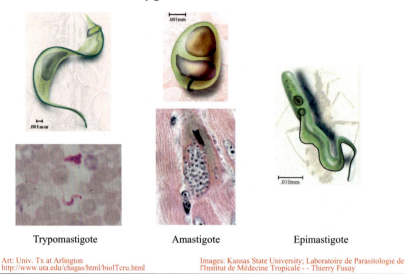

| Trypomastigote | Amastigote | Epimastigote |

The triatomine insect is shown:

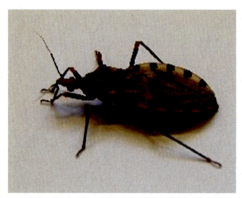

Triatomine insects (aka reduviid or kissing bugs)

Chagas disease is rare in most of the United States. However, as early as the 1990s, an experimental blood donor screening question for Chagas would have caused 7%–14% of potential donors in Miami and Los Angles to be deferred.[12] Meanwhile, seroprevalence has continued to increase.

Blood testing for Chagas is by enzyme-linked immunosorbent assay (ELISA), which was licensed by FDA on December 13, 2006. Radioimmunoprecipitation Assay (RIPA) is the confirmatory test. Screening protocols typically test donations using ELISA, and if repeatedly reactive, confirmation is by RIPA.

On May 22, 2015, FDA made it mandatory to test West Nile virus and Chagas disease for every donation.[7] In the case of West Nile virus, a mini-pool that contains the donor's sample qualifies as testing each donation.

Babesia—A Potential Candidate for Mandatory Donor Testing?

Babesiosis is the most common tick-borne, transfusion-transmitted infection in the United States. It is transmitted by the deer tick in the Northeastern United States, often in coastal regions such as Cape Cod, Martha's

Vinyard, and Long Island, but it has also expanded significantly into the upper Midwest. Indeed, Babesia's geographic range is extensive and growing.[13] Babesiosis is most commonly caused by *Babesia microti*, but it may also be due to infection by WA1-type Babesia. In the United States, more than 160 cases of transfusion-transmitted babesiosis have been identified, causing at least 28 deaths.[14]

Babesia are obligate intraerythrocytic protozoan parasites. As shown in Figure 3, Babesia organisms can be observed both intra- and extracellularly in the bloodstream. They tend to be numerous in the bloodstream. The "Mercedes Benz" tetrad seen on the right of Figure 3 is pathognomonic. Laboratory diagnosis of Babesia is made by a blood smear, molecular (NAT) testing, or visualization of parasites in an inoculated animal.

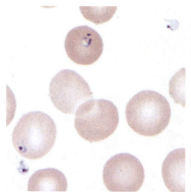
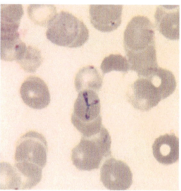

Babesia: Intra- and extra-erythrocytic, pleomorphic, and vacuolated

The tetrad is pathognomonic for *Babesia*

Babesiosis is classically a febrile illness resembling malaria, and associated with hemolytic anemia 1–4 weeks after being infected. However, the infection is also sometimes clinically silent. Untreated, Babesia may easily persist for several months, in some cases even longer. Thus, the blood-borne infection can be clinically silent as well as persistent, making clinically occult infections a risk to the blood supply.

Making Babesia even more dangerous, the organism can survive in blood products for over 40 days.[13] Thus, the organism is able to persist for extended amounts of time not only in donors' bloodstreams, but also in blood units. A single episode of babesiosis causes a blood donor to be permanently deferred from donating blood (i.e., deferred for life).

Several companies are developing screening assays for Babesia. However, there is currently no FDA approved screening test for Babesia. Without an FDA-cleared diagnostic test, the organism cannot be included among the infectious diseases that are subject to screening in each blood donation. The additional cost per unit for Babesia screening would likely be about $20, so FDA might consider requiring screening only in regions of the country in which Babesia is endemic.[15]

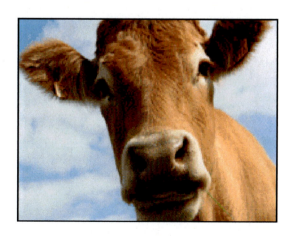

How would Babesia get on the mandatory donor testing list? What process does FDA use? FDA defines "transfusion-transmitted infection" (TTI) at 21 CFR §630.3(l) as a disease or disease agent, transmissible by blood, that could be fatal or life threatening, or could result in permanent impairment of a body function or body structure, or could require medical or surgical intervention to preclude permanent impairment of a body function or body structure.[16] The Agency then defines "relevant" transfusion-transmitted infections. A relevant transfusion-transmitted infection is a TTI, as defined earlier, with one of two additional features. One option is to be an infectious organism on the list of established TTIs, which presently include HIV, HBV, HCV, HTLV, syphilis, West Nile virus, Chagas disease, CJD, vCJD, Plasmodium spp. (malaria), West Nile virus, Chagas disease, and Zika virus (a newcomer to the list). The second alternative is to meet the following criteria: (1) a screening measure has been developed—screens such as questions in a medical history or an FDA-cleared screening test; and (2) the agent has sufficient incidence and/or prevalence to affect the donor population.

Thus, additional organisms can be added to the list of relevant TTIs, according to the criteria stated earlier. In the example of Zika virus, there was no cleared screening test for Zika virus when the May 22, 2015 Guidance was issued, so it was not listed as a relevant TTI. The IND for Zika virus NAT was approved in 2016. In August 2016, FDA officially recognized Zika virus as a relevant TTI with mandatory screening under 21 CFR §630.3(l).[9] Thus, Babesia would be placed on the mandatory screening list if an IND was approved for Babesia and FDA considered it appropriate to initiate screening.

Transmissible Spongiform Encephalopathies

Undetectable, it incubates for years. It kills by eating holes in people's brains, so that they stagger and collapse and lose their minds. It's one hundred percent fatal.

RICHARD RHODES, DEADLY FEASTS[17]

Primum non nocere (First, do no harm).

ANON

Transmissible spongiform encephalopathies are caused by prions, which are in essence, infectious proteins. Prions are abnormal isoforms of a normal CNS protein. If the prion folds correctly, it is harmless. If it folds incorrectly, it triggers a series of prion misfoldings in otherwise normal prions, forming β-pleated sheets, leading to clumps of protein, cellular injury, and amyloid deposition in the brain.

Transmissible spongiform encephalopathies include scrapie in sheep; bovine spongiform encephalopathy ("mad cow disease") in cattle; kuru in humans (supposedly due to funerary practices); sporadic CJD in humans; and vCJD in humans, a condition in which prions are transmitted to humans via consumption of infected beef.

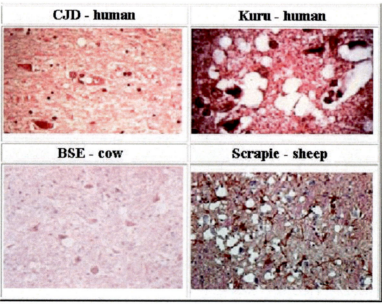

Viral Informatics Resource Center & Viral Informatics-Canada

There are presently no licensed, approved, or cleared donor screening tests for CJD and vCJD. FDA has stated that, if donor screening tests do become available, testing would be made mandatory only if testing was necessary to adequately and appropriately reduce the risk of transmitting CJD or vCJD, taking into account the risks presented by donated blood.[18] At present, the risk of vCJD transmission via blood transfusion is low and continuing to decrease as infectious cattle are eliminated.

Permanent deferrals are mandated for blood donors with vCJD or CJD, and their family members, as well as individuals who have received dura matter grafts, insulin from bovine sources, or travel/residence for 3 months in the United Kingdom between 1980 and 1996 (when the United Kingdom destroyed all of their cattle); 5 years in France/Europe since 1980; and certain military and their dependents.

Malaria Deferrals

Plasmodium species cause malaria, specifically *P. falciparum*, *P. malariae*, *P. ovale*, and *P. vivax*. Some European countries rely on antibody detection assays, usually enzyme-linked immunosorbant assays (EIA), as the best choice for laboratory screening. The United Kingdom, France, and other countries employ antibody-based assays. Such testing is usually combined with deferral periods to allow time for seroconversion. For example, a policy for allowing donation after a visit to an endemic area may include a 3-month deferral from the date of return from the endemic country, followed by testing negative for malaria, before being eligible to donate blood. Nucleic acid–based tests may not be a good option for malaria screening. The infectious dose of malaria in humans is probably fewer than 10 parasites. Therefore, a donor with very few organisms in their body could be a source of transfusion-associated malaria. Similarly, direct assays such as immunofluorescence microscopy may not be sufficiently sensitive for screening purposes. Thus, automatic deferral of those returning from indigenous areas may remain the most reliable approach.

In 2009, FDA sought a strategy for minimizing donor loss due to malaria. FDA found that travel to Mexico was a very significant source of donor deferrals (FDA estimated about 41%). However, malaria transmission in Mexico was shown to be very low, particularly in Quintana Roo, which is the state that includes Cancun and Cozumel. Quintana Roo was responsible for 70% of all malaria deferrals for Mexico. FDA calculated that, if Quintana Roo were treated as a nonendemic area, the increase in risk would be only 1.1%, while the donor pool would increase by 79,000 units of blood. The FDA Blood Products Advisory Committee (BPAC) approved the proposal to declare the state of Quintana Roo to be a nonendemic area, 17-1 in favor. The recommendations went into effect in August 2014.[19]

FDA also adjusted the length of travel deferrals for malaria-endemic countries. Malaria-endemic areas are, by definition, areas where CDC recommends antimalarial chemoprophylaxis, as published in the most current version of CDC's *The Yellow Book*. The deferral rules at the time of this writing are as follows:

Travel to a malaria-endemic area means being in the area for more than 24 h to less than 5 years. **Residence** in a malaria-endemic country is a continuous stay for greater than 5 years. Thus, it is possible to "travel" to a malaria-endemic country by taking more than 24 h to pass through the country on a trip. One can also travel to a country for 4 years and 51 weeks and still be considered a traveler. If a donor spent greater than 5 years, however, the donor is considered a resident.

The deferral rule for "residence" (>5 years) in a malaria-endemic country is to defer the individual from giving blood for 3 years. For "travel" to a malaria-endemic area, defer for 1 year.

The 3-year deferral for residents reflects the possibility of low-grade parasitemia in individuals with clinical immunity, meaning that a new infection may be asymptomatic while parasites are in the bloodstream. Immunity is thought to wane absent restimulation, so continued exposure to malaria parasites is necessary to maintain clinical immunity.

A **"history of malaria"** means actually contracting malaria. Prospective donors with a history of malaria should be deferred for 3 years. If a donor is symptom-free and has been exclusively in nonendemic areas for 3 years, the donor may be accepted for donation.

NATIONAL DONOR DEFERRAL REGISTRIES

National donor deferral registries were intended to provide an important layer of redundancy for keeping blood free of infectious agents. The registries were envisioned as a repository of names of potential blood donors who were deferred from donating blood. The plan was for blood establishments to consult the registry every time a potential donor presented for a donation. Unfortunately, this layer of protection has not yet lived up to hopes due to the inability to construct the necessary infrastructure. FDA sought input regarding the feasibility of sharing donor deferral lists among licensed and registered establishments. Connectivity (e.g., with bloodmobiles), computer reliability, time burden, and lack of buy-in have caused the initiative to be delayed.[7]

QUARANTINE

Quarantine is a simple concept, but very powerful. The essence of the principle is that all donated blood and blood products must be quarantined until they have been tested completely and been demonstrated to be free of infectious agents. One essential aspect of effective quarantine is to have the quarantined area meaningfully separated from the rest of the inventory. Blood should be quarantined if it is subject to a recall, of course, but quarantine should also be practiced whenever uncertainty arises relative to a unit. If a product is part of a lookback, it must be quarantined. Another example might be a patient who anticipates surgery, and wishes to use his or her own dedicated blood, perhaps due to a rare antibody. If that patient is positive for Hepatitis C, the blood bank would need to quarantine the unit. In fact, many transfusion services would not permit the unit to be brought into the facility, due to concerns that, if the unit is anywhere near in the inventory, a technologist could inadvertently release the unit to another patient by accident.

PROBLEMS AND DEFICIENCIES

Recall the notion that a near miss is a gift: No actual harm occurred, but the event revealed a risk that needed to be shored up. The same attitude should be carried into addressing all problems and deficiencies. It is inevitable that deficiencies are demoralizing, but they should also be embraced. All deficiencies should be corrected, and the corrective action must be documented. As appropriate, a plan for effective monitoring should be put in place to confirm the problem has been corrected. It is also important to notify FDA when deviations occur in products that are distributed.

REMARKS

Transfusion-transmitted infectious diseases is a vast field. Guidance documents, Standards, updates from professional organizations, and a vast literature on the science, public policy, and practice can ensure ample opportunity for intellectual and professional growth, while doing a great deal of good for patients. It is important not to lose the big picture. How safe is safe? How much should it cost—or how much can it cost? How do we address emerging infections, with better testing or better surveillance, or a combination of both? Currently, our tolerances in risk reduction are impossibly thin, as we attempt to achieve near perfection. Where life-saving blood meets life-threatening infectious agents, everything we do is risk management and to a certain extent, everything we do is policy-making.

The pathogens demand a response, and our responses in today's world must be both international and local. More and more, we need to be strategic beyond our borders, and for that we need good allies, and we need to *be* good allies.

REFERENCES

1. Cserti CM, Dzik WH. The ABO blood group system and *Plasmodium falciparum* malaria. *Blood.* 2007;110:2250–2258.
2. Kwiatkowski DP. How malaria has affected the human genome and what human genetics can teach us about malaria. *Am J Hum Genetics.* 2005;77:171–192.
3. *Keeping Blood Transfusions Safe: FDA's Milti-layered Protections for Donated Blood.* 2018. https://www.fda.gov/BiologicsBloodVaccines/SafetyAvailability/BloodSafety/ucm095522.htm.
4. Stramer SL, Wend U, Candotti D, et al. Nucleic acid testing to detect HBV infection in blood donors. *N Engl J Med.* 2011;364:236–247.
5. http://www.fda.gov/cber/faq/msmdonor.htm. No longer available.
6. *Guidance for Industry, Revised Recommendations for Reducing the Risk of Human Immunodeficiency Virus Transmission by Blood and Blood Products.* December 2015, finalizing 80 FR 27973, May 15, 2015. https://www.fda.gov/downloads/BiologicsBloodVaccines/GuidanceComplianceRegulatoryInformation/Guidance/Blood/UCM446580.pdf.
7. Requirements for blood and blood components intended for transfusion or for further manufacturing use; Final Rule. 21 CFR Part 606, 610, 630, et al., Fed Regist. 80(9)/Friday, May 22, 2015, at 29,857.
8. *AABB Association Bulletin #13-02 – West Nile Virus Nucleic Acid Testing – revised Recommendations.* 2018. http://www.aabb.org/programs/publications/bulletins/Pages/ab13-02.aspx.
9. Guidance for Industry. *Revised Recommendations for Reducing the Risk of Zika Virus Transmission by Blood and Blood Components.* July 2018. https://www.fda.gov/BiologicsBloodVaccines/GuidanceComplianceRegulatoryInformation/Guidances/default.htm.
10. Williard C. In the blood. *Nature.* 2017;549:S19–S21.
11. MMWR Weekly. 2007;56(07):141–143.
12. Leiby DA, Herron RM, Read EJ, et al. *Trypanosoma cruzi* in Los Angeles and Miami blood donors: impact of evolving donor demographics on seroprevalence and implications for transfusion transmission. *Transfusion.* 2002;42:549–555.
13. Centers for Disease Control and Prevention. *National Notifiable Infectious Conditions.* Babesiosis. Atlanta, GA, 2013. https://wwwn.cdc.gov/nndss/conditions/notifiable/2013/infectious-diseases/.
14. Herwaldt BL, Linden JV, Bosserman E, et al. Transfusion-associated babesiosis in the United States: a description of cases. *Ann Intern Med.* 2011;155:509–519.
15. Williard C. In the blood. *Nature.* 2017;549:S19–S21.
16. 21 CFR 630.3(l).

17. Rhodes R. *Deadly Feasts: Tracking the Secrets of a Terrifying New Plague.* New York: Simon & Schuster, Inc; 1997.

18. Guidance for Industry. *Revised Recommendations for Reducing the Risk of Human Immunodeficiency Virus Transmission by Blood and Blood Products, at 29857*; December 2015. https://www.fda.gov/downloads/BiologicsBloodVaccines/GuidanceComplianceRegulatoryInformation/Guidance/Blood/UCM446580.pdf.

19. Guidance for Industry. *Recommendations for Donor Questioning, Deferral, Reentry and Product Management to Reduce the Risk of Transfusion-Transmitted Malaria.* 2018. https://www.fda.gov/downloads/BiologicsBloodVaccines/GuidanceComplianceRegulatoryInformation/Guidances/Blood/UCM080784.pdf.

CHAPTER 6

Transfusion Review: Monitoring Transfusion Practice

JOSEPH D. SWEENEY, MD, FACP, FRCPATH

INTRODUCTION

Blood centers are concerned with the collection, processing, testing, storage, inventory management, and shipping of blood components, and hospital blood banks are concerned with ensuring the compatibility of blood components with recipients. As discussed in Chapter 3, the processes in the blood center are regulated in the United States mostly by the Food and Drug Administration (FDA). Extramural oversight of blood banks is performed by accrediting organizations, in particular the American Association of Blood Banks (AABB), the College of American Pathologists (CAP), and The Joint Commission (TJC). The focus of both regulatory agencies and accrediting organizations has been, and largely continues to be, the quality of manufactured components and the integrity of the processes, which determine compatibility. By and large, there has been less emphasis on monitoring the utilization of blood components. The primary reasons that account for this are as follows: First, the FDA does not concern itself with the practice of medicine; second, most blood banks are administratively part of the clinical laboratory; and third, the focus of the clinical laboratory is often good laboratory practice rather than good clinical practice. Pathologists, who provide medical direction for most blood banks in the United States, can sometimes be uncomfortable inserting themselves into clinical decision making, which can potentially antagonize their clinical colleagues. Only the larger academic institutions have transfusion medicine specialists on staff. In the past decade, there has been increasing interest in blood transfusion avoidance (bloodless medicine and surgery) and promoting evidence-based good transfusion practice, sometimes referred to as patient blood management (PBM). The leadership of PBM[1-8] programs has been provided as often by internists, anesthesiologists, and surgeons, as much as by pathologists. This has the effect of disconnecting the blood bank

personnel from active involvement in blood transfusion practice. This is regrettable because the blood bank knows *how much* blood is transfused overall and *who* is getting transfused, and the clinicians (in theory, at least) know *why* the blood is being prescribed. Connecting the *who* to the *why* is at the core of effective prospective monitoring and can be the basis for a highly effective PBM program.[9,10] PBM is linked to risk management because PBM tends to decrease the volume of blood transfused and the fewer units transfused, the less the potential for an adverse event. This chapter will concern itself with these important concerns, discuss approaches to monitoring transfusion practice, and describe ways of engaging with physicians to effect changes in prescribing practices.

How Much Blood Is Transfused?

There are different ways to report how much blood is transfused. At the level of a community, state, or entire country, this is most commonly reported as units collected and transfused per 1000 population. The accuracy of these data will depend on an accurate census of the population and accurate information from collection organizations and transfusing hospitals, each of which could be prone to error. In the United States, in recent years, the National Collection and Blood Utilization Survey (NCBUS) report has been regarded as the most reliable source.[11] More recently, this survey has been conducted with the AABB, generating the most recent data for 2014–15.[12] These data show approximately 12.8 million units of red cells collected and 11 million transfused, or 36.8 units per 1000 population (2015). This continues the decline in red blood cell utilization, which started nationally in 2009, and likely indicates the impact of PBM programs, promoting a more conservative approach to red cell transfusion.[13] A more important number, however, is the amount of blood transfused within any individual hospital

Risk Management in Transfusion Medicine. https://doi.org/10.1016/B978-0-323-54837-3.00006-7

or system of hospitals. This can be described as an absolute amount, but this gives very little insight into appropriate usage or good transfusion practice. However, it is a number readily available in nearly all blood banks. This number can be modified in a number of ways, using the number of discharges or inpatient days in the denominator to account for patient volume.[14] The problem with this modification is that as many as 20%–30% of all red blood cells are transfused to outpatients, mainly in the support of oncology patients with hypoproliferative anemia. Hence, a better statistic would be total red blood cells transfused to inpatients per 1000 discharges.[15] This may be more challenging for the blood bank because separation of inpatient versus outpatient transfusions may not be readily available and require data extraction, even manual extraction, which is awkward. This modification takes patient volume into account but not patient acuity. Fig. 6.1 represents total red blood cell use adjusted for patient volume with discharges in the denominator tracked over a 20-year period in a tertiary care teaching hospital. This allows for year to year comparison and documents the impact of a PBM program in reducing red blood cell usage over time. The fluctuation in the past few years indicates that a plateau may have been reached.

Fig. 6.2 from the same hospital shows a change in nonapheresis plasma transfused in the same period. A dramatic decline is evident, approximately 95%, consistent with current thinking that much of plasma transfused is nonevidence based.[16] Similar to the red cells, a plateau is evident.

A method to take patient acuity into account (sicker patients are more likely to be transfused) is required for interinstitutional comparison. Consider three hospitals within a system: hospital A, a tertiary care center with 719 beds; hospital B, a 247-bed hospital; and hospital C, a small community hospital with 129 beds. Because the absolute number of red cells transfused per hospital will differ substantially related to patient volume and acuity, adjusting the total red cell usage for both could allow for a more valid comparison of usage. Table 6.1 shows data collected for a 4-year period, 2013 through 2016, for all three hospitals. The mean case mix index (CMI) was used as a measure of patient acuity. The CMI is a value representing the clinical complexity and case diversity of all patients in a hospital. As it is used to allocate resources appropriately, it is readily available and accurate, because there

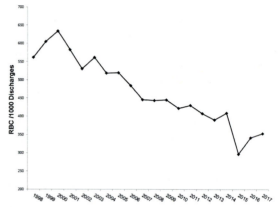

FIG. 6.2 Decrease in plasma transfusions over a 20-year period.

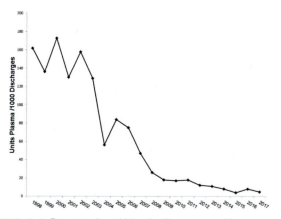

FIG. 6.1 Decrease in red blood cell use over a 20-year period.

TABLE 6.1
Red Blood Cell Transfusion in Three Hospitals, Adjusted for Patient Volume and Acuity

	Hospital A	Hospital B	Hospital C
Total red blood cell units over 4 years	54,500	21,055	6333
Total discharges over 4 years	140,025	65,576	18,113
Mean CMI for 4 years	1.67	1.49	1.41
Red cell units/1000 discharges	389	323	350
Red cell units/1000 discharges/mean CMI	233	215	250

are stiff financial penalties for inaccurate reporting. In general, the CMI varies from 0.5 to 18 per discharge; patients with more complex medical problems, complications, or surgery have higher CMIs. The CMI was used in this calculation to account for the complexity of cases seen in each hospital, as a surrogate for acuity. The higher the CMI, the more complex the cases, and therefore it is expected that more blood would be used. The comparison of usage was performed first by calculating usage of red cells per 1000 discharges. A further calculation took the usage per 1000 discharges and divided that ratio by the CMI. As is evident, when adjusted for acuity, the small community hospital appears to have the higher transfusion rate, not the bigger academic hospital. This would not have been evident using the unadjusted units per 1000 discharges ratio.

WHO IS BEING TRANSFUSED?

Having determined *how much* blood is being transfused, the second relevant question is *who* is being transfused. This question seeks to identify the patient

subpopulation(s) that receive blood components and the types of components they receive. This is useful data because it provides a picture of where, within the healthcare facility, the blood components are being administered, and has the potential to project future needs for blood. Obviously, a list can be generated of all patients transfused for any given period, but such a list requires manipulation: Patients have to be put into categories to analyze the data. It is possible to categorize transfusion recipients in a number of ways, and each individual institution will have to assess the most useful way to categorize its patient subpopulations. Suggestions are offered in Table 6.2.

Age or gender may be useful as an initial descriptive and will probably show that most recipients are older (>65 years) and predominantly female. The probability of receiving a blood transfusion below the age of 40 years is estimated to be about 0.26%, but above the age of 65 years, the probability of transfusion on an annual basis is approximately 5%.[17] Although a fraction of the population over the age of 65 years is approximately 13% in the United States, they account for 50% of all red cells transfused. More useful information will be derived by "drilling down" further into broad categories. The initial broad categories could be medicine and surgery: There are often different transfusion practices between these core services. If most of the blood is transfused in one broad category or the other, focusing on that category initially might be more useful. Drilling down further into specific services will begin to yield information, which can be used for comparative purposes against some benchmark, for example, looking at blood usage in cardiac surgery.[18] Table 6.3 shows an audit of blood usage by cardiac surgery patients over a 3-month period. More detailed data on this cohort will be given later.

These data could be further broken into elective versus emergency surgery, CABB versus non-CAGG, etc. A similar data capture could be performed for orthopedic

---

TABLE 6.2
Different Methods for Classifying Transfusion Recipients

1. Age, gender, or both
2. Broad categories (medical, surgical, obstetrics, pediatrics)
3. Specific services (oncology, orthopedic, surgery, cardiac surgery, trauma)
4. Individual physician
5. Disease grouping: (DRG—diagnosis-related group—links discharge diagnosis to a disease category; ICD-9 codes)
6. Hospital location (intensive care unit, emergency department, etc.)

TABLE 6.3
Total Blood Component Use in Cardiac Surgery (n = 185 Cases)

	Total Transfused	Percent of Patients Transfused (%)	Mean for all Patients	Mean per Transfused Case
Red blood cells (units)	284	46	1.5	3.3
Platelets (doses)	56	19	0.3	1.6
Fresh frozen plasma (units)	84	13	0.4	3.5
Cryoprecipitate (pools)	52	13	0.3	2.2

TABLE 6.4
Audit of Blood Transfusion in Cardiac Surgery Over a 4-Month Period

Surgeon	Cases	Percent Transfused	Total RBC Transfused	Mean RBC per Transfused case	Admitting Hemoglobin (g/dL)	Discharge Hemoglobin (g/dL)
4-Month Period: 2016						
A	106	37 (35%)	124	3.4	12.3	9.2
B	49	17 (35%)	54	3.2	10.6	8.8
C	67	44 (66%)	322	7.3	12.0	9.0
Total	222		500			

TABLE 6.5
Audit of Blood Transfusion in Cardiac Surgery Over a Subsequent 3-Month Period

Surgeon	Cases	Percent Transfused	Total RBC Transfused	Mean RBC per Transfused Case	Admitting Hemoglobin (g/dL)	Discharge Hemoglobin (g/dL)
3-Month Period: 2017						
A	57	24 (42%)	67	2.8	11.7	8.6
B	13	6 (46%)	28	4.7	11.1	9.1
C	37	21 (57%)	75	3.6	12.9	9.3
D	78	37 (49%)	114	3.0	12.3	8.8
Total	185		284			

surgery, with subdivision into elective versus urgent, hip replacement versus knee replacement, and spinal fusion surgery. Such a data capture will show that elective knee surgery is rarely associated with red cell transfusion, elective hip to a greater degree, and urgent hip replacement will have the highest probability of transfusion. Furthermore, although a significant amount of transfusion in cardiac surgery is performed intraoperatively or in the immediate postoperative period, nearly all orthopedic surgery transfusion occurs on postoperative day 2–4. Another service that uses a significant fraction of all blood components is oncology. However, this service differs in that most of the transfusions are outpatient, in the context of hypoproliferative anemia and thrombocytopenia. Hence, there are differences between services that are important to understand because this information will potentially be used to affect changes in practice.

Data capture and tabulation by individual physician can also be an important step in affecting practice change. Consider the following two time periods in a cardiac surgery service:

Inspection of these two tables shows significant differences for surgeon C, who was an outlier in Table 6.2.

The mean red blood cell per transfused case for this surgeon decreased from 7.3 units (Table 6.4) to 3.6 units (Table 6.5) without any material change in the admitting hemoglobin and discharge hemoglobin. This is a useful illustration of the use of retrospective data to influence individual physician practice.

Categorizing transfusion recipients into diagnosis-related groups (DRGs) can also be useful. DRGs are readily available, and a report can be run electronically. A small number of DRGs capture the majority of the blood being transfused (Table 6.6). As might be expected, the major hospital procedures and services that use blood are well represented. Note that tracheotomy, DRG483, is used for ICU patients during their stay, which is why this DRG accounts for the large volume of blood transfused. In the aggregate, these DRGs account for 70% of all red blood cells transfused.

Hospital location is another way to examine transfusion practices. Particular areas of high transfusion are the ICU (all components), outpatients (red blood cells and platelets), operating room (all components), and interventional radiology (plasma mainly). Questionable practices can be uncovered, which, when challenged, can result in a reduction in component usage.

TABLE 6.6
Blood Transfused in Different DRGs

Procedure	DRG#	Total RBCs Transfused
Cardiac services	104–111, 116,127	3615
Bowel surgery	148, 149	267
GI hemorrhage	174, 175	572
Orthopedic—1	209–211	435
Coagulation/RBC disorder	395–397	229
Tracheotomy	483	752

TABLE 6.7
Reasons for Physicians to Prescribe Blood Components

1. Historical precedent: "This is the way I have always done it and I have never had a problem."
2. Eminence-based medicine: The practice is based on the opinions of perceived experts or groups. This is especially the case with physicians trained in a prestigious hospital or medical school. A variant of eminence-based medicine is the publications of guidelines by professional societies based on consensus rather than high-quality data. Such guidelines are generated typically by experienced and respected physicians. They are well intentioned, but often there are inadequate data available to reach a conclusion. The group, regardless, may make recommendations, which then become enshrined as "standards of care."[19]
3. Fear of litigation. This can be a powerful motivating force. It can be seen in the practice of prophylactic plasma transfusion based on arbitrary INRs by interventional radiologists or surgeons before an invasive procedure.
4. Evidence-based transfusion medicine. This is increasingly being applied, but high-quality data on many transfusion practices are unfortunately lacking.

WHY IS BLOOD TRANSFUSED?

This is really the key question in blood utilization, and it is here that the true potential of transfusion practice monitoring can be realized to make a material intrainstitutional difference, not just in terms of the prescribing patterns of individual physicians, but for groups of physicians as a whole. At the simplest level, a physician prescribes a blood product because he/she believes that the transfusion is efficacious and will improve the clinical outcome of his/her patient. This type of prescription is largely based on the judgment of the physician and his/her previous experiences. Physician judgment is fashioned by observations or knowledge, which is subjected to varying degrees of objective analysis. Physicians have a tendency to learn patterns of practice early in their career and to perpetuate such practices. Physician practices can be resistant to change even with objective data, and that resistance is especially strong when that data are at variance with previously learned patterns. Several reasons why physicians prescribe blood components are shown in Table 6.7.

EARLY STEPS TO IMPROVE PHYSICIAN PRESCRIBING PRACTICES

The initial step in any institution for blood utilization control is to develop a set of intrainstitutional guidelines reflecting good transfusion practice.[20] These guidelines can be developed within the context of a transfusion committee or similar transfusion practice group. Involvement of key stakeholders is critical at this stage. These guidelines need to be blood component specific. It is likely that the initial engagement of different groups of prescribing physicians will result in some (maybe considerable!) disagreement, as established practices become challenged. Once a set of guidelines

can be agreed to, they should be ratified by the different groups of physicians involved and approved by the medical executive committee. This now provides a framework within which to conduct audits and monitoring. These guidelines need to be available to the medical staff in printed or electronic formats and available in the blood bank for monitoring purposes. Education of staff physicians, trainee physicians, and other transfusing personnel such as nurses, nurse anesthetists, and perfusionists is important at this stage. This can take the form of formal presentations such as Grand Rounds[21] or informal clarifications at meetings such as morbidity and mortality conferences, tumor boards, etc. Supportive brochures, in print or electronic format, can also be made available. An example of such a brochure is shown in the appendix.

AUDITING AND MONITORING PHYSICIAN PRESCRIBING PRACTICES

The development of guidelines, in itself, is unlikely to make changes in practice, so some form of monitoring will be required to promote adherence to good transfusion practices. Monitoring can be applied in a number of ways and can be categorized as retrospective, early retrospective, or prospective.[22,23] The monitoring can be electronic, with or without embedded clinical decision support (CDS),[24] or nonelectronic, with either manual gathering of retrospective data or engaging with the prescribing physician at the time of ordering.

Retrospective monitoring (RM): RM is one of the most widely used methods. RM has the advantage of being capable of being performed as time becomes available and does not entail physician engagement during the data gathering phase. It is really an audit of practice focused on an individual physician or groups of physicians. RM can identify patterns of practice that are at variance with intrainstitutional guidelines or national benchmarks, or it can identify specific physicians as outliers (see Tables 6.4 and 6.5). The data need to be tabulated and summarized and presented as feedback. This can occur at a Transfusion Committee meeting or a departmental meeting. RM does not prevent any unnecessary transfusions because of its retrospective nature, and the success of RM in changing practice can be unpredictable.[20,22,23]

Early retrospective monitoring (ERM): ERM differs from RM in that the feedback is presented shortly after the prescription, typically within 24 h to a few weeks. In ERM, the prescribing physician is contacted after the transfusion of the blood component, and the prescription is challenged, usually in written form or by email. The prescribing physician may or may not be asked to respond. ERM has the potential to antagonize the prescribing physician, depending on the content (and tone) of the challenge, possibly setting up an adversarial situation with an acrimonious exchange. In some situations, the prescription may be within guidelines, but this was not immediately evident from the available clinical information, which can result in a sarcastic response. In general, ERM should be embarked upon with caution.

Prospective monitoring (PM): PM is the ideal form of monitoring, as it provides the opportunity to interdict the questionable transfusion. PM can be performed in a number of ways. Most commonly, it is performed electronically at the point of physician order entry (POE).[24] There are many variations, but, in essence, the physician prescribes the blood component and either the physician is required to enter additional laboratory data or the application will search for the most recent laboratory information. The option of by-passing in the event of an emergency transfusion or bleeding must be available to the ordering physician. Some systems require entry of clinical information either as a dropdown menu or radio buttons, and there may also be a free text field. Some POEs indicate that the transfusion may

be inappropriate based on laboratory data. For example, requesting a red blood cell unit for a patient with a hemoglobin of 9 g/dL or a plasma transfusion with an INR of 1.8 could result in a pop-up questioning the prescription (note: the author does not endorse these thresholds, they are provided only as examples). Other systems will offer hyperlinks to guidelines, which are typically within the hospital intranet. Some POEs will have a hard-stop (prescription is prevented) if a form is not completed or certain fields are not populated. For example, the prescription is not submitted if relevant clinical information is not provided or a radio button is not checked indicating that consent has been obtained. There has been much interest in the use of clinical decision support (CDS) at the point of POE.[25,26] CDS generally provides pointers to best practices and is a useful tool for physician education as well as interdicting unnecessary transfusions. Electronic ordering provides the opportunity to generate physician-specific reports or prescribing pattern reports for different groups of physicians, e.g., departments or service lines.

The resulting order either appears on a screen in the blood Bank or is printed out from a printer located in the blood bank. The printed order to transfuse allows the technologist to make sure that all is in place to dispense the blood component (compatibility testing completed, plasma thawed, etc.). The technologists will next ascertain whether they have an historic or current type for plasma or platelets or have a current in-date specimen for a red blood cell. At this point, the blood bank technologist may perhaps examine the order for appropriateness.[10] Typically, however, the order is simply fulfilled without question at this point, taking the technologist out of the screening chain. There can be a reluctance on the part of the technologists to screen, because of the need to fulfill orders in a timely manner or a perception that this is not the responsibility of technologists or that they are underqualified to engage in this task. At this point, if the prescription appears questionable, the technologist can either refer the order to the blood bank medical director or directly engage the prescribing physician. The latter is, in general, preferable because it allows for a more timely resolution (whether to go ahead with the order, put on hold for more information or cancel). This contact, however, is often not without difficulty. Physicians may not respond to a pager or cell phone, causing frustration and delay, or the physician responds indicating that he/she is not the doctor of record and that contact with a second physician is required. Thus, a chain of communications occurs for a single order! After contact is made, however, and in case of doubt, the technologist can provide the medical director's contact information and the matter can be discussed physician to physician. In urgent clinical situations, such engagement is discouraged, as it may cause needless delay in providing blood component to bleeding patients.

It is the author's point of view that these interactions between technologists and physicians and between the medical director and prescribing physicians, while time-consuming, yield a rich reward.[10,14,15] First, the physician is challenged (perhaps for the first time) with regard to his/her decision. Physicians react differently to this challenge. The younger physicians tend to be appreciative and will often modify or cancel the order. Older physicians, as might be expected, see this challenge as an affront to their professional competence, and a heated verbal exchange may ensue. Despite the potential difficulties, we have observed that physicians, once questioned about an order, will contact the blood bank directly with subsequent orders to ask regarding appropriateness. We also find that physicians talk among themselves, and after a few interventions, the senior residents or older physicians will monitor how their junior colleagues prescribe. Furthermore, these interactions provide immediate feedback to ordering physicians. Finally, these interventions help promote a conservative approach to transfusion and shift the institution from a transfusion-prone culture (perception that blood transfusion is generally efficacious and that risk is low) to a transfusion-averse culture (skepticism regarding the efficacy of blood transfusion in many situations and an awareness that there is risk associated with transfusion). For example, requests for prophylactic plasma are now rare at one hospital with such a PBM program, and this most likely reflects the anchoring of a transfusion-averse culture (see Fig. 6.2). This kind of intervention is uncommon, however. As discussed in the introduction, medical direction of blood banks is commonly performed by general-practice pathologists, whose training may provide minimal exposure to acting as a consultant in transfusion medicine decision making.

Providing Physician Feedback

As discussed above, POE monitoring and especially prospective monitoring provides early feedback. However, there is an important role for examining transfusion practice for groups of physicians or service lines for limited time periods (audits).[22,23] Examples are seen in Tables 6.4 and 6.5. These data are optimally presented at department meetings but should also be presented at Transfusion Committee meetings. The

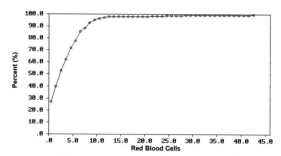

FIG. 6.3 Cumulative distribution curve of red blood cell transfusion in 328 patients who underwent cardiac surgery with sternotomy.

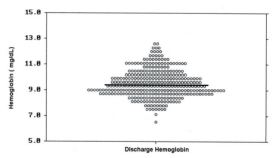

FIG. 6.4 Distribution of discharge hemoglobins in the 328 patient cohorts.

mode of presentation is important and data need to be summarized. This can be done as descriptive statistics (mean, medians, some measure of variance) in tabular form, but graphical representation is recommended and a display of data distribution is useful. This can be a histogram, a dot plot, or a cumulative distribution curve. Consider a cohort of 328 patients who had cardiac surgery (Figs. 6.3 and 6.4). From the cumulative distribution curve, slightly less than 30% of patients received no red cells. The median is about 2 (half the patients received 2 units or less), but the mean (±1SD) is 3.3 ± 4.3 (data not shown). The tail at the top is interesting, representing a subpopulation of patients, each of whom received a large volume of red blood cells (>5 units). Fig. 6.4 shows a dot plot of the discharge hemoglobins in the same cohort. A large fraction of patients is seen with a high hemoglobin on discharge (arbitrarily > 9 g/dL). Taken together, these figures indicate that there is needless over transfusion of red blood cells and an opportunity for improvement.

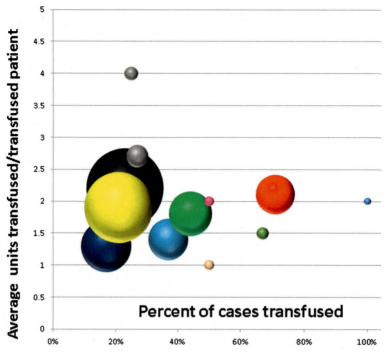

FIG. 6.5 Bubble graph of transfusion by surgeon in elective orthopedic surgery.

Another example is shown in Fig. 6.5. This is a bubble graph of an audit of both autologous and allogeneic red blood cell transfusion in elective orthopedic surgery (hips and knees) over a 6-month period. The axes are self-evident. Each bubble represents a single orthopedic surgeon, and the size of the bubble represents the number of cases performed per surgeon. As is evident, there is considerable variation between surgeons and even those surgeons performing the most procedures transfuse a high percentage of patients. In the years following this graph, predeposit autologous red blood cells were eliminated,[27] the use of tranexamic acid (both intravenous and intraarticular) became widespread, and postoperative transfusion thresholds for allogeneic red blood cells were decreased to 8 g/dL,[28] consistent with the FOCUS study.[29] The prevalence of transfusion (allogeneic only) in this population is currently 4%–5%.

CONCLUSION

The modern blood bank must continue to have policies, practices, and procedures in place to ensure the integrity of compatibility testing. Beyond this, there is a need to engage in monitoring the appropriateness of blood transfusion and to promote good transfusion practice. Both these activities are interlinked and are essential for risk minimization. The former ensures that the patient gets the *right blood* and the latter for the *right reason*.

REFERENCES

1. Goodnough LT, Shander A. Patient blood management. *Anesthesiology*. 2012;116:1367–1376. Erratum in: Anesthesiology 2013;118:224.
2. Yazer MH, Waters JH. How do I implement a hospital based blood management program? *Transfusion*. 2012;52:1640–1645.
3. Shander A, Javidroozi M. Strategies to reduce the use of blood products: a US perspective. *Curr Opin Anaesthesiol*. 2012;25:50–58.
4. Carson JL. The shifting paradigm for transfusion of red blood cells. *Clin Adv Hematol Oncol*. 2015;13:152–154.
5. Carson JL, Kuriyan M. What should trigger a transfusion? *Transfusion*. 2010;50:2073–2075.
6. Goodnough LT, Shander A. Patient blood management. *Anesthesiology*. 2012;116:1367–1376.
7. Thakkar RN, Kenlee KH, Ness PM, et al. Relative impact of a patient blood management on utilization of all three major blood components. *Transfusion*. 2016;56:2212–2220.

8. Frank SM, Savage WJ, Rothschild JA, et al. Variability in blood and blood component utilization as assessed by an anesthesia information management system. *Anesthesiology*. 2012;117:99–106.

9. Sweeney JD. The blood bank physician as a hemostasis consultant. *Transfus Apher Sci*. 2008;39:145–150.

10. Nixon CP, Tavares MF, Sweeney JD. How do we reduce plasma transfusion in Rhode Island? *Transfusion*. 2017;57: 1863–1873.

11. *National Blood Collection & Utilization Survey [Internet]*. Washington, DC: US Department of Health and Human Services; 2011. Available from: http://www.hhs.gov/ash/bloodsafety.

12. The 2014-2015 AABB Blood Collection and Survey Report; 2016. Available at. http://www.aabb.org/research/hemovigilance/bloodsurvey/Docs/2014-2015-AABB-Blood-Survey-Report.pdf.

13. Klein HG. Blood collection and use in the United States: you can't manage what you can't measure. *Transfusion*. 2016;56:2157–9.

14. Tavares M, DiQuattro P, Nolette N, Conti G, Sweeney JD. Reduction in plasma transfusion after enforcement of transfusion guidelines. *Transfusion*. 2011;51:754–761.

15. Tavares M, DiQuattro P, Sweeney JD. Reduction in red cell usage associated with engagement of the ordering physician. *Transfusion*. 2014;54:2625–2630.

16. Puetz J. Fresh frozen plasma: the most commonly prescribed hemostatic agent. *J Thromb Haemostas*. 2013;11:1794–1799.

17. Vamvakas EC, Taswell HF. Epidemiology of blood transfusion. *Transfusion*. 1994;34:464–470.

18. Snyder-Ramos SA, Mohnle P, Wang YS, et al. The on-going variability in blood transfusion practice in cardiac surgery. *Transfusion*. 2009;48:1284–1299.

19. Malloy PC, Grassi CJ, Kundu S, et al. Standards of Practice Committee with Cardiovascular and Interventional Radiological Society of Europe (CIRSE) Endorsement. Consensus guidelines for peri-procedural management of coagulation status and hemostasis risk in percutaneous image-guided interventions. *J Vasc Interv Radiol*. 2009;20:S240–S249.

20. Guyatt G, Heddle NM, et al. Aabb red blood cell transfusion guidelines. Something for almost everyone. *J Am Med Assoc*. 2016;316:1984–1985.

21. Sarode R, Refaai MA, Matevosyan K, et al. Prospective monitoring of plasma and platelet transfusions in a large teaching hospital results in significant cost reduction. *Transfusion*. 2010;50:487–492.

22. Tinmouth A, MacDougall L, Fergusson D, et al. Reducing the amount of blood transfused. *Arch Intern Med*. 2005;165:845–852.

23. Wilson K, MacDougall L, Fergusson D, et al. The effectiveness of interventions to reduce physicians' levels of inappropriate transfusion: what can be learned from a systematic review of the literature. *Transfusion*. 2002;42: 1224–1229.

24. Frank SM, Rothschild JA, Masear CG, et al. Optimizing preoperative blood ordering with data acquired from an anesthesia information management system. *Anesthesiology*. 2013;118:1286–1297.

25. Kassakian SZ, Yackel TR, Keloughery T, et al. Clinical decision support reduces overuse of red blood cell transfusions: interrupted time series analysis. *Am J Med*. 2016;129. 636.e13-636.e20.

26. Goodnough LT, Baker SA, Shas N. How I use clinical decision support to improve red blood cell utilization. *Transfusion*. 2016;56:2406–2411.

27. Roberts LD, Krohto S, Sweeney J. Elimination of predeposit autologous donation for joint replacement surgery. *Transfusion*. 2016;56:S4. 112 A.

28. Layton J, Rubin L, Sweeney JD. Advanced blood management strategies for elective joint arthroplasty. *Rh I Med J*. 2013;96:23–25.

29. Jeffrey L, Carson MD, Terrin ML. Liberal or restrictive transfusion in high-risk patients after hip surgery. *N Engl J Med*. 2011;365:2453–2462.

Appendix: Red Cell Transfusion in Normovolemic Anemia

Joseph D. Sweeney, MD, FACP, FRCPath

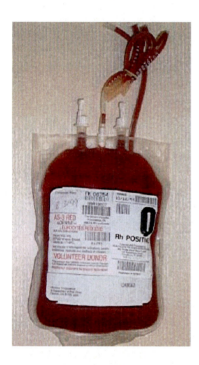

RED CELL TRANSFUSION IN NORMOVOLEMIC INPATIENTS

For many decades, it has been a practice to routinely transfuse red blood cells to a patient with a hemoglobin of less than 10 g/dL or a hematocrit of less than 30.[1] This practice is appealing since the 10/30 rule is simple; however, it is without empiric clinical justification, exposes the patients to potentially fatal adverse events and incurs wasteful use of a scarce resource.

WHAT IS NORMOVOLEMIC ANEMIA?

These are patients, who are hemodynamically stable, not actively bleeding nor immediately at risk for hemorrhage. Although any hemoglobin less than 12.5 g/dL is anemia, in practice this often refers to patients with hemoglobin of 10 g/dL or less. Note an important effect of posture on anemia which can change hemoglobin by as much as 1 g/dL.[2]

I'VE SEEN OTHER PHYSICIANS ORDER 2 UNITS OF RED CELLS FOR THESE PATIENTS. WHAT WRONG WITH THIS?

First, the decision to transfuse red cells should be based on the clinical state of the patient and *not just the measured hemoglobin or hematocrit*. Data from Jehovah's Witness patients show that hemoglobins as low as 5 g/dL are tolerated in acute blood loss anemia, and in chronic anemia, a hemoglobin as low as 3 g/dL is tolerable.[3-5] This is, of course, in otherwise healthy patients capable of increasing cardiac output. In patients with compromised cardiac function, cerebrovascular disease, or pulmonary disease, the threshold level would be higher, but no absolute threshold level of hemoglobin is appropriate for all patients.[6-8] One observational study using hospital admission data suggests that a threshold hemoglobin of 10 g/dL is appropriate for transfusion in older patients (over 65 years) with acute myocardial infarction in that 30-day patient mortality is favorably affected, but this data is controversial and must not be extrapolated to other patient populations.[9] A small recent randomized control trial suggested a benefit of red cell transfusion in patients presenting with acute coronary syndrome, but the age difference between the liberal versus restrictive groups rendered the data statistically inconclusive.[10] In general, patients with clinical symptomatology of hypoxemia (fatigue, dyspnea on exertion, tachycardia, tachypnea, impaired mentation, postural hypotension, angina, transient ischemic attack) and who have low hemoglobin could be considered candidates for red cell transfusion. This will likely occur when the hemoglobin falls below 7.0 g/dL and possibly below 8 g/dL, but many patients with a hemoglobin of 8–10 g/dL are well compensated and not symptomatic.[11-15] The second consideration is the dose of red cells. Avoid routinely ordering "2 units". It is acceptable to request "1 unit." Transfuse this unit and look for objective improvement in symptoms and hemoglobin at 4–6 h. One unit may well be sufficient, especially in low weight elderly patients.[16] If improvement is not adequate, transfuse a second unit.

WHY SHOULD I WAIT 4–6 H?

The increase in hemoglobin can be assessed as early as 30 min post transfusion.[17,18] However, it takes at least 4–6 h (maybe longer) for the 2,3 DPG levels to be partially restored in the red blood cells.[19] This will improve off-loading of oxygen to hypoxemic organs. Evaluation at 24 h would be even better, but the clinical situation may make this impractical.

WHAT ABOUT OUTPATIENTS?

For outpatients with hypoproliferative anemia, this approach is impractical and prescribing a dose of red cells to achieve a post-transfusion hemoglobin of 10 g/dL or more is reasonable in symptomatic patients or in asymptomatic patients in whom an anticipated decrease in hemoglobin is likely, as with chemotherapy treatment.

WHAT ARE THE DATA?

There are several studies addressing this question of the threshold hemoglobin/Hct for red cell transfusion. The Jehovah Witness's studies are very important[3–5]; however, other clinical studies have failed to demonstrate objective benefit in patients routinely transfused to maintain a hemoglobin of 10 g/dL or greater.[11–14,20–22] More recently, a retrospective observational study,[23] two randomized control trials,[24,25] meta-analyses of recent reports[26,27] and data from the PCI registry[28] confirm the lack of efficacy of red cell transfusion and show an association of red cell transfusion with worse outcomes–typically an increase in nosocomial infections in surgical patients[26] and an increase in thrombotic events in medical patients.[27,28] The thrombotic events may be related to prothrombotic red cell microparticles which accumulate during red cell storage.[29]

THIS DOESN'T MAKE SENSE. IF I TRANSFUSE A PATIENT WHO HAS A HEMOGLOBIN LESS THAN 10 G/DL, I MUST BE DOING SOME GOOD SINCE OXYGEN CARRIAGE IS INCREASED AND THAT WILL IMPROVE TISSUE OXYGEN DELIVERY

Transfusing red cells will increase oxygen carriage and the potential to deliver (DO_2) more oxygen but the critical measure is oxygen consumption (VO_2), not delivery. There is no general agreement that increasing the DO_2 by transfusing stored allogeneic red cells will increase the VO_2,[30,31] although other strategies to increase DO_2 may be helpful in a subpopulation of patients.[32,33] This

can be explained in a number of ways: (1) transfused red cells often have undetectable 2,3 DPG–this means that oxygen pick-up at the lungs is normal, but oxygen off-loading at the tissue is minimal[19]; (2) the increase in hematocrit post-transfusion increases whole blood viscosity and therefore the work-load on the myocardium; (3) transfused red cells have a very distorted shape (spheroecchinocytic),[29] at least initially immediately after transfusion, and this may cause difficulty traversing the microcirculation; (4) scavenging of nitric oxide (NO) by the transfused red cells may result in vasoconstriction thereby preventing the red cells from delivering oxygen to the hypoxemic microcirculation.[34] These may explain why red cell transfusion may actually **HARM** rather than **HELP** some normovolemic patients with minimal reductions in hemoglobin (8–10 g/dL).[35,36]

ARE THERE PATIENTS WHOM I SHOULD TRANSFUSE PROPHYLACTICALLY?

Yes. Data from post-operative vascular surgery patients suggests a transfusion threshold of 9.0 g/dL (Hct 27)[37] but a similar threshold does not appear appropriate for all post-operative, elderly patients, even those with known coronary artery disease.[22,25]

IS THIS APPROACH SUPPORTED BY EXPERT OPINION?

Yes. Several national groups have addressed this question over the past 15 years and are largely in agreement with the use of a conservative (restrictive) approach to red cell transfusion with the possible exception of patients with acute myocardial infraction.[38]

REFERENCES

1. Adam RC, Lundy JS. Anesthesia in cases of poor risk: some suggestions for decreasing the risk. *Surg Gynecol Obstet.* 1942;74:1011–1101.
2. Jacob G, Raj SR, Ketch T, et al. Postural pseudoanemia: posture dependent change in hematocrit. *Mayo Clin Proc.* 2005;80:611–614.
3. Viele MK, Weiskopf RB. What can we learn about the need for transfusion for patients, who refuse blood? The experience with Jehovah's Witnesses. *Transfusion.* 1994;34:396–401.
4. Mann MC, Votto J, Kanike J, et al. Management of the severely anemic patient who refused transfusion: lessons learned during the care of a Jehovah's Witness. *Ann Int Med.* 1992;117:1042–1048.
5. Kitchens CS. Are transfusions overrated? Surgical outcome of Jehovah's Witnesses. *Am J Med.* 1993;941:117–119.

6. Welch HG, Meehan KR, Goodnough T. Prudent strategies for elective red blood cell transfusion. *Ann Int Med.* 1992;116:392–402.

7. Greenburg AG. A physiologic basis for red blood cell transfusion decisions. *Am J Surg.* 1995;170(Suppl):325–365.

8. Stehling L, Simon TL. The red blood cell transfusion trigger. *Arch Pathol Lab Med.* 1994;118:429–434.

9. Wu WC, Saif S, Rathore MPH, et al. Blood transfusion in elderly patients with acute myocardial infarction. *N Eng J Med.* 2001;345:1230–1236.

10. Carson JL, Brooks MM, Abbott JD, et al. Liberal versus restrictive transfusion thresholds for patients with symptomatic coronary artery disease. *Am Heart J.* 2013;165:964–971.

11. Kim DM, Brecher ME, Estes TJ, et al. Relationship of hemoglobin level and duration of hospitalization after total hip arthroplasty: implications for the transfusion target. *May Clin Proc.* 1993;68:37–41.

12. Vuille-Lessard E, Yoshitake I, Wakui S, et al. Postoperative anemia does not impede functional outcome and quality of life early after hip and knee surgery. *Transfusion.* 2012;52:261–270.

13. Hebert PC, Wells G, Marshall J, et al. Transfusion requirements in critical care. *J Am Med Assoc.* 1995;273:1439–1444.

14. Babineau TJ, Dzik WH, Borlase BC, et al. Re-evaluation of current transfusion practices in patients in surgical intensive care units. *Am J Surg.* 1992;164:22–25.

15. Simon TJ, Alverson DC, AuBuchon J, et al. Practice parameter for the use of red blood cells. *Arch Pathol Lab Med.* 1998;122:130–138.

16. Tavares M, DiQuattro P, Sweeney JD. Reduction in red cell usage associated with engagement of the ordering physician. *Transfusion.* 2014;54:2625–2630.

17. Elizalde JI, Clemente J, Marin JL, et al. Early changes in hemoglobin and hematocrit levels after packed red cell transfusion in patients with acute anemia. *Transfusion.* 1997;37:573–576.

18. Wiesen AR, Hospenthal DR, Byrd JC, et al. Equilibration of hemoglobin concentration after transfusion in medical inpatients not actively bleeding. *Ann Intern Med.* 1994;121:278–280.

19. Heaton A, Keegan T, Holme S. In vivo regeneration of red cell 2,3 DPG following transfusion of DPG depleted AS-1, AS-3 and CPDA-1 red cells. *Br J Haematol.* 1989;71:131–136.

20. Hebert PC, Wells G, Blajchmann MA, et al. A multicenter, randomized, controlled clinical trial of transfusion requirements in critical care. *N Eng J Med.* 1999;340:409–417.

21. Hebert PC, Fergusson DA. Red cell transfusions in critically ill patients. *J Am Med Assoc.* 2002;288:1525–1526.

22. Carson JL. Liberal or restrictive transfusion in high risk patients after hip surgery. *N Eng J Med.* 2011;365:2453–2462.

23. Rao SV, Jollis JG, Harrington RA, et al. Relationship of blood transfusion and clinical outcomes in patients with acute coronary syndromes. *J Am Med Assoc.* 2004;292:1555–1562.

24. Cooper HA, Rao SV, Greenberg MD, et al. Conservative versus liberal red cell transfusion in acute myocardial infarction. *Am J Cardiol.* 2011;108:1108–1111.

25. Hajjar LA, Vincent JL, Galas FR, et al. Transfusion requirements after cardiac surgery: the TRACS randomized controlled trial. *J Am Med Assoc.* 2010;304:1559–1567.

26. Chatterjee S, Wetterslev J, Sharma A, et al. Association of blood transfusion with increase mortality in myocardial infarction: meta-analysis and diversity adjusted study sequential analysis. *JAMA Intern Med.* 2013;173:132–139.

27. Rohde JM, Dimcheff DE, Blumberg N, et al. Health care: associated infection after red blood cell transfusion. *J Am Med Assoc.* 2014;311:1317–1326.

28. Sherwood MW, Sherwood MN, Wang Y, et al. Patterns and outcomes of red blood cell transfusion in patients undergoing percutaneous coronary intervention. *J Am Med Assoc.* 2014;311:836–843.

29. Sweeney JD, Kouttab N, Kurtis JD. Stored red cell supernatant facilitates thrombin generation. *Transfusion.* 2009;49:1569–1579.

30. Menk RB, Pollack MM. Effect of blood transfusion on oxygen consumption in pediatric septic shock. *Crit Care Med.* 1990;18:1087–1091.

31. Marik PE, Sibbald WJ. Effect of stored blood transfusion on oxygen delivery in patients with sepsis. *J Am Med Assoc.* 1993;269:3024–3029.

32. Tuchschmidt J, Fried J, Astiz M, et al. Elevation of cardiac output and oxygen delivery improves outcome in septic shock. *Chest.* 1992;102:216–220.

33. Yu M, Levy M, Smith P, et al. Effect of maximizing oxygen delivery on morbidity and mortality in critically ill patients: a prospective randomized, controlled trial. *Crit Care Med.* 1993;21:830–838.

34. Reynolds JD, Ahearn GS, Angelo M, nitrosohemoglobin deficiency S-. A mechanism for loss of physiological activity in banked blood. *Proc Natl Acad Sci Unit States Am.* 2007;104:17058–17062.

35. Ward N, Levy M. Blood transfusion practice today. *Crit Care Clin.* 2004;20:179–186.

36. Roubinian NH, Escobar GJ, Liu V, et al. Decreased red blood cell use and mortality in hospitalized patients. *JAMA Intern Med.* 2014;174:1405–1407.

37. Nelson AH, Fleischer LA, Rosenbaum SH. Relationship between postoperative anemia and cardiac morbidity in high risk vascular patients. *Crit Care Med.* 1993;21:860–866.

38. Carson JL, Stanworth SJ, Alexander JH, et al. Clinical trials evaluating red blood cell transfusion thresholds: an updated systematic review and with additional focus on patients with cardiovascular disease. *Am Heart J.* 2018;200:96–101.

EXPERT OPINION

1. Hill SR, Carless PA, Henry DA, et al. Transfusion thresholds and other strategies for guiding all2ogeneic red blood cell transfusion. *Cochrane Library.* 2003;(3).
2. Carson JL, Grossman BJ, Keinman S, et al. Red blood transfusion : a clinical practice guideline from the AABB. *Ann Intern Med.* 2012;157:49–58.
3. Carson JL, Carless PA, Hebert PC. Outcomes using lower vs higher hemoglobin thresholds for red cell transfusion. *J Am Med Assoc.* 2013;309:83–84.
4. Qasseem A, Humphrey LL, Fitterman N, et al. Treatment of anemia in patients with heart disease : a clinical practice guideline from the American College of physicians. *Ann Intern Med.* 2013;159:770–779.

CHAPTER 7

Patient Blood Management: Reducing Risk by Reducing Inappropriate and Avoidable Transfusions

JOSEPH D. SWEENEY, MD, FACP, FRCPATH

INTRODUCTION

An important aspect of risk reduction in Transfusion Medicine is to identify physician practices that result in unnecessary transfusion. Unnecessary transfusions are transfusions in which the transfusion is prescribed and administered in the context of an absence of data with regard to efficacy (inappropriate transfusions) or in which there may be evidence or a consensus for efficacy but transfusion avoidance might have been possible if an alternative approach had been applied in a timely manner (avoidable transfusions). Although the majority of unnecessary transfusions do not result in any observed patient harm, they are wasteful of resources. If harm should ensue, unnecessary transfusions result in a substantial risk to the organization and prescribing physicians. This chapter will focus on this aspect of transfusion medicine, providing actual examples of unnecessary transfusions, some of which resulted in morbidity or mortality. The overall fraction of blood components that are prescribed unnecessarily is unknown and will likely vary from institution to institution and be different for different components. Alarmingly, it is possible that a substantial percentage of blood components are unnecessarily transfused. In the case of plasma transfusions, for example, intrainstitutional reduction in the range of 90%–95% has been achieved without any evidence of patient harm.[1]

Unnecessary Red Blood Cell Transfusions
Inappropriate red blood cell transfusions
Red blood cells are transfused in two clinical contexts. First, red cells are transfused to patients who are actively bleeding and exhibiting clinical features of hypovolemia. Here, the purpose is twofold: to restore normovolemia and provide hemoglobin to alleviate microcirculatory hypoxemia. The dose of red cells transfused in this situation will depend on the extent of the bleed, which will vary from patient to patient. Clinical judgment remains the most useful approach in gaging the need to transfuse in the first place and the continuing need to transfuse going forward. Attempting to assess the appropriateness or otherwise of red cell transfusion in this situation can be complicated and the default status is to consider such transfusions largely appropriate. However, there is variation in physician thresholds for transfusion. One trial of acute gastrointestinal bleeding in the context of liver cirrhosis randomized subjects presenting with acute gastrointestinal hemorrhage to a liberal versus a restrictive arm, after the administration of a single unit of red cells.[2] This study was therefore a *red cell dose study* and enrolled 921 participants. The liberal group received red blood cells when the hemoglobin decreased to less than 9 g/dL to maintain a hemoglobin between 9 and 11 g/dL, and the restrictive arm received RBCs if the hemoglobin decreased to less than 7 g/dL, to maintain a hemoglobin between 7 and 9 g/dL. The primary outcome measure was all cause 45-day mortality, with secondary outcomes being in-hospital complications and further rebleeding. There was a statistically significant difference favoring the restrictive group ($P = .02$), which was evident regardless of stage of cirrhosis or site of bleeding (variceal vs. peptic ulceration). This finding, which might appear to be contra-intuitive, lacked a clear explanation but it was hypothesized that the liberal group who received more transfusions maintained higher portal pressures favoring bleeding. The conclusion is important however, as it provides data to support a conservative approach to red cell transfusion in the context of acute gastrointestinal hemorrhage: whether this finding can be generalized to acute spontaneous bleeding from other anatomic sites is unclear but in the absence of such data, a conservative approach would appear justifiable.

Risk Management in Transfusion Medicine. https://doi.org/10.1016/B978-0-323-54837-3.00007-9

69

The second context in which RBCs are transfused involves patients who are not actively bleeding, but who have normovolemic anemia. Although by definition any hemoglobin less than 13 g/dL is anemia, this generally refers to patients with a hemoglobin less than 10 g/dL. These patients are hemodynamically stable, without evidence of bleeding. The mechanism of the anemia may be multifactorial, spanning hematinic deficiency, anemia of inflammation, acute-on-chronic or chronic blood loss anemia, hemolytic anemia, hypoproliferative anemia or anemia due to ineffective erythropoiesis. In some such patients the cause for the anemia may be apparent, in others not so. If the cause is readily identifiable, such as hematinic deficiency, that should be corrected promptly with iron, B12, and/or folate. Patients with very low levels of hemoglobin (arbitrarily <5 g/dL) are most likely to benefit from red blood cells but it is less clear whether patients with hemoglobins between 5 g/dL and 10 g/dL achieve any useful improved clinical outcome. The decision to transfuse generally takes into consideration the level of hemoglobin and any associated clinical features,[3] although the level of hemoglobin, in itself, often may drive the decision to transfuse. This is well illustrated by a 70-year old male who developed an unexpected blood loss posthernia surgery. The surgeon was concerned and wished to transfuse, but the patient was asymptomatic and reluctant. A transfusion medicine consultation recommended observation rather than transfusion, as the pattern of hemoglobin levels suggested stabilization. In this case, the patient was discharged without transfusion (Fig. 7.1).

The controversy in these patients is the hemoglobin threshold at which an improvement in clinical outcome is achieved by transfusion. In the past 20 years, there have been numerous randomized controlled trials involving different populations of patients which have examined this threshold. The earliest trial was the Transfusion Requirements in Critical care (TRICC) study published in 1999 which equally randomized 834 patients in the Intensive Care Unit (ICU0) to a restrictive arm (transfusion threshold <7 g/dL) and a liberal arm (transfusion threshold <9 g/dL).[4] Red blood cell dosage was titrated to maintain a hemoglobin between 7 and 9 g/dL in the restrictive arm and 9–11 g/dL in the liberal arm. The outcome was 30-day mortality. Overall, there was no difference in 30-day mortality, but in a subpopulation with low Acute Physiology and Chronic Health Evaluation (APACHE) scores, a benefit was seen in the restrictive arm. Of considerable interest, Table 7.3 of the manuscript showed a difference in myocardial infarction between the two arms (0.7% for the restrictive arm and 2.9% for the liberal arm, $P = .2$). This was not commented upon, yet might be considered to be surprising. However, recent data suggests that stored red blood cells may contain prothrombotic red cell microvesicles, providing some insight into the observation.[5] Since the TRICC trial, there have been several other randomized control trials examining the hemoglobin threshold for transfusion in different populations: the Transfusion Requirement after Cardiac surgery (TRACS) trial,[6] a Brazilian study in postoperative cardiac surgery patients; the Transfusion requirements in Septic Shock (TRISS) trial,[7] a study in patients with sepsis; the conservative versus liberal transfusion in acute myocardial infarction (CRIT) study[8] in patients with acute myocardial infarction; and the Functional Outcomes in Cardiovascular Patients Undergoing Surgical Hip Fracture Repair (FOCUS) study[9] in postoperative hip fracture surgery patients These studies have shown that restrictive policies to transfuse at a threshold of 7 g/dL (in patients without cardiac disease) or 8 g/dL (in patients with cardiac disease) are appropriate and may be associated with a better outcome, as supported by a recent meta-analysis.[10] There is ongoing controversy regarding acute myocardial infarction (AMI) and a two arm randomization to hemoglobin thresholds of 8 g/dL or 10 g/dL is ongoing (Myocardial ischemia and Transfusion [MINT] study). This study could be problematic however: a three-arm study with randomization at 8 g/dL, 9 g/dL or 10 g/dL might have been a better design if the critical threshold for decision in this population is close to 9 g/dL. Currently, red cell transfusion at hemoglobin thresholds of 7 g/dL for noncardiac patients and 8 g/dL for patients with cardiac disease would appear reasonable.[11] The threshold of 8 g/dL may need to be reconsidered in AMI[12] or very elderly patients.[12,13] Furthermore, a restrictive policy was shown to be inferior in oncology patients undergoing surgery[14] and in oncology patients in the ICU.[15] It may be that a threshold of 8.0 g/dL, or even higher, is appropriate in these populations. It should be emphasized that, in general, a single-unit red cell transfusion should be the dose prescribed in nonbleeding patients, with reevaluation of the clinical situation and posttransfusion hemoglobin performed prior to a second or third unit.[16] This is well illustrated in Fig. 7.1(Fig. 7.2) in which a low weight recipient with a pretransfusion hemoglobin less than 8 g/dL received a single unit of red cells containing a red cell mass of approximately 190 mL. A posttransfusion hemoglobin of greater than 10 g/dL is evident 8 h posttransfusion and a repeat sample 12 h later verified the hemoglobin increase (Fig. 7.2).

Avoidable red blood cell transfusion

Red blood cell substitutes have never become a clinical reality despite decades of research. However, the availability of erythrocyte stimulating agents (ESAs) has

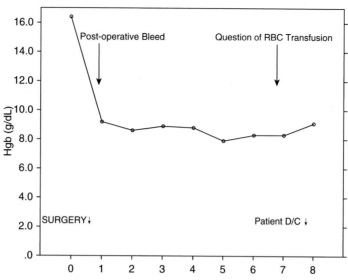

FIG. 7.1 The decision to transfuse or not transfuse in a hemodynamically stable 70-year old male with postoperative acute blood loss anemia.

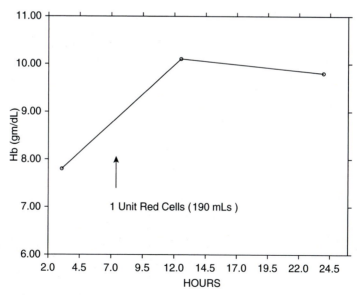

FIG. 7.2 Increase in hemoglobin after the transfusion of a single unit of red cells to a low weight (45 kg) female recipient.

impacted transfusion in a few clinical areas, mostly the management of anemia in patients with chronic renal failure (CRF) and to some extent in oncology.[17–19] Iron deficiency is the most common cause of anemia worldwide and timely correction with iron repletion can frequently avoid a red cell transfusion.[20] Included in this category are younger women with iron loss from menorrhagia or older patients scheduled for elective surgery. Younger females who develop severe iron deficiency due to menorrhagia may present to the emergency room with fatigue and are not infrequently transfused. The use of intravenous iron in this context can result in red cell transfusion avoidance but requires education of both Obstetricians and Emergency Department physicians.[21] Another scenario is elective surgery in elderly patients, especially orthopedic surgery.[22] Anemia is common (20%–30%) in elderly patients (>65 years) and related to impaired iron absorption due to reduced gastric acidity. This is illustrated in Fig. 7.3, which shows preoperative hemoglobin levels in 268 patients scheduled for elective hip or knee replacement. The probability of transfusion is determined mostly by the preoperative hemoglobin, and a hemoglobin of less than 11 g/dL was associated with a 60% chance of postoperative red cell transfusion in this cohort. A substantial number of preoperative patients have such a low hemoglobin level, and correction preoperatively could greatly mitigate red blood cell transfusion in this population.

Another strategy in orthopedic surgery is the use of tranexamic acid, either intravenously at induction or intracapsular during the operation, or both. This approach has been shown to reduce blood loss and the likelihood of red cell transfusion.[22]

Unnecessary Plasma Transfusion
Inappropriate plasma transfusion
Plasma is transfused in two clinical situations: prophylactically, prior to an invasive procedure in patients with evidence of clotting factor deficiency; and therapeutically, in patients who are actively bleeding with a known coagulopathy or who develop a hemodilutional coagulopathy after a large volume red blood cell transfusion. The coagulation test most commonly used to determine the presence and extent of a coagulopathy is the prothrombin time (PT), often resulted as its derivative, the International Normalized Ration (INR). The problem is that the prothrombin time was originally described as an assay of prothrombin, although we now know it measures a number of clotting factors in the extrinsic system.[23] It is especially sensitive to FVII, although FVII deficiency is not, in general, associated with clinical bleeding,[24] Many retrospective observational studies[25–39] and one randomized control trial[40] have failed to see any relationship between clinical bleeding and the PT or INR. The transfusion of plasma justified on the basis of a prolonged PT or elevated INR has come under considerable criticism.[41–44] Despite this, plasma continues to be prescribed in this context and guidelines continue to use this test as a justification for prophylactic plasma transfusion.[45] Consider the following patient: A 56-year old female with endometrial carcinoma was scheduled for a radical hysterectomy. A preoperative INR was 1.4. The anesthesiologist was concerned that such an INR could be associated with clinical bleeding and transfused five units of plasma

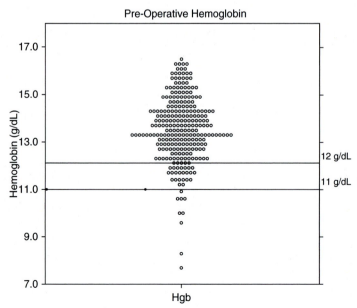

FIG. 7.3 Preoperative hemoglobins in a cohort of 268 patients scheduled for elective hip or knee replacements.

preoperatively (day 0). Approximately 30 min later, the patient developed fever, with chills and facial flushing. One to 2 h later, she developed increasing dyspnea and surgery was cancelled. She was transferred to the ICU. Three of the five donors were multiparous females. The dyspnea improved over a few days. She returned for surgery 7 days later. No plasma was given and surgery was performed uneventfully. The sample from the initially intended day of surgery (day 0) was not available for clotting factor assays, but the sample on day 7 (day of surgery) was available. As is seen in the table, there was no change in the INR and there is no clotting factor deficiency. Hence, the rationale for plasma transfusion (clotting factor deficiency) is erroneous, the transfusion of plasma was inappropriate and furthermore, the patient suffered a nonfatal TRALI reaction as a result of the inappropriate plasma transfusion (Table 7.1).

The mechanism of the elevated INR in this patient is likely the increase in D-dimer associated with the malignant condition. Inappropriate plasma transfusion appears particularly common in patients with liver disease. An elevated INR is typical of patients with advanced liver disease and is generally due to a low FV and/or hypofibrinogenemia or dysfibrinogenemia. However, patients with liver disease have a high FVIII and a low antithrombin III and a low protein C. Hence, on balance, these patients may be hypercoagulable, not hypocoagulable.[46] Furthermore, patients with a mildly elevated INR do not respond to plasma transfusion with a material shortening of the INR. This is well

illustrated (Fig. 7.4) in a series of 46 patients with an INR of <2.0 who received plasma and had measures of the INR within 6 h of plasma infusion. The mean (±1SD) pre-INR is 1.55 ± 0.3 and post-INR is 1.43 ± 0.3. This poor response of the INR to plasma transfusion has also previously been reported.[47]

Whether patients with very high INRs (>3.0) benefit from plasma transfusion is unclear. However, retrospective studies even in this population give no support to the practice of prophylactic plasma transfusion,[48] and

TABLE 7.1 Clotting Tests in a 56-year Old Female With Endometrial Carcinoma Who Received Plasma (Day 0) and Had a TRALI Reaction		
	Day 0	**Day 7**
PT (s)	15.3	15.3
INR	1.4	1.4
aPTT (s)	27	25
Fibrinogen (mg/dL)		696
D-dimer (µg/mL)	>4	>4
FII (%)		80
FV (%)		85
FVII (%)		58
FX (%)		102

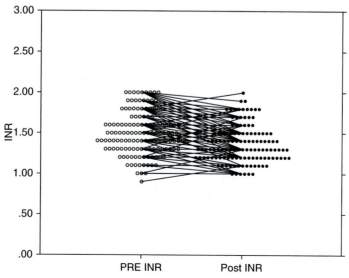

FIG. 7.4 Joined dot plot of 46 patients with an INR of <2.0 pretransfusion. The post-INR was within 6 h of the plasma transfusion.

many patients with such INRs have vitamin K deficiency or are taking a vitamin K antagonist, which should be managed with intravenous vitamin K,[49,50] restricting the use of 4-factor prothrombin complex concentrates for the most urgent cases.[51]

Avoidable plasma transfusion

There are many situations in which prophylactic plasma transfusion can be avoided if the cause of the prolonged INR is understood and potentially can be reversed or does not need to be reversed. Consider the following scenario: A request is received at 2320 h for 1 unit of FFP for a patient with an INR of 2.4 prior to surgery on the following day. A preoperative INR of <2.0 is desired. The technologist calls the surgeon and suggests giving vitamin K intravenously. The surgeon responds that the patient has liver disease and that vitamin K would not be helpful. Regardless, she agrees to administer 5 mg vitamin K intravenously that was given at 2345 h. At 0545, the INR has declined to 1.5. However, the surgeon fails to note the new test result and 1 unit of FFP is issued at 0645 immediately prior to surgery. The samples from the evening before surgery (day 0) and immediately pre-surgery (day 1) were available for clotting factor assays that are shown in Table 7.2:

TABLE 7.2
Response to Intravenous Vitamin K

	Day 0	Day 1
Time	1756	0545
Fibrinogen (mg/dL)	552	479
FV (%)	144	138
FVIII (%)	>200	>200
FVII (%)	25	55
FX (%)	18	48

As is evident, the patient has vitamin K deficiency that responded to intravenous vitamin K. This could have been predicted from the fibrinogen level, as patients with vitamin K deficiency have normal to high fibrinogen levels while patients with liver disease have low normal or low fibrinogen levels.

Another scenario is a request from the Emergency Department for two units of plasma for a 30-year old male with headache and fever prior to a lumbar puncture (LP). There is no personal or family history of a bleeding or clotting. However, the aPTT was 30 s (normal: 24–37) and the INR was 2.1. The physician is reluctant to perform the LP. Clotting factor assays to clarify the elevated INR revealed a selective FVII deficiency and a mixing study corrected the INR to 1.1. The LP was performed without plasma and without any bleeding complications (day 0). Infusion of vitamin K on the following day showed no responsiveness in the vitamin K dependent factors, confirming heterozygous FVII deficiency, an hereditary disorder not considered to be associated with clinical bleeding.[24] In this case, the transfusion of plasma was avoided.

The failure to administer vitamin K in a timely manner prior to an invasive intervention can also have dire consequences, as illustrated by the following case: A 78-year old female on warfarin for atrial fibrillation required endoscopy for rectal bleeding. The INR is 4.3. Two units FFP are requested. The chronology of events is shown in Table 7.4.

Both of these units were from female donors. The first unit was from a multiparous female who returned for testing. No HLA antibodies were present in the plasma. The second unit was from a female who had a single live pregnancy in 1981 and was transfused with one unit of red blood cells. This donor returned for testing and had class I and class II anti-HLA antibodies (anti-A_2, anti-A_{68}, anti B_{44}, anti-B_{45}). The recipient was DNA typed as A_2, B_{44}, DRB1*0401, confirming the TRALI mortality.

TABLE 7.3
Confirmation of Hereditary Heterozygous FVII Deficiency and Avoidance of Plasma Transfusion

	Time	INR	aPTT (s)	Fibrinogen (mg/dL)	FVII (%)	FX (%)	FV (%)	FVIII (%)
Day 0	0100	2.0	30		19	106	87	>200
Day 1	0308	1.8	31		23	99	78	>200
Day 1	1030	1.9	30	464	22	91	72	>200

TABLE 7.4
Chronology of Events in a Patient With a Fatal TRALI Reaction

- 1143: Specimen received in the Blood bank and types as Group O Rh (D) positive
- 1222: 1st unit FFP dispensed and transfused
- 1245: 2nd unit FFP dispensed and transfused
- 1315: Arrives in endoscopy suite
- 1320: Complains of slight dyspnea
- 1330: Procedure cancelled; more severe dyspnea; CXR shows bilateral pulmonary edema
- 1330–1400: O_2 saturation declines progressively over 30 min as follows: 86%, 77%, 66%, 32%
- Patient expires at 1404

TABLE 7.5
Myths Regarding Intravenous Vitamin K

- Oral vitamin K acts as rapidly as intravenous vitamin K
- Subcutaneous vitamin K is more rapid in onset of action and more consistent in lowering the INR than oral vitamin K
- Intravenous vitamin K has a high risk of an anaphylactoid reaction
- Intravenous vitamin K does not lower the INR for at least 6 h
- Intravenous vitamin K will cause difficulty in reestablishing anticoagulation with warfarin

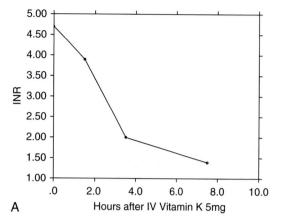

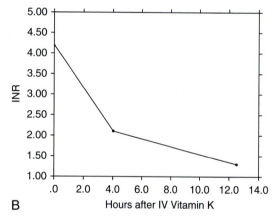

FIG. 7.5 (**A** and **B**) Rapid response to intravenous vitamin K in two patients requiring urgent partial warfarin reversal.

These cases illustrate patients with an elevated INR in which the diagnosis is unclear (heterozygous FVII deficiency), not suspected because of the context (erroneously considered to be due to liver disease) or known but not managed correctly (failure to administer vitamin K intravenously on the evening before endoscopy). In each case, plasma was prescribed in doses that would be considered ineffective. Physician education by Transfusion specialists in this area of coagulopathy is critical to avoid plasma transfusion.[52] Intravenous vitamin K has an important role in management[49,50] but there has been a bias against the use of vitamin K based on certain myths (Table 7.5).

Of particular concern is the myth that intravenous vitamin K takes at least 6 h to decrease the INR to approximately 2.0 or less. Fig. 7.5A and B demonstrates that intravenous vitamin K successfully achieves such an INR in less than 4 h. The rapid response of FVII is evident in Fig. 7.6, which is the main driver of the decrease in INR. Importantly, these changes are achieved at doses of 5 mg IV, which would not be expected to complicate the reintroduction of warfarin postprocedure.

Plasma is also used as an exchange fluid in thrombotic thrombocytopenic purpura (TTP) and in tertiary care centers, this can account for a significant fraction of all plasma transfused. The pathophysiology of sporadic TTP is a deficiency of ADAMTS13, a metalloprotease involved in the cleavage of ultra-large multimers of von Willebrand factor. Implementation of an ADAMTS13 assay with rapid turnaround time has been shown to be extremely useful in separating TTP from other thrombotic microangiopathies thus avoiding the unnecessary use of plasma in this context.[53] Taken together, avoidance of plasma transfusion in patients with mild (<2.0) or moderate (<3.0) elevation of the INR, careful

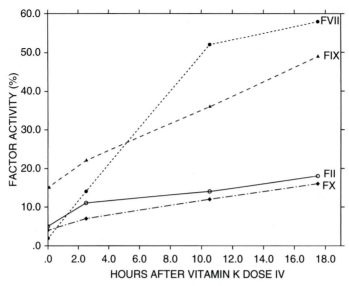

FIG. 7.6 Changes in clotting factors in response to 5 mg vitamin K.

assessment of the cause of any elevated INR, correction of an elevated INR with vitamin K where appropriate, and timely diagnosis of patients with TTP can greatly impact plasma use.[1,54]

Unnecessary Platelet Transfusion
Inappropriate platelet transfusion
Platelets are transfused in three clinical situations: prophylactically, to prevent spontaneous bleeding; prophylactically, prior to an invasive diagnostic or therapeutic procedure; and therapeutically, in thrombocytopenic patients or patients with thrombocytopathy who are actively bleeding. Most of the platelet transfusions are administered to thrombocytopenic patients to prevent spontaneous bleeding. These patients have a hypoproliferative thrombocytopenia due to a marrow disorder (acute leukemia, myeloproliferative neoplasm, myelodysplastic syndrome, or chemotherapy or radiation therapy). In general, there is reasonable agreement regarding appropriate platelet transfusion to prevent spontaneous bleeding for this category of recipients.[55–57] Platelet transfusions are appropriate for stable patients with single digit thrombocytopenia (platelet count $<10 \times 10^9$/L); unstable patients with clinical evidence of an inflammatory process with a platelet count $<15 \times 10^9$/L; patients with platelet counts of $10–20 \times 10^9$/L who are exhibiting a rapid decline in the platelet count in association with chemotherapy; patients with a de novo venous thrombosis requiring full anticoagulant therapy with heparin and a platelet

count of $<30 \times 10^9$/L. Stable autologous adult bone marrow transplant patients are now managed with therapeutic only transfusions,[58–60] reserving prophylactic transfusion for those patients who are unstable. The dose is considered a standard adult dose[61] or approximately $2.5–4.0 \times 10^{11}$. Transfusing platelets outside of these guidelines should be rare, as they are based on good data.[62]

There are a few clinical scenarios where platelet transfusion to this category of patients can be questioned: (1) Patients with stable single digit thrombocytopenia who are not on any treatment. These patients typically are out-patients with MDS or aplastic anemia and despite the severe thrombocytopenia have long bleeding-free intervals without transfusion. It may be appropriate *not* to transfuse such patients prophylactically as there are always risks of transfusion.[60] Consider the following: A 68-year old male with MDS, not on any treatment nor any overt bleeding, was transfused as an out-patient with a pretransfusion platelet count of 14×10^9/L. The patient was Group O, Rh negative and received prepooled whole blood derived platelets, all Group O, Rh negative. The pool was 5 days old. The transfusion occurred in clinic without any adverse event observed and he was discharged. About 1–2 h later, he stared to experience chills, followed by dry wrenching. Approximately 3 h after discharge, he returned to clinic where he was noted to be febrile. A reaction was called and the container, which had been discarded, was retrieved. The gram stain showed

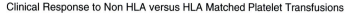

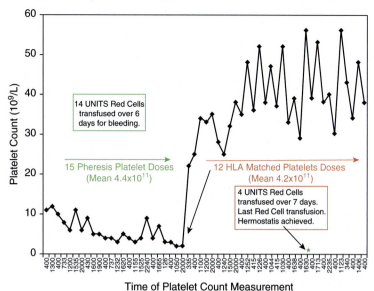

FIG. 7.7 Changes in the post transfusion platelet count after transfusion of non-HLA matched and HLA-matched platelets.

numerous gram positive coagulase negative cocci. He was admitted and started on intravenous cefazolin 2 G every 8 h. He was discharged 3 days later, to continue the intravenous antibiotics for another week. In retrospect, a decision to not transfuse this patient could have been a better overall approach. (2) Patients who are refractory due to broad spectrum HLA alloimmunization. These patients should be left untransfused until a suitable high grade HLA match is available, unless a life-threatening bleed ensues. This is illustrated by the following: A 69-year old female underwent allogeneic bone marrow transplant for MPN. She developed lower gastrointestinal bleeding requiring red cell transfusion. Despite the HLA alloimmunization, non-HLA matched platelets were transfused, as shown (Fig. 7.7), without any benefit as measured by platelet increments, and the clinical bleeding continued. The treating physician desired a platelet count of 30×10^9/L, which was largely unattainable with non-HLA matched platelets. After HLA matched platelets were procured, better increments were seen and the bleeding ameliorated.

(3) Overdosing. In stable patients with very severe single digit thrombocytopenia (platelet counts < 5 × 10^9/L), there may be a request for a double adult dose on the basis that this will protect further against spontaneous bleeding. There is no evidence that such

a treatment strategy decreases the risk, if any, of clinical bleeding.[61] Consider this 36-year old patient with AML undergoing induction therapy who developed neutropenic sepsis. The course of platelet transfusions is shown in Fig. 7.8. Noteworthy is the double dose of platelets given when the platelet count was approximately zero. While this achieved a higher increment, the increment was short lived and likely represents unnecessary overdosing.

(4) Patients with immune thrombocytopenia. These patients have severe single digit thrombocytopenia and are frequently transfused in the emergency department. Such transfusions are largely futile as the platelet increment is short lived. Platelet transfusion in this context is only appropriate for life-threatening bleeding. (5) Lastly, patients with thrombotic microangiopathy (TMA) or posttransfusion purpura (PTP). Platelet transfusions are largely considered to be contra-indicated in these clinical situations.

The second prophylactic use of platelets is to prevent bleeding in association with an invasive diagnostic or therapeutic intervention. Regrettably, there are no randomized controls in this setting, only retrospective observational reports which neither support nor refute any specific platelet threshold. It is commonly believed that the bleeding risk in this scenario is higher than the risk of spontaneous bleeding, but no predetermined

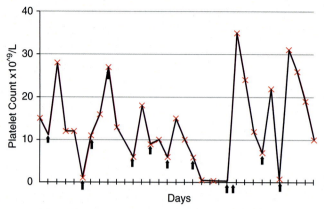

FIG. 7.8 Multiple platelet transfusions in AML induction complicated by sepsis. Upward arrows indicate a platelet transfusion. Most of the transfusions are appropriate (pretransfusion platelet count < 10 × 10⁹/L). A double dose (two contiguous *arrows*) is administered on one occasion when the platelet count is very low.

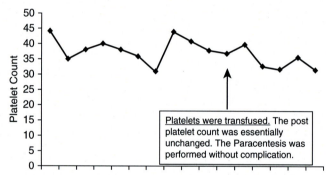

FIG. 7.9 Platelet transfusion in an 84-year old patient with ascites. The platelet count is 41 × 10⁹/L. The notches in the X-axis represent days.

threshold can be justified based on good data. However, guidelines are available,[60,62] and it has become a common practice to transfuse prophylactically when the platelet count is <50 × 10⁹/L. However, some recent data would support a lower threshold for central line placement and also lumbar puncture for diagnostic purposes or intrathecal therapy.[60] This is an important area for study. Consider an 84-year old patient with a platelet count of 41 × 10⁹/L requiring paracentesis. The interventional radiologist insisted on a prophylactic platelet transfusion. The platelets were administered as shown. No meaningful change occurred in the platelet count as would be anticipated (Fig. 7.9).

A slightly different case is a 23-year old male newly diagnosed with B-Cell ALL. A diagnostic LP was planned

and a target platelet count of 50 × 10⁹/L arbitrarily desired. His pretransfusion platelet count was 14 × 10⁹/L. He was prescribed two apheresis doses of platelets with the intention of a performing the LP after the second dose. The first dose was dispensed at 1400h and was uneventful. The second dose was dispensed at 1800h and the administration commenced at 1805h. At 1835h, after 111 mL of a 162 mL product had been transfused, the patient complained of difficulty breathing, which became progressively worse over the next hour. The respiratory rate increased to 44/min and oxygen saturation was 88% on room air. The LP was not performed and he was transferred to ICU, intubated and ventilated. He slowly improved over the next 24 h, was extubated and transferred out of the ICU. Fig. 7.10 shows the chest

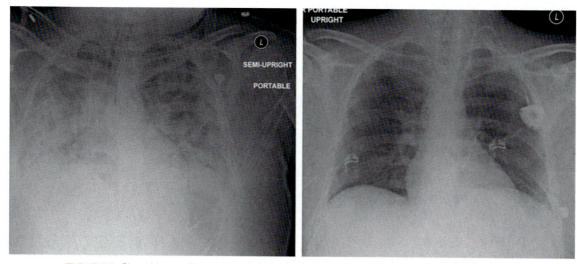

FIG. 7.10 Chest X-rays after receipt of the second unit of platelets and 2 days later postrecovery.

X-ray shortly after the second dose and several days later. This is an example of overdosing prior to an invasive procedure and illustrates the undesired consequences of a well-intentioned but unsubstantiated policy.

These cases illustrate the problems confronting the blood bank with regard to prophylactic platelets prior to an invasive procedure. It is unlikely that randomized controlled trials will be performed as the sample size required to reach a conclusion would be large, and the bleeding risk is low. In practice, a large number of participants would have to be enrolled. Furthermore, patient heterogeneity would likely raise confounders in interpretation. Therefore, a patient registry approach might be more suitable. Given the uncertainty, identifying "inappropriate" platelet transfusions in this context is difficult. The recent ASCO guidelines are helpful in this respect but evidence to justify the guidelines is lacking.[60]

The third indication for platelet transfusion is therapeutic platelet transfusions in thrombocytopenic patients or patients with thrombocytopathy who are actively bleeding. With regard to thrombocytopenia, no threshold can be defined: as a practical matter, a threshold of 50×10^9/L is commonly used, but this has no empiric justification and may be unnecessary, even with intracranial hemorrhage (ICH). In this respect, an interesting retrospective observational study was reported from MD Anderson of ICH in patients with leukemic or MDS over a 3-year period between 2007 and 09.[63] A total of 76 adult patients with ICH were reported: 42 with subdural hematoma, 9 subarachnoid bleeds, 18 intraparenchymal bleeds, and 7 intraventricular bleeds. The median platelet count at presentation was 17×10^9/L (range 0–178).

Moreover, 8 of 76 patients had platelet count $>50 \times 10^9$/L and 3 had platelet count $>100 \times 10^9$/L. The management objective was to achieve and maintain a platelet count $>50 \times 10^9$/L. Only 24/68 achieved a platelet count $>50 \times 10^9$/L (responders). Evaluation was performed at 72 h and 30 days. At 72 h, mortality (15/76, 20%) was related to Glasgow Coma Score (GCS) score <10, but not initial platelet count, achievement of platelet count $>50 \times 10^9$/L, or the number of platelet transfusions administered. Death due to ICH at 30 days was related to age and platelet responsiveness but not to GCS, the peak platelet count achieved, or number of days with a platelet count $>50 \times 10^9$/L. This study indicates that the outcome of ICH in these patients is determined by factors other than the platelet count, and platelet transfusions, early platelet transfusion responsiveness, or achievement of a platelet count $>50 \times 10^9$/L did not influence clinical outcome at 72 h or 30 days. This report casts doubt on the use of any platelet threshold or target in ICH and calls into question the use of large doses of platelets in the management of these patients.

There is some better data on the use of platelet transfusions in patients on antiplatelet therapy. The recent Platelet Transfusion Versus Standard Care After Acute Stroke due to Spontaneous Cerebral Haemorrhage Associated with Antiplatelt Therapy (PATCH) study is a randomized control study in which patients on antiplatelet therapy (APT) with spontaneous (nontrauma) intracranial bleeding were randomized to either receive platelet transfusion or placebo.[64] This study involved 60 hospitals in the UK, Netherlands, and France. Patients were randomized within 6 h of the bleed to receive therapeutic platelets or

TABLE 7.6
Agents That Promote Better Hemostasis in Thrombocytopenia or Thrombocytopathy

Antifibrinolytics: Aminocaproic Acid and Tranexamic Acid[66–71]
Desmopressin[72]
Recombinant human FVIIa[73–76]
Thrombopoietic agents[71–82]
Red blood cell transfusion[83–85]

standard of care. Outcomes were death-or-dependence, measured by a modified Rankin score adjusted for stratification variables, and clinical hemorrhagic score. There were 190 participants: 97 received platelet transfusion and 91 received standard of care. The odds of death-or-dependence were 2.05 in the platelet transfused group. Furthermore, 42% of the platelet transfused group had an adverse event and 24% died. In the standard of care group, 29% had an adverse event and 17% died. The conclusion was that platelet transfusion did NOT favorably affect clinical outcome in this population. The use of therapeutic platelet transfusions in patients on APT has not been advocated by the AABB Guidelines.[62]

Avoidable platelet transfusion
As yet, there is no substitute available as an alternative to platelet transfusion. The general approach has been to attempt to use agents that could augment or work in concert with platelets to promote better hemostasis. A general list is given in Table 7.6. The subject has been reviewed elsewhere[65] but there is no consensus that these agents are efficacious.

Conclusion: Inappropriate transfusions are commonplace in-hospital and occur on account of the continuation of outdated, nonevidence-based practices. Avoidable transfusions occur because patient management is not optimized. Addressing intrainstitutional inappropriate practices and promoting good transfusion management can be a highly effective risk reduction strategy.

REFERENCES

1. Nixon CP, Tavares MF, Sweeney JD. How do we reduce Plasma Transfusion in Rhode Island? *Transfusion.* 2017;57:1863–1873.
2. Villanueva C, Colomo A, Bosch A, et al. Transfusion strategies for acute upper gastrointestinal bleeding. *N Engl J Med.* 2013;368:11–21.
3. Vincent JL. Indications for blood transfusions: too complex to base on a single number? *Ann Intern Med.* 2012;157:71–72.
4. Hebert PC, Wells G, Blajchman MA, et al. A multicenter, randomized, controlled clinical trial of transfusion requirements in critical care. Transfusion Requirements in Critical Care Investigators, Canadian Critical Care Trials Group. *N Engl J Med.* 1999;340:409–417.
5. Sweeney JD, Kouttab N, Kurtis JD. Stored red cell supernatant facilitates thrombin generation. *Transfusion.* 2009;49:1569–1579.
6. Hajjar LA, Vincent JL, Galas FR, et al. Transfusion requirements after cardiac surgery: the TRACS randomized controlled trial. *J Am Med Assoc.* 2010;304:1559–1567.
7. Holst LB, Haase N, Wetterslev J, et al. Lower versus higher hemoglobin threshold for transfusion in septic shock. *N Engl J Med.* 2014;371:1381–1391.
8. Cooper HA, Rao SV, Greenberg MD, et al. Conservative versus liberal red cell transfusion in acute myocardial infarction (the CRIT Randomized Pilot Study). *Am J Cardiol.* 2011;108:1108–1111.
9. Carson JL, Terrin ML, Noveck H, et al. Liberal or restrictive transfusion in high-risk patients after hip surgery. *N Engl J Med.* 2011;365:2453–2462.
10. Salpeter SR, Buckley JS, Chatterjee S. Impact of more restrictive blood transfusion strategies on clinical outcomes: a meta-analysis and systematic review. *Am J Med.* 2014;127(2):124–131.
11. Carson JL, Guyatt G, Heddle NM, et al. Clinical practice guidelines from the AABB: red blood cell transfusion thresholds and storage. *J Am Med Assoc.* 2016;316:2025–2035.
12. Carson JL, Stanworth SJ, Alexander JH, et al. Clinical trials evaluating red blood cell transfusion thresholds: an updated systematic review and with additional focus on patients with cardiovascular disease. *Am Heart J.* 2018;200:96–101.
13. Simon GI, Graswell A, Thom O, Fung YL. Outcomes of restrictive versus liberal transfusion strategies in older adults from nine randomized controlled trials: a systematic review of and met-analysis. *Lancet Haematol.* 2017;4: e465–e474.
14. de Almeida JP, Vincent JL, Galas FR, et al. Transfusion requirements in surgical oncology patients: a prospective, randomized controlled trial. *Anesthesiology.* 2015;122:29–38.
15. Bergamin FS, Almeida JP, Landoni G, et al. Liberal versus restrictive transfusion strategy in critically ill oncologic patients: the transfusion requirements in critically ill oncologic patients randomized controlled trial. *Crit Care Med.* 2017;45:766–773.
16. Tavares M, DiQuattro P, Sweeney JD. Reduction in red cell usage associated with engagement of the ordering physician. *Transfusion.* 2014;54:2625–2630.
17. Folkert VW, Meyer TW, Holster TH. Anemia therapy in ESRD: time to move on. *Clin J Am Soc Nephrol.* 2010;5:1163–1164.

18. Goodnough LT, Shander AS. Erythropoiesis stimulating agents, blood transfusion, and the practice of medicine. *Am J Hematol.* 2010;85:835–837.
19. Goodnough LT, Shander A. Update on erythropoiesis-stimulating agents. *Best Pract Res Clin Anaesthesiol.* 2013;27:121–129.
20. Litton E, Xiao J, Ho KM. Safety and efficacy of intravenous iron therapy in reducing requirement for allogenic blood transfusion: systematic review and meta-analysis of randomized clinical trials. *BMJ.* 2013;347:F4822.
21. Nixon CP, Sweeney JD. Severe iron deficiency anemia: red blood cell transfusion or intravenous iron. *Transfusion* (in press). 2018;58:1824–1826.
22. Layton J, Rubin L, Sweeney JD. Advanced blood management strategies for elective joint arthroplasty. *Rh I Med J.* 2013;96:23–25.
23. Caldwell S, Shah N. The Prothrombin time derived international normalized ratio: great for warfarin, fair for prognosis and bad for bleeding risk. *Liver Internat.* 2008;28:1325–1327.
24. Barnett JM, Demel KC, Mega A, et al. Lack of bleeding in patients with severe factor VII deficiency. *Am J Hematol.* 2005;78:134–137.
25. Spector I, Corn M, Ticktin HE. Effect of plasma transfusion on the prothrombin time and clotting factors in liver disease. *N Eng J Med.* 1966;275:1032–1037.
26. Ewe K. Bleeding after liver biopsy does not correlate with indices of peripheral coagulation. *Digest Dis Sc.* 1981;26:388–393.
27. Ragni MV, Lewis JH, Spero JA, et al. Bleeding and coagulation abnormalities in alcoholic cirrhotic liver disease. *Alcohol Clin Exp Res.* 1982;6:267–274.
28. Friedman EW, Sussman II . Safety of invasive procedures in patients with the coagulopathy of liver disease. *Clin Lab Hematol.* 1989;11:199–204.
29. McVay PA, Toy PTC. Lack of increased bleeding after liver biopsy in patients with mild hemostatic abnormalities. *Am J Clin Pathol.* 1990;94:747–753.
30. Zins M, Vilgrain V, Gayno S, et al. U.S. guided percutaneous liver biopsy with plugging of the needle track: a prospective study in 72 high-risk patients. *Radiology.* 1992;184:841–843.
31. Squillante CE, Siena A, Cellerino C, et al. Fine needle liver biopsy in patients with severely impaired coagulation. *Liver.* 1993;13:270–273.
32. Inabnet W, Deziel D. Laparoscopic liver biopsy in patients with coagulopathy, portal hypertension and ascites. *Amer Surg.* 1995;61:603–606.
33. McVay PA, Toy PTC. Lack of increased bleeding after paracentesis and thoracentesis in patients with mild coagulation abnormalities. *Transfusion.* 1991;31:164–171.
34. Foster PF, Moore LR, Sankary HN, et al. Central venous catheterization in patients with coagulopathy. *Arch Surg.* 1992;127:273–275.
35. Doerfler ME, Kaufman B. Central venous catheter placement in patients with disorders of hemostasis. *Chest.* 1996;110:185–188.
36. Goldfard G, Lebrec D. Percutaneous cannulation of the internal jugular vein in patients with coagulopathies: an experience based on 1,000 attempts. *Anesthesiology.* 1982;56:321–323.
37. Mumtaz H, Williams V, Hauer-Jensen M, et al. Central venous catheter placement in patients with disorders of hemostasis. *Am J Surg.* 2000;180:503–506.
38. DeLoughery TG, Liebeer JM, Simonds VH. Invasive line placement in critically ill patients: do hemostatic defects matter? *Transfusion.* 1996;36:827–831.
39. Kozak EA, Brath LK. Do "screening" coagulation tests predict bleeding in patients undergoing fiber optic bronchoscopy with biopsy? *Chest.* 1994;106:703–705.
40. Muller MC, Arbous MS, Spoelstra-deMan AM, et al. Transfusion of fresh frozen plasma in critically ill patients with a coagulopathy before invasive procedures: a randomized clinical trial. *Transfusion.* 2015;55:26–35.
41. Stanworth SJ, Brunskill SJ, Hyde CJ. Is fresh frozen plasma clinically effective? A systematic review of randomized controlled trials. *Br J Haematol.* 2004;126: 139–154.
42. Segal JB, Dzik WH. Paucity of studies to support that abnormal coagulation test results predict bleeding in the setting of invasive procedures: an evidence based review. *Transfusion.* 2005;45:1413–1425.
43. Roback JD, Caldwell S, Carson J, et al. Evidence based practice guidelines for plasma transfusion. *Transfusion.* 2010;50:1227–1239.
44. Yang L, Stanworth S, Hopewell S, et al. Is fresh frozen plasma clinically effective? An update of a systematic review of randomized controlled trials. *Transfusion.* 2012;52:1673–1686.
45. Malloy PC, Grassi CJ, Kundu S, et al. Standards of Practice Committee with Cardiovascular and Interventional Radiological Society of Europe (CIRSE) Endorsement. Consensus guidelines for peri-procedural management of coagulation status and hemostasis risk in percutaneous image-guided interventions. *J Vasc Interv Radiol.* 2009;20:S240–S249.
46. Tripodi A, Mannucci PM. The coagulopathy of chronic liver disease. *N Eng J Med.* 2011;365:147–156.
47. Abdel-Wahab OI, Healy B, Dzik WH. Effect of fresh-frozen plasma transfusion on prothrombin time and bleeding in patients with mild coagulation abnormalities. *Transfusion.* 2006;46:1279–1285.
48. Carino GP, Tsapenko AY, Sweeney JD. Central line placement in patients with coagulopathy with or without prophylactic plasma. *J Crit Care.* 2012;27: 529e9–529e13.
49. Meehan R, Tavares M, Sweeney JD. Clinical experience with oral versus intravenous vitamin K for warfarin reversal. *Transfusion.* 2013;53:491–498.
50. Sahai T, Tavares MF, Sweeney JD. Rapid response to intravenous vitamin K may obviate the need to transfuse prothrombin complex concentrates. *Transfusion.* 2017;57:1885–1890.

51. Sarode R, Milling Jr TJ, Refaai MA, et al. Efficacy and safety of a 4-factor prothrombin complex concentrate in patients on vitamin K antagonists presenting with major bleeding: a randomized, plasma-controlled, phase IIIB study. *Circulation.* 2013;128:1234–1243.

52. Sweeney JD. The blood bank physician as a hemostasis consultant. *Transfus Apher Sci.* 2008;39:145–150.

53. Connell NT, Cheves TC, Sweeney JD. Effect of ADAMTS13 activity turnaround time on plasma utilization for suspected thrombotic thrombocytopenic purpura. *Transfusion.* 2016;56:354–359.

54. Tavares M, DiQuattro P, Nolette N, Conti G, Sweeney JD. Reduction in plasma transfusion after enforcement of transfusion guidelines. *Transfusion.* 2011;51:754–761.

55. Rebulla P, Finazzi G, Marangoni F, et al. The threshold for prophylactic platelet transfusions in adults with acute myeloid leukemia. *N Engl J Med.* 1997;26:1870.

56. Wandt H, Frank M, Ehninger G, et al. Safety and cost effectiveness of a 10 x 10^9/L trigger for prophylactic platelet transfusion compared with the traditional 20 x 10^9/L trigger: a prospective comparative trial in 105 patients with acute myeloid leukemia. *Blood.* 1998;91:3601–3606.

57. Heckmann KD, Weiner GJ, Davis CS, et al. Randomized study of prophylactic platelet transfusion threshold during induction therapy for adult acute leukemia: 10,000/uL versus 20,000/uL. *J Clin Orthod.* 1997;15:1143–1147.

58. Stanworth SJ, Estcourt LJ, Powter G, et al. A no-prophylaxis platelet-transfusion strategy for hematologic cancers. *N Engl J Med.* 2013;368:1771–1780.

59. Wandt H, Schaefer-Eckart K, Frank M, Birkmann J, Wilhelm M. A therapeutic platelet transfusion strategy is safe and feasible in patients after autologous peripheral blood stem cell transplantation. *Bone Marrow Transplant.* 2006;37: 387–392.

60. Schiffer CA, Bohlke K, Delaney M, et al. Platelet transfusion for patients with cancer: American society of clinical oncology clinical practice guideline update. *J Clin Oncol.* 2018;36:283–299.

61. Slichter SJ, Kaufman RM, Assmann SF, et al. Dose of prophylactic platelet transfusions and prevention of hemorrhage. *N Engl J Med.* 2010;362:600–613.

62. Kaufman RM, Djulbegovic B, Gernsheimer T, et al. Platelet transfusion: a clinical practice guideline from the AABB. *Ann Intern Med.* 2015;162:205–213.

63. Chern JJ, Tsung AJ, Humphries W, Sawaya R, Lang FF. Clinical Outcome of leukemia patients with intracranial hemorrhage. *J Neurosurg.* 2011;115:268–272.

64. Baharoglu MI, Cordonnier C, Al-Shahi Salman R, et al. Platelet transfusion versus standard care after acute stroke due to spontaneous cerebral haemorrhage associated with antiplatelet therapy (PATCH): a randomised, open-label, phase 3 trial. *Lancet.* 2016;387:2605–2613.

65. Lozano M, Sweeney JD. Alternatives to platelet transfusion. In: Sweeney JD, Lozano M, eds. *Platelet Transfusion Therapy.* Bethesda, MD: AABB Press; 2013:567–589.

66. Dunn CJ, Goa KL. Tranexamic acid - a review of its use in surgery and other indications. *Drugs.* 1999;57: 1005–1032.

67. Gardner FH, Helmer III RE. Aminocaproic acid. Use in control of hemorrhage in patients with amegakaryocytic thrombocytopenia. *J Am Med Assoc.* 1980;243:35–37.

68. Garewal HS, Durie BG. Anti-fibrinolytic therapy with aminocaproic acid for the control of bleeding in thrombocytopenic patients. *Scand J Haematol.* 1985;35:497–500.

69. Bartholomew JR, Salgia R, Bell WR. Control of bleeding in patients with immune and nonimmune thrombocytopenia with aminocaproic acid. *Arch Intern Med.* 1989;149:1959–1961.

70. Ben Bassat I, Douer D, Ramot B. Tranexamic acid therapy in acute myeloid leukemia: possible reduction of platelet transfusions. *Eur J Haematol.* 1990;45:86–89.

71. Fricke W, Alling D, Kimball J, et al. Lack of efficacy of tranexamic acid in thrombocytopenic bleeding. *Transfusion.* 1991;31:345–348.

72. Kobrinsky NL, Tulloch H. Treatment of refractory thrombocytopenic bleeding with 1-desamino-8-D-arginine vasopressin (desmopressin). *J Pediatr.* 1988;112:993–996.

73. Hedner U. Recombinant FVIIa. *Vox Sang.* 2004;87(suppl 2):25–28.

74. Poon MC. The evidence for the use of recombinant human activated factor VII in the treatment of bleeding patients with quantitative and qualitative platelet disorders. *Transfus Med Rev.* 2007;21:223–236.

75. Kristensen J, Killander A, Hippe E, et al. Clinical experience with recombinant factor VIIa in patients with thrombocytopenia. *Haemostasis.* 1996;26(supp 1):159–164.

76. Savani BN, Dunbar CE, Rick ME. Combination therapy with rFVIIa and platelets for hemorrhage in patients with severe thrombocytopenia and alloimmunization. *Am J Hematol.* 2006;81:218–219.

77. Stasi R, Bosworth J, Rhodes E, et al. Thrombopoietic agents. *Blood Rev.* 2010;24:179–190.

78. Kaser A, Brandacher G, Steurer W, et al. Interleukin-6 stimulates thrombopoiesis through thrombopoietin: role in inflammatory thrombocytosis. *Blood.* 2001;98:2720–2725.

79. McHutchison JG, Dusheiko G, Shiffman ML, et al. Eltrombopag for thrombocytopenia in patients with cirrhosis associated with hepatitis C. *N Engl J Med.* 2007;357:2227–2236.

80. Afdhal NH, Giannini EG, Tayyab G, et al. Eltrombopag before procedures in patients with cirrhosis and thrombocytopenia. *N Engl J Med.* 2012;367:716–724.

81. Kantarjian H, Fenaux P, Sekeres MA, et al. Safety and efficacy of romiplostim in patients with lower-risk myelodysplastic syndrome and thrombocytopenia. *J Clin Oncol.* 2010;28:437–444.

82. Olnes MJ, Scheinberg P, Calvo KR, et al. Eltrombopag and improved hematopoiesis in refractory aplastic anemia. *N Engl J Med.* 2012;367:11–19.

83. Boneu B, Fernandez F. The role of the hematocrit in bleeding. *Transfus Med Rev.* 1987;1:182–185.

84. Ch H. The hemostatic effect of packed red cell transfusion in patients with anemia. *Transfusion.* 1998;38:1011–1014.

85. Escolar G, Garrido M, Mazara R, et al. Experimental basis for the use of red cell transfusion in the management of anemic-thrombocytopenic patients. *Transfusion.* 1988;34: 406–411.

CHAPTER 8

Transfusion Risk Management in Children and Neonates

STUART P. WEISBERG, MD, PHD • SARAH VOSSOUGHI, MD

INTRODUCTION TO PEDIATRIC TRANSFUSION MEDICINE

Children are known to have distinct health considerations from adults and are generally treated as a unique category in both medicine and pathology.[1] Compared to adults, there continues to be a lack of high quality clinical studies for pediatric patients, with evidence-based medicine often extrapolated from adult studies.[2] However, each developmental transition during childhood is associated with distinct changes in physiology, hematological parameters, immune function, and body composition that influence transfusion decisions and responses to transfusion. In addition, pediatric disease states requiring frequent transfusion therapy, such as prematurity and cyanotic heart disease, display unique physiology that cannot be easily extrapolated from adult studies. The distinct biology of pediatric patients necessitates a specialized approach to transfusion risk management in the pediatric patient population. Evidence from multiple observational studies show that children receiving therapeutic transfusions have increased morbidity, independent of other risk factors. Specifically, transfusion therapy in children has been linked with longer duration of ventilation postoperatively, prolonged hospitalizations, and an increased risk for infections.[3-6] Several observational studies, both in the United States and internationally, have shown an increased rate of transfusion reactions in pediatric patients compared to adults.[7-9] Although these results are drawn from observational data and thus subject to potential bias, these risks necessitate expanded pediatric-specific transfusion medicine and risk management research and practices.

CONSERVATION AND STEWARDSHIP

Given the association of transfusion with poor outcomes in pediatric patients, the first step in managing transfusion risks should be avoidance of unnecessary transfusion. Unfortunately, very few high quality studies are currently available defining the clinical criteria for determining transfusion necessity in specific pediatric patient populations, although this is an active and dynamic area of research. Most randomized controlled trials conducted to date do not show adverse outcomes in pediatric patients on restrictive transfusion regimens; however, the use of restrictive transfusion remains an area of controversy and conflicting data, especially when applied to the pediatric patient groups most susceptible to hypoxia such as those with cyanotic heart disease and premature infants.[10,11]

Two trials with conflicting results illustrate the difficulties in arriving at consensus regarding when to transfuse pediatric patients. Premature infants frequently require transfusion during their hospital stay, however the optimal clinical and laboratory criteria for initiating transfusion are not well defined, nor are the short- and long-term risks of transfusing too much or too little. In a single-center trial at the University of Iowa that randomized very low birth weight infants to liberal or restrictive transfusion, increased incidence of brain hemorrhage, periventricular leukomalacia, and apnea were observed in the restrictive transfusion arm.[12] However, upon long-term follow-up of these subjects, neurocognitive outcomes were inferior in the liberal transfusion arm at age 7–10.[13] In contrast, the Premature Infants in Need of Transfusion (PINT) study showed no difference in short-term morbidity or mortality in patients assigned to liberal versus restrictive red blood cell (RBC) transfusion, but follow-up at 18–24 months showed increased incidence of cognitive delay in the restrictive arm.[14,15] Additional randomized trials are now underway to help clarify optimal transfusion thresholds for premature infants, and as the results of these trials become available for both long- and short-term outcomes, having pediatric specialists involved on the institutional transfusion committee will be essential for rapidly interpreting these data and responding with improved standardized transfusion practices that minimize transfusion risks to neonates.

Risk Management in Transfusion Medicine. https://doi.org/10.1016/B978-0-323-54837-3.00008-0

Further confounding the ability to understand pediatric outcomes related to transfusion is the significant variability in practice and lack of agreed-upon standards. There is even demonstrated variability within individual institutions by day of the week. For example, pediatric patients admitted for surgeries on the weekend are more likely to receive a blood transfusion despite no difference in rates of hemorrhage intraoperatively.[16] Despite these limitations, several concrete measures that can decrease transfusion risks by minimizing patient blood loss are available.

Conservation

Among possible interventions to conserve the use of blood products are the avoidance of phlebotomy and the prevention of blood loss intraoperatively. One current method of blood conservation implemented by blood banks includes limiting pretransfusion testing in infants under 4 months of age. After initial testing that includes ABO and D typing of the infant's red cells and screening for unexpected red cell antibodies in the infant's or mother's serum or plasma, AABB *Standards* allows omission of repeated ABO grouping and Rh typing until the age of 4 months, provided the initial antibody screen is negative, the transfused RBCs are ABO identical or compatible, and the transfused RBCs are D negative or matched to the infant.[17] However, before issuing non group O RBCs, passively acquired maternal anti-A and anti-B must be ruled out in the infant's serum or plasma in antiglobulin phase. In the event of a positive antibody screen, repeat antibody testing with crossmatching and selection of antigen negative blood is required until the maternal antibody is no longer detected.

Avoiding Phlebotomy

Iatrogenic blood loss, particularly in critically ill patients, remains a significant obstacle to inpatient blood conservation with significant variation among different practice settings that are not reflective of any known evidence-based practice guidelines.[18]

Blood loss due to admission blood draws has been found to be predictive of the need for transfusions during hospital stays, and anemia is an independent risk factor for death in sick patients.[19] Unwarranted laboratory testing can be reduced by moving away from preselected order sets; instead only ordering those specific tests clinically indicated for a given patient and only on the specific dates they are necessary, with no automatic repeat ordering (daily orders).[20] In addition to avoiding unnecessary testing or excessive testing that will not change the clinical decision making or outcome, it is also important to consider the volume required for testing. Phlebotomy in excess of requested blood volumes from the

lab potentially increases the amount drawn by as much as 55%–375% over the volume required to perform testing.[21] Using pediatric blood collection tubes preferentially can decrease phlebotomy-associated blood loss by as much as half without compromising the integrity of the test.[20] One of the highest causes of absolute blood volume wastage in laboratory testing, even with the use of pediatric culture bottles, is the reflex blood culture order in febrile pediatric patients. Reducing the frequency of blood cultures for sepsis workups by using comprehensive treatment algorithms developed by multidisciplinary teams, which require more than just the presence of a fever, have the potential to significantly reduce iatrogenic blood loss without affecting mortality or readmission rates.[22]

Preventing Intraoperative Blood Loss

Intraoperative blood conservation strategies can be used to decrease transfusion requirements during major surgery. Pediatric patients with congenital heart disease often require transfusion during cardiopulmonary bypass surgery. Higher volumes of blood product transfusion during cardiopulmonary bypass is independently associated with excessive postoperative bleeding even when controlling for multiple other variables including age, weight, complexity, and time on bypass, among others.[23] Data from small clinical trials have shown that cell salvage and restrictive transfusion thresholds can be used safely in children during bypass procedures with no increase in 30-day mortality. Children undergoing surgeries requiring cardiopulmonary bypass have also been shown to have a decreased incidence of postoperative renal dysfunction when cell salvaged blood was used compared to allogeneic blood transfusions.[24] However, these studies are small and heterogeneous, so additional trials are needed to fully understand the impact of these interventions.[25] In addition to cell salvage, circuit miniaturization and ultrafiltration are also frequently implemented to reduce blood loss intraoperatively, resulting in decreased postoperative transfusion requirements.[26] Bloodless surgical techniques, often applied to individuals who decline transfusion for religious reasons, have also been successful in the neonatal population, including practices such as changing the position of the bypass console closer to the table, using smaller sized oxygenators, shorter tubing, smaller diameter tubing, and priming of circuits with electrolyte solutions.[27]

Stewardship

The utilization of blood products and transfusion management are among the most relevant and highest priority of concern among many laboratory professionals.[28]

To meet safety and quality improvement goals for pediatric patients, a discussion of patient blood management and the current state of pediatric transfusion guidelines is necessary.

Patient Blood Management

Patient blood management (PBM) begins before the patient enters the hospital, with the aim to improve safety and clinical outcomes by "managing" the patient's blood with a proactive multidisciplinary approach including basing transfusion decisions on best practices.[29] The *Society for the Advancement of Blood Management* offers guidelines for patient blood management programs, including guidance on pediatric patients that encourages utilizing restrictive transfusion thresholds, having pediatric-specific massive transfusion protocols, limiting donor exposure, reducing blood sampling, and basing transfusion volumes on not only weight, but also desired hemoglobin increment change.[30] However, pediatric-specific PBM literature is otherwise sparse and few hospitals have a pediatric-specific program.[31]

Transfusion Guidelines

Transfusion guidelines in children are largely based on a scaled-down (size-based dosing) version of what is given to adults, with as many as 50% of US pediatric intensive care (PICU) patients receiving transfusions.[32] Unfortunately, due to the lack of high quality evidence, this is currently the only option available for transfusion medicine services to recommend. An otherwise healthy pediatric patient can tolerate significant anemia with hemoglobin levels of 6–7 g/dL, and transfusion is not indicated for patients who can be treated with alternative measures.[26] For pediatric patients who are not otherwise healthy, such as in the PICU, there is evidence that restrictive transfusion strategies may be appropriate. The 2007 TRIPICU noninferiority trial established that decreasing the transfusion threshold in stable PICU patients without cyanotic heart disease to 7 g/dL did not increase adverse outcomes when compared to a 9.5 g/dL threshold.[33]

Need for Standardization

Despite increasing evidence supporting more restrictive practices in pediatric transfusion, and the need for evidence-based practices, a number of studies have shown significant variation in transfusion practices at pediatric treatment centers, often due to providers' failing to follow the guidelines provided by the transfusion and PBM services.[34–36] This is not unique to pediatric providers, nor is it specific to transfusion threshold guidelines. Both confusion and variability in practice exist in a number of areas of transfusion medicine among clinical teams at the bedside, including massive transfusion protocols and even informed consent practices.[37,38] Regardless of the strategy used at an institution when approaching transfusion guidelines, it is evident that pediatric patients represent a unique population, and an individualized approach may be necessary more often than in the adult setting, necessitating more targeted pediatric-specific transfusion medicine training and research. However, developing a set of clear evidence-based guidelines appropriate to the pediatric setting, that are easily accessible to providers and understandable to non blood bankers, is necessary for safe and effective component therapy in pediatric patients.

PRODUCT SELECTION AND SPECIAL PROCESSING

Product selection in pediatric patients must account for a number of factors, depending on the specific situation and desired outcome. While often not clinically relevant for adult patients, seemingly small issues such as the age of the product, potassium content, the size and preparation of aliquots, timing of leukoreduction, additive solution types and volume, special products, and dosing take on much more significance in pediatric patients.

Storage Lesion

The term "storage lesion" refers to the cumulative damage done to RBCs during refrigerated storage, leading to decreased posttransfusion recovery and/or function. The observable and repeatedly proven effects of storage on RBCs include a decreased pH, shape changes, decreased available 2,3-diphosphoglycerate (DPG), decreased glutathione, decreased adenosine triphosphate (ATP), and decreased nitric oxide (NO); with resulting increases in extracellular hemoglobin, heme, potassium, and lactate dehydrogenase.[39] Levels of 2,3-DPG in RBCs rapidly decline after 1–2 weeks in storage, which increases the affinity of their hemoglobin for oxygen, thereby reducing their oxygen delivery to tissues. For most transfusion recipients, transient depletion of 2,3-DPG is clinically insignificant. However, infants less than 4 months of age have diminished capacity to replete 2,3-DPG and compensate for hypoxemia. Thus, for large volume transfusions or exchange transfusions where a large proportion of the infant's hemoglobin will be replaced with donor blood, use of red cell units less than 14 days old is recommended for infants under 4 months of age. However, for routine, smaller volume RBC transfusions (15 cc/kg) in these patients, using exclusively fresh units necessitates increasing donor exposure. Prospective randomized trials have shown that small volume transfusion from single RBC units stored in AS-1 for up to 42 days is safe for very low birth weight neonates and decreases donor exposure compared to transfusing from fresh CPDA-1 units.[40,41]

In adults and pediatric patients, the storage lesion also leads to damaged RBC clearance after transfusion by extravascular hemolysis, with release of non-transferrin bound iron that can potentially promote bacterial growth and oxidative stress.[42–44] Prospective randomized trials have, thus far, not detected significant increases in adverse events following fresh versus old RBC transfusion in pediatric patients; however, this research field remains a rapidly evolving work in progress. The Age of Red Blood Cells in Premature Infants (ARIPI) trial compared fresh and standard RBC transfusion in low birth weight premature infants and found no improvement of outcome with the use of fresh (7 days of less) RBCs compared to standard practice, but the mean age of RBCs in the "standard" group was less than 15 days with a median of only 13 days.[45] The applicability of these results has been questioned, because the conditions tested do not reflect the neonatal transfusion practices of many centers where the same RBC unit is reserved for individual hospitalized infants to prevent multiple donor exposures. Additional studies are needed to assess the safety of RBCs older than 2 weeks in premature infants.[46]

The TOTAL randomized trial examined a broader range of storage times (1–10 days vs. 25–35 days) in older children. Specifically, it found no differences in the efficacy of stored versus fresh RBCs for improving tissue oxygenation in Ugandan children aged 6–60 months with severe malaria. No differences were found in secondary safety endpoints, adverse events at 24 h, and survival and health at 30 days posttransfusion.[47] Thus, while prolonged storage of RBCs does lead to increased hemolysis and iron release in pediatric patients, a causal relationship with specific adverse clinical outcomes remains to be established.

Irradiation to Prevent Transfusion-Associated Graft Versus Host Disease

Transfusion-associated graft versus host disease (TAGVHD) is caused by engraftment of alloreactive donor T-cells within the recipient and has a mortality of >90%. It is of particular concern in infants due to incompletely developed cellular immune responses, and newborns with congenital immunodeficiency syndromes are at increased risk.[29] A definitive diagnosis requires demonstration of donor white blood cell (WBC) chimerism with the absence of alternative diagnoses.[48] However, given the almost universally fatal nature of TAGVHD, prevention is of the utmost importance. Prevention requires irradiation of cellular blood components (RBCs, platelets and granulocytes) at 15–50 Gy, and many pediatric hospitals have gone to universal irradiation of their blood supplies to minimize risk of TAGVHD.

Strategies to Prevent Transfusion-Transmitted Cytomegalovirus Disease

Cytomegalovirus (CMV) is a β Herpes virus subfamily that causes a mild, transient illness in immunocompetent individuals. CMV remains dormant within infected individuals with a likely reservoir in mononuclear leukocytes. CMV seroprevalence ranges between 50% and 85% in adults in the United States, and cellular blood components (RBCs, platelets, and granulocytes) containing intact WBCs have the capacity to transmit CMV to immunologically naïve recipients. Populations at greatest risk for transfusion transmitted CMV (TT-CMV) include fetuses (intrauterine transfusion), premature low-birth weight infants (<1250–1500 g) born to seronegative mothers (who cannot provide passive immunity), seronegative recipients of seronegative allogeneic or autologous hematopoietic stem cell (HSC) transplants, seronegative recipients of seronegative solid organ transplants, and seronegative patients with human immunodeficiency virus (HIV)-infection. Primary infection in these patients can lead to serious end organ damage or failure, including CMV hepatitis, retinitis, colitis, interstitial pneumonitis, esophagitis, polyradiculopathy, transverse myelitis, and subacute encephalitis.

Blood banks are required to have a risk reduction policy in place to prevent product-related CMV transmission.[17,49] Selection of blood from CMV seronegative donors reduces the risk of CMV transmission.[50,51] As the virus is carried by mononuclear leukocytes, use of leukoreduction at the time of collection also can prevent TT-CMV.[29,52] Prestorage leukoreduction also carries the additional benefit of preventing febrile nonhemolytic transfusion reactions.[53] The vast majority (>90%) of institutions report universal leukoreduction of blood products to prevent TT-CMV, but variation still exists in the practice of seronegative product use. Many centers with neonatal intensive care units (NICUs) report providing leukoreduced blood that is also CMV negative to neonates under 4 months of age.[54] Cases of possible TT-CMV have been reported in infants receiving blood with leukoreduction alone; however, these cases cannot be definitively linked to transfusion due to extensive CMV transmission from other sources such as breastmilk.[55,56] Current evidence does not favor the dual prevention strategy over leukoreduction alone; however, additional high quality clinical studies are needed to determine if CMV seronegativity further reduces CMV transmission from leukoreduced blood.[54,57,58] One potential drawback to institutional dependence on universal leukoreduction as a primary TT-CMV mititgation strategy is vulnerability to leukoreduction filter failure. In the event of a widespread leukoreduction filter recall, as occurred in June 2016, supplies of CMV seronegative blood will be severely limited, and institutions should have policies in place to provide CMV seronegative products only to those patients at highest risk of TT-CMV disease.

Strategies to Prevent Complications From Potassium

Extracelluar potassium levels in RBC products rise in a linear fashion with increasing storage time, and irradiation further increases potassium release from red cells during storage.[26] This is not generally of concern in adult patients as the extracellular potassium load is less than 7 mEq even in expired units, and no preventative measures are recommended for routine RBC transfusions.[29] It is also possible that there is no clinically significant increase in serum potassium in pediatric patients when receiving routine transfusions.[59] However, transfusion-associated hyperkalemic cardiac arrest has been demonstrated in infants and neonates and has been associated with high rates of RBC infusion, prolonged RBC storage, and transfusion through central venous catheters.[60] Patients at high risk for complications from transfusion-induced hyperkalemia include infants receiving high volumes of red cells due to exchange transfusion, extra corporeal membrane oxygenation (ECMO), or massive blood loss. Mitigation strategies in these cases include correcting pretransfusion hyperkalemia, selecting fresher RBC units, and avoiding irradiated units that are stored for more than 24 h. Washing RBCs close to the time of administration can help mitigate this risk if large amounts of products (>20 mL/kg) are expected to be transfused, such as with cardiac surgery or exchange transfusion. In addition, RBC units in additive solution (AS) or saline-adenine-glucose-mannitol (SAGM) both deliver less potassium than citrate-phosphate-dextrose-adenine (CPDA)-1 units.[29] Standard washing removes approximately 98% of the plasma containing the free potassium, and resuspension in sterile saline is the recommended and standard practice when washing is necessary for pediatric transfusions.[17,26]

Pathogen Inactivation Technology

Pathogen inactivation technologies for plasma, platelets, and RBCs utilize solvent-detergent (for plasma) or photochemical treatment (for platelets and RBCs) to eliminate a broad range of infectious organisms. The United States Food and Drug Administration (FDA) approved a solvent detergent-treated pooled plasma product in 2013. A prospective observational study on critically ill children showed that the use of solvent/detergent-treated plasma may be associated with improved survival, however no randomized controlled trials have been performed.[61] Solvent/detergent-treated plasma has also been shown to be safe in large volume exchanges for thrombotic microangiopathy (TMA), but no subjects under age 15 years were included in this study.[62]

In 2014 the FDA approved a photochemical treatment for pathogen inactivation (PI) in apheresis platelet components. Little is known about the long-term consequences for pediatric patients exposed to the psoralen-based compounds used for pathogen inactivation, but short-term effects are assumed to be similar to that of adults. Randomized trials have focused on adult thrombocytopenic hematology/oncology patients and show noninferiority of PI versus conventional platelets; however, studies also show decreased corrected count increments and increased platelet use in patients receiving PI platelets.[63–65] For pediatric patients, the benefits of broad spectrum pathogen inactivation need to be weighed against the risks of increased platelet requirements and donor exposure to achieve therapeutic benefit.

When using psoralen-based pathogen reduction, consideration must be given to patients undergoing phototherapy and the interactions that may occur. Psoralens intercolate nonspecifically into DNA or RNA. Once in place, psoralens are activated by UV-A light, causing the psoralen to nonspecifically cross-link DNA or RNA pyramidine bases, rendering infectious organisms incapable of replication. In the process of pathogen reduction, UV-A exposure is performed in the laboratory, then compound adsorption is performed to remove the psoralen prior to transfusing the unit. However, for patients undergoing phototherapy, there is a theoretical risk that psoralens remaining in the unit might cross-link the patient's own DNA or RNA. As DNA and RNA damage would be nonspecific, it would be very difficult to identify harms in postmarketing surveillance should they occur. The only current guidance relating to this is a contraindication in neonatal patients treated with phototherapy at wavelengths less than 425 nm due to the risk of erythema.[66,67] One randomized trial showed an increased incidence of acute respiratory distress syndrome (ARDS) in recipients of psoralen-processed platelets compared to conventional platelets, so the product carries a labeling warning to monitor patients for signs and symptoms of ARDS.[66–68] The trials for postmarket surveillance and safety of amotosalen-treated pathogen reduced platelets in the United States are ongoing as of 2018, and results for pediatric safety data have not yet been published.[69] Previous clinical trials included only 30 patients under the age of 16 but showed a similar incidence of adverse events.[68,70–75] Safety data from France and Switzerland include 59 patients under the age of 1 year with 185 patients aged 1–18 years, and they show that the frequencies of adverse events were not increased compared to conventional platelet transfusions.[76,77] This is consistent with a larger hemovigilance study from Europe, which included 242 pediatric patients as part of postmarketing surveillance showing a similar rate of transfusion reactions and adverse events with none of the pediatric cohort experiencing a serious adverse event.[78]

Pathogen reduction using riboflavin and UV light is unique in that riboflaven is considered a nontoxic compound and nonmutagenic, therefore it is not necessarily removed at the end of the treatment, but performance and safety trials did not include patients under 20 years old.[79]

Aliquoting to Minimize Donor Exposure

Often in pediatric patients, smaller volumes ordered in milliliters are needed compared to those given to adults as units or doses. Dividing RBC units into small volume aliquots for these transfusions prevents blood wastage and allows pediatric patients to receive multiple transfusions from the same donor, thus decreasing overall donor exposures. Some blood suppliers can prepare an RBC unit divided into four equal volumes in a closed sterile system. These "quad packs" can be easily separated by the hospital transfusion service leaving the remaining aliquots intact for future transfusions. The primary risk with preparing aliquots at the hospital transfusion service is contamination of the product. Hospital transfusion services with a sterile connecting device can create customized aliquots of RBCs or platelets in small bags or syringes.[17,26] When syringes are prepared, it is important to note whether an in-line filter was used during preparation. Use of such a syringe set with an in-line 150-μm filter eliminates the need for bedside manipulation and is preferable to avoid mislabeling or contamination.[29]

Additive Solutions

Red cell additive solutions (AS) provide buffering capacity and nutrients allowing for prolonged storage of RBCs for up to 42 days. Prolonged storage of RBC units along with careful aliquoting can significantly decrease donor exposures in pediatric patients.[40,41] Safety considerations when selecting components in AS are the addition of adenine, which can cause renal toxicity at very high doses, and mannitol, a potent diuretic. Clinical studies have shown that these additives are safe for individual transfusion amounts in children.[26,41,80,81] However, there is little evidence on the safety of various additive solutions in pediatric patients when transfused above 20 mL/kg. In pediatric patients with hepatic or renal insufficiency receiving high volume RBC transfusions, use of CPDA-1 RBC units or washing of AS RBC units can be considered.

Platelet additive solution (PAS) may be used to replace approximately two-thirds of human plasma for the storage of apheresis platelets. Platelets stored in 65% PAS/35% plasma maintain functional integrity for up to 5 days and substantially reduce recipient exposure to potentially damaging human plasma components such as plasma proteins that can trigger allergic reactions, isohemagglutinins that can cause hemolysis in ABO incompatible platelet transfusions, and anti-HLA antibodies which have been linked to transfusion-related acute lung injury (TRALI).[82,83] Indeed, clinical studies have shown decreased overall transfusion reaction rates, and specifically decreased allergic transfusion reactions, in both adult and pediatric patients transfused with PAS platelets compared to conventional plasma platelets.[84–86] Studies powered to detect differences in TRALI incidence or hemolysis have not been performed. Although some studies show 1–4 h CCIs are lower after PAS platelet transfusion, the 12–24 h CCIs are similar to plasma platelets and, unlike PI platelets, PAS platelets are not associated with increased bleeding events or platelet transfusion requirements.[85–87] In the United States, the FDA-approved PAS consists of an isotonic solution composed of phosphate buffers with citrate as an anticoagulant and acetate as a platelet energy source, and these components do not pose specific safety concerns for pediatric patients.[88] With equal efficacy compared to plasma platelets and lower risk for transfusion reactions, selection of PAS platelets is becoming increasingly common for pediatric patients, particularly those with a history of transfusions interrupted by allergic reactions. Indeed, PAS has become the platelet storage medium of choice for pediatric transfusion in the United Kingdom.[89,90]

Strategies to Prevent Hemolysis From ABO Incompatible Platelets

Transfusion of ABO incompatible platelet units is a common practice in adults, and clinically significant hemolysis from the passively acquired anti-A and/or anti-B antibodies from the plasma is only rarely reported.[91] Because of their smaller blood and plasma volume, children and infants are considered to be at higher risk for hemolysis with ABO incompatible platelet transfusion and it is generally accepted that transfusion of platelets containing ABO incompatible plasma should be avoided in these patients.[92] Institutions may limit incompatible plasma exposure based on weight or restrict ABO incompatible platelet transfusion below a certain age. In the event that incompatible platelet transfusion becomes necessary in an infant, plasma can be removed by volume reduction or plasma removal followed by saline resuspension.[93,94]

Granulocytes

Infections are a major cause of morbidity and mortality in patients undergoing hematopoietic stem cell transplant (HSCT), and transfusion of donor granulocytes has been used for both prevention and treatment in these situations.[95,96] However, the efficacy of granulocyte transfusions in both the pediatric and adult patient populations remain a hotly debated topic. Most data in pediatric patients are based on single-center studies with lower patient weight being associated with better survival outcomes.[95,97] This is presumably due to dose dependence with the higher dose/kg available in a single transfusion with smaller versus larger patients, but there remains no high quality data to demonstrate efficacy of this product.[29,95,98,99] The most common complication of granulocyte infusion is fever; however, severe respiratory distress can occur in approximately 5% of patients, possibly due to neutrophil sequestration in the pulmonary vascular bed. Due to questionable efficacy of this component and risk for severe adverse events, institutional policy should carefully monitor pediatric granulocyte requests and restrict the use of granulocytes to only those patients with severe infection unresponsive to appropriate antibiotics in the setting of severe neutropenia or neutrophil dysfunction (absolute neutrophil count<500/μL or chronic granulomatous disease or leukocyte adhesion deficiency).[29,100] Granulocyte donors must be ABO and D compatible with the recipient due to the high red cell content in granulocyte products, and they should be CMV seronegative for CMV seronegative recipients. The granulocyte product also must be irradiated to prevent TA-GVHD.[29]

Directed Donations

Directed donations, also known as dedicated donations, are an often-provided service of many blood collection services, despite the increased costs and logistical burden. Parents may have concerns over their child receiving blood products from an unknown allogeneic donor. However, families should be counseled about the risks of such donations, as directed blood donations have been shown to have higher rates of HIV, hepatitis C virus (HCV), hepatitis B virus (HBV), and human T-lymphotropic virus (HTLV).[101] In addition to the risk of viral infection, a related donor is more likely to have shared HLA haplotypes and an associated increased risk of transfusion-associated graft versus host disease (TA-GVHD). Therefore, when directed donation is used from a blood relative, irradiation is required.[17] In pediatrics, another source of directed donation is the donation of antigen-negative platelets for treatment of neonatal alloimmune thrombocytopenia (NAIT), which is the treatment of choice. In this instance, the platelets should be washed to remove maternal antiplatelet antibodies and irradiated to prevent TA-GVHD.[49]

Dosing

Often a cookie-cutter approach of 10–15 mL/kg is used (with 5–10 mL/kg for platelets), which does not take into account unique pediatric physiology as these numbers are extrapolated from adult studies; nor does it take into account the specific goals of treatment with component therapy in the pediatric population.[26,29] Both a patient's age and disease can alter pharmacokinetics of drugs in different ways from adults, therefore extrapolation dosing needs significantly more attention and study to truly understand the appropriate approach.[102] Growth is known to not be linear, and allometric (size based) dosing has potential problems due to changes in organ function, body composition, and biochemical parameters as children mature.[103–105]

Approaches to Dosing

Unfortunately, there is no available high quality data on pediatric component dosing, so transfusion services are left with the allometric approach. However, not all components are created equal. It is important to educate providers on the guidelines in the institution and to stay up to date on current clinical practice guidelines, and the guidelines from different professional societies are not always concordant with each other.[106–108] Although a developmentally based approach to component dosing may be preferable in the pediatric population, no such guidelines exist, and universal guidelines are the current best option. In addition, it will be necessary for transfusion committees to develop disease-specific guidelines with the input of pediatric specialists as findings from studies on pediatric transfusion risks continue to emerge.

UNIQUE CONSIDERATIONS
Obesity

Obesity has reached epidemic proportions in western countries, and the magnitude of the associated risks are just beginning to be understood. Obese patients have a higher risk of a number of morbidities including longer hospital stays, increased numbers of postoperative complications, wound complications, infections, and postpartum hemorrhage.[109–112] In transfusion medicine, this is concerning due to the fact that these patients may also have increased component needs. For example, in orthopedic surgeries, elevated BMI is associated with increased estimated blood loss and the need for transfusions, even when adjusting for age and types of fractures, and this pattern holds true for trauma and surgical procedures as well.[113–115] This is not entirely surprising given that larger-sized patients have larger predicted blood volumes. However, in pediatrics, where transfusion volumes are often based on estimates from body weight and desired end hemoglobin, this can be problematic. Increased body mass is not necessarily linearly related to increased blood volume as body composition may vary depending on the cause of obesity, the distribution of the adipose tissue, and the bone mass.[116–118] When estimating total blood volume in obese children for transfusion purposes, a lower estimate of 65 mL/kg may be used.[119]

Frequently or Chronically Transfused

Although transfusions can prevent many complications from blood disorders such as hemoglobinopathies, iron overload in chronically transfused pediatric patients is common. Liver iron monitoring should be done noninvasively with magnetic resonance imaging when possible, in addition to laboratory monitoring and chelation therapy when necessary.[120] In addition to iron overload, frequent exposure to blood products carries the risk of alloimmunization that increases with each subsequent transfusion.[121] Additionally, patients with sickle cell disease are shown to have a disproportionately higher rate of alloimmunization, with a mean rate of 25% before the implementation of phenotype matching.[122]

Phenotype Matching

Alloantibody formation can result in both acute and delayed hemolytic transfusion reactions, and the symptoms can mimic a sickle cell crisis, making diagnosis difficult in some situations.[123] Hyperhemolysis syndrome can result from alloimmune hemolysis leading to a severe life threatening anemia.[124] Therefore, prevention of alloimmunization in the chronically transfused pediatric population is the primary mitigation strategy. Antigen-matched units can prevent alloimmunization, and these patients should receive units matched for C, E, and K at a minimum, with extended matching for Kidd and Fy(a) when possible.[26,125,126] This method is not perfect, and even patients who are phenotypically matched develop antibodies due to altered alleles and donor-recipient mismatch of these variants.[127] There is great genetic diversity within the *RH* gene that cannot be distinguished by serologic testing alone, and genotyping of important immunogenic minor blood group antigen loci may soon be employed to select blood that minimizes alloimmunization risk in chronically transfused patients.[128,129]

ADMINISTRATION STRATEGIES
Monitoring

Pediatric patients treated in specialized PICUs have lower associated morbidity and mortality than those treated in mixed adult-child ICUs.[130] When transfusing a pediatric patient, it is important to keep in mind that this is a unique specialty where appropriately trained nurses are extremely valuable to improve the safety and decrease the risk of complications. Monitoring a blood transfusion should be performed by trained specialty-specific nurses, preferably certified in pediatric nursing. Given that there are a number of considerations like specialty products, syringe pump delivery, and pediatric infusion devices, a nurse familiar with available equipment in the pediatrics ward is best suited for this type of patient.

INFUSION
Equipment

It is important to use infusion equipment specifically designed for pediatric patients rather than "retrofitting" tubing on the fly, as added connections and unnecessary additions to a circuit substantially decrease the flow delivered to the patient.[131] Blood warmers are often used in pediatrics when large amounts of products are needed to maintain core temperatures, and attention should be paid to the manufacturer's instructions on minimum intravenous (IV) catheter size, as some products require an 18 g or larger whereas slower infusion systems may be necessary when using smaller catheters.[132] Infusion pumps are now equipped with "smart pump" technology where limits for different medications can be programmed into the device, and these are becoming the standard of care in a number of settings.[133,134] Newer syringe pumps are equipped with programmable weight-based parameters to aid in dosing error prevention, and these should be used where available.[135,136]

Administration

Infusion of blood too rapidly can result in transfusion-associated circulatory overload (TACO) in both adults and in children with associated decompensated heart failure.[48,137] The rate of administration should be specified by the ordering physician, as it is highly dependent on the indication for transfusion and clinical condition of the patient. Infusion rates as fast as 3 mL/kg/h have been shown to be safe in a small retrospective review, and a 10–15 mL/kg dose can be given over 2–4 h in most pediatric patients.[26,137] If a transfusion will require more than 4 h to maintain slower rates, the dose can be split into two separate transfusions by the blood bank staff before issue, and calculating the time needed to obtain the desired volume ahead of time can prevent wastage or unnecessary additional donor exposure. Just as with adults, transfusion of blood components rapidly or in large volumes can result in adverse events such as TACO or hyperviscosity if dosing is not appropriate.

Strategies to Prevent Citrate Toxicity

Blood products are anticoagulated with citrate, which binds to and chelates calcium causing transient hypocalcemia during transfusions. This is generally not of clinical significance in adult patients. However, citrate toxicity can be a risk for pediatric patients receiving exchange transfusions and massive transfusions, where hypocalcemia can become severe. In patients unable to report symptoms of citrate toxicity, strategies to prevent citrate toxicity should be implemented for large volume transfusions, for example, prophylactic addition of a weight-based infusion of 10% calcium gluconate solution in a separate line could be considered in addition to slowing the rate of citrate containing products to <1 mL/kg/min.[26,138] Children have also been shown more likely to have gastrointestinal complaints rather than traditional symptoms of tingling paresthesia with citrate toxicity commonly seen in adults.[139] This may make identifying this potentially dangerous complication more difficult in children.

ADVERSE EVENTS

Guidelines on transfusion reaction criteria for diagnosis, severity of different reactions, and the imputability of the reaction (likelihood that the reaction was due to the transfusion) are available from the Centers for Disease Control (CDC) National Healthcare Safety Network (NHSN).[48] However, these guidelines are not age specific and some symptoms may be difficult to identify in young children or infants. Literature on transfusion reaction reporting using both retrospective approaches and prospective surveillance and expert consensus indicates that reactions and adverse events are likely underreported.[140-142] Development of pediatric-specific transfusion reaction guidelines and increased education of bedside providers on types and symptoms of reactions in this population could be beneficial, but no consensus yet exists on the best approach. Close monitoring and early identification of most reactions remains the best practice.

REACTIONS

Febrile and Allergic Transfusion Reactions

The most commonly reported reactions in the pediatric population are febrile nonhemolytic transfusion reactions (FNHTR) and allergic reactions.[7,8] Both reaction types often have readily identifiable symptoms that do not depend on the patient's ability to communicate such as hives or a temperature increase. Platelets stored in additive solution contain less plasma and subsequently have a lower associated rate of allergic reactions and have been shown to be noninferior with respect to FNHTRs.[84] One differential always to consider in the pediatric age group is sepsis, as temperature changes and blood pressure changes can be seen not only with allergic and FNHTR reaction types but also in sepsis. In addition, sepsis may present with decreased body temperatures rather than fevers or as compensated shock rapidly devolving into a critical situation if not treated early.[143]

TRALI AND TACO

Reaction types such as TACO or TRALI may be more difficult to identify early in a patient unable to report symptoms. The majority of literature on TRALI in children is limited to case reports, but there are studies showing that the incidence is likely similar to that of adults.[144,145] As little as 10–20 mL of residual plasma has been associated with case reports of TRALI.[146]

Necrotizing Enterocolitis

Necrotizing enterocolitis (NEC) is a severe intestinal disease in premature neonates characterized by ischemic necrosis of the intestinal mucosa and mortality >50% for those patients requiring surgery.[147] Several retrospective studies have shown an increased risk of NEC within 48 h of RBC transfusion with the severity of anemia preceding transfusion further increasing the risk of NEC.[148,149] Given the close relationship between severe anemia and the need for transfusion, discerning the causal factors in transfusion-associated NEC has been challenging. A recent multicenter prospective observational study indicates that severe anemia and not RBC transfusion was associated with increased risk of NEC.[150] Although it remains unclear whether transfusion or anemia or some interaction between the two risk factors leads to NEC, several potential mitigation strategies are available. Data from small retrospective studies indicate that reducing or withholding feeds around the time of transfusion may be associated with lower incidence of NEC.[151,152] In addition, measures to prevent severe anemia in premature neonates such as delayed cord clamping, cord "milking", and limiting phlebotomy losses have been effective in preventing NEC.[153]

CONCLUSIONS

Transfusion decisions in pediatric patients carry uniquely complex and high impact risks. For example, the decision to transfuse RBCs in a very low birth weight neonate may lead to NEC within 48 h but the decision not to transfuse that same neonate could lead to neurocognitive impairment a decade later. An incompletely antigen-matched RBC unit given to a sickle cell patient at age 2 could cause alloimmunization to an immunogenic Rh variant and severely restrict his options for transfusion therapy for the remaining decades of his life. Based on current knowledge, making the correct decision for such children may be difficult or impossible. However, in the coming years, a deluge of new technologies and data from clinical trials will become available to better define and mitigate transfusion risks in pediatric patients. Institutions must be prepared to meet the challenge of parsing and interpreting these new products and data and then applying it to create standardized transfusion practices that improve pediatric patient care. Concrete steps to improve pediatric risk management include installing pediatric specialists on institutional transfusion committees or creating pediatric-specific transfusion committees; collecting extensive internal data on pediatric blood product use and outcomes and analyzing it in a way that takes into account age, patient blood volume, and disease state; and carefully monitoring the medical literature for new evidence that may call for institution-wide practice changes.

REFERENCES

1. Maitra A. Diseases of infancy and childhood. In: Kumar V, Abbas AK, Aster JC, eds. *Robbins and Cotran: Pathologic Basis of Disease.* 9th ed. Philadelphia, PA: Elsevier-Saunders; 2015:451–482.
2. Klassen TP, Hartling L, Craig JC, Offringa M. Children are not just small adults: the urgent need for high-quality trial evidence in children. *PLoS Med.* 2008;5(8):e172.
3. Willems A, Van Lerberghe C, Gonsette K, et al. The indication for perioperative red blood cell transfusions is a predictive risk factor for severe postoperative morbidity and mortality in children undergoing cardiac surgery. *Eur J Cardio Thorac Surg.* 2014;45(6):1050–1057.
4. Szekely A, Cserep Z, Sapi E, et al. Risks and predictors of blood transfusion in pediatric patients undergoing open heart operations. *Ann Thorac Surg.* 2009;87(1):187–197.
5. Kipps AK, Wypij D, Thiagarajan RR, Bacha EA, Newburger JW. Blood transfusion is associated with prolonged duration of mechanical ventilation in infants undergoing reparative cardiac surgery. *Pediatr Crit Care Med.* 2011;12(1):52–56.
6. Salvin JW, Scheurer MA, Laussen PC, et al. Blood transfusion after pediatric cardiac surgery is associated with prolonged hospital stay. *Ann Thorac Surg.* 2011;91(1):204–210.
7. Vossoughi S, Perez G, Whitaker BI, Fung MK, Stotler B. Analysis of pediatric adverse reactions to transfusions. *Transfusion.* 2018;58(1):60–69.
8. Oakley FD, Woods M, Arnold S, Young PP. Transfusion reactions in pediatric compared with adult patients: a look at rate, reaction type, and associated products. *Transfusion.* 2015;55(3):563–570.
9. Akalin Akkok C, Seghatchian J. Pediatric red cell and platelet transfusions. *Transfus Apher Sci.* 2018.
10. Goel R, Josephson CD. Recent advances in transfusions in neonates/infants. *F1000Res.* 2018:7.
11. Guzzetta NA. Benefits and risks of red blood cell transfusion in pediatric patients undergoing cardiac surgery. *Paediatr Anaesth.* 2011;21(5):504–511.
12. Bell EF, Strauss RG, Widness JA, et al. Randomized trial of liberal versus restrictive guidelines for red blood cell transfusion in preterm infants. *Pediatrics.* 2005;115(6):1685–1691.

13. McCoy TE, Conrad AL, Richman LC, Lindgren SD, Nopoulos PC, Bell EF. Neurocognitive profiles of preterm infants randomly assigned to lower or higher hematocrit thresholds for transfusion. *Child Neuropsychol.* 2011;17(4):347–367.

14. Kirpalani H, Whyte RK, Andersen C, et al. The Premature Infants in Need of Transfusion (PINT) study: a randomized, controlled trial of a restrictive (low) versus liberal (high) transfusion threshold for extremely low birth weight infants. *J Pediatr.* 2006;149(3):301–307.

15. Whyte RK, Kirpalani H, Asztalos EV, et al. Neurodevelopmental outcome of extremely low birth weight infants randomly assigned to restrictive or liberal hemoglobin thresholds for blood transfusion. *Pediatrics.* 2009;123(1):207–213.

16. Goldstein SD, Papandria DJ, Aboagye J, et al. The "weekend effect" in pediatric surgery - increased mortality for children undergoing urgent surgery during the weekend. *J Pediatr Surg.* 2014;49(7):1087–1091.

17. AABB. Standards for blood banks and transfusion services. In: *Process Control.* 30th ed. Bethesda, Maryland: AABB; 2016.

18. Ullman AJ, Keogh S, Coyer F, Long DA, New K, Rickard CM. 'True Blood' the Critical Care Story: an audit of blood sampling practice across three adult, paediatric and neonatal intensive care settings. *Aust Crit Care.* 2016;29(2):90–95.

19. Bateman ST, Lacroix J, Boven K, et al. Anemia, blood loss, and blood transfusions in North American children in the intensive care unit. *Am J Respir Crit Care Med.* 2008;178(1):26–33.

20. Fischer DP, Zacharowski KD, Meybohm P. Savoring every drop - vampire or mosquito? *Crit Care.* 2014;18(3):306.

21. Valentine SL, Bateman ST. Identifying factors to minimize phlebotomy-induced blood loss in the pediatric intensive care unit. *Pediatr Crit Care Med.* 2012;13(1):22–27.

22. Woods-Hill CZ, Fackler J, Nelson McMillan K, et al. Association of a clinical practice guideline with blood culture use in critically ill children. *JAMA Pediatr.* 2017;171(2):157–164.

23. Agarwal HS, Barrett SS, Barry K, et al. Association of blood products administration during cardiopulmonary bypass and excessive post-operative bleeding in pediatric cardiac surgery. *Pediatr Cardiol.* 2015;36(3):459–467.

24. Ye L, Lin R, Fan Y, Yang L, Hu J, Shu Q. Effects of circuit residual volume salvage reinfusion on the postoperative clinical outcome for pediatric patients undergoing cardiac surgery. *Pediatr Cardiol.* 2013;34(5):1088–1093.

25. Wilkinson KL, Brunskill SJ, Doree C, Trivella M, Gill R, Murphy MF. Red cell transfusion management for patients undergoing cardiac surgery for congenital heart disease. *Cochrane Database Syst Rev.* 2014;(2):Cd009752.

26. *Pediatric Transfusion: A Physician's Handbook.* 4th ed. Bethesda, Maryland: AABB; 2015.

27. Boettcher W, Sinzobahamvya N, Miera O, et al. Routine application of bloodless priming in neonatal cardiopulmonary bypass: a 3-year experience. *Pediatr Cardiol.* 2017;38(4):807–812.

28. Waibel E, Garcia E, Kelly M, Soles R, Hilborne L. Systematic review of non-ASCP choosing Wisely recommendations relevant to pathology and laboratory medicine. *Am J Clin Pathol.* 2018;149(3):267–274.

29. Fung MK, Eder A, Spitalnik SL, Westhoff CM. In: *Technical Manual.* 19th ed. Bethesda, Maryland: AABB; 2017.

30. Management SftAoB. In: *Administrative and Clinical Standards for Patient Blood Management Programs.* 4th ed. SABM; 2017.

31. Goel R, Cushing MM, Tobian AA. Pediatric patient blood management programs: not just transfusing little adults. *Transfus Med Rev.* 2016;30(4):235–241.

32. Josephson CD, Mondoro TH, Ambruso DR, et al. One size will never fit all: the future of research in pediatric transfusion medicine. *Pediatr Res.* 2014;76(5):425–431.

33. Lacroix J, Hebert PC, Hutchison JS, et al. Transfusion strategies for patients in pediatric intensive care units. *N Engl J Med.* 2007;356(16):1609–1619.

34. New HV, Grant-Casey J, Lowe D, Kelleher A, Hennem S, Stanworth SJ. Red blood cell transfusion practice in children: current status and areas for improvement? A study of the use of red blood cell transfusions in children and infants. *Transfusion.* 2014;54(1):119–127.

35. Bahadur S, Sethi N, Pahuja S, Pathak C, Jain M. Audit of pediatric transfusion practices in a tertiary care hospital. *Indian J Pediatr.* 2015;82(4):333–339.

36. Parker RI. Transfusion in critically ill children: indications, risks, and challenges. *Crit Care Med.* 2014;42(3):675–690.

37. Vossoughi SR, Macauley R, Sazama K, Fung MK. Attitudes, practices, and training on informed consent for transfusions and procedures: a survey of medical students and physicians. *Am J Clin Pathol.* 2015;144(2):315–321.

38. Tran MH, Vossoughi S, Harm S, Dunbar N, Fung M. Massive transfusion protocol: communication ordering practice survey (MTP COPS). *Am J Clin Pathol.* 2016;146(3):319–323.

39. Hod EA, Spitalnik SL. Stored red blood cell transfusions: iron, inflammation, immunity, and infection. *Transfus Clin Biol.* 2012;19(3):84–89.

40. Jain R, Jarosz C. Safety and efficacy of AS-1 red blood cell use in neonates. *Transfus Apher Sci.* 2001;24(2):111–115.

41. Strauss RG, Burmeister LF, Johnson K, et al. AS-1 red cells for neonatal transfusions: a randomized trial assessing donor exposure and safety. *Transfusion.* 1996;36(10):873–878.

42. Hod EA, Francis RO, Spitalnik SL. Red blood cell storage lesion-induced adverse effects: more smoke; is there fire? *Anesth Analg.* 2017;124(6):1752–1754.

43. Kalhan TG, Bateman DA, Bowker RM, Hod EA, Kashyap S. Effect of red blood cell storage time on markers of hemolysis and inflammation in transfused very low birth weight infants. *Pediatr Res.* 2017;82(6):964–969.

44. L'Acqua C, Bandyopadhyay S, Francis RO, et al. Red blood cell transfusion is associated with increased hemolysis and an acute phase response in a subset of critically ill children. *Am J Hematol.* 2015;90(10):915–920.

45. Fergusson DA, Hebert P, Hogan DL, et al. Effect of fresh red blood cell transfusions on clinical outcomes in premature, very low-birth-weight infants: the ARIPI randomized trial. *Jama.* 2012;308(14):1443–1451.

46. Belpulsi D, Spitalnik SL, Hod EA. The controversy over the age of blood: what do the clinical trials really teach us? *Blood Transfus.* 2017;15(2):112–115.

47. Dhabangi A, Ainomugisha B, Cserti-Gazdewich C, et al. Effect of transfusion of red blood cells with longer vs shorter storage duration on elevated blood lactate levels in children with severe anemia: the TOTAL randomized clinical trial. *J Am Med Assoc.* 2015;314(23):2514–2523.

48. National Healthcare safety Network biovigilance component hemovigilance module surveillance protocol. In: *Atlanta, GA: Centers for Disease Control and Prevention.* v2.5.2 ed. 2018.

49. *Neonatal Transfusion Practices.* Switzerland: Springer; 2017.

50. Bowden RA, Sayers M, Flournoy N, et al. Cytomegalovirus immune globulin and seronegative blood products to prevent primary cytomegalovirus infection after marrow transplantation. *N Engl J Med.* 1986;314(16):1006–1010.

51. Yeager AS, Grumet FC, Hafleigh EB, Arvin AM, Bradley JS, Prober CG. Prevention of transfusion-acquired cytomegalovirus infections in newborn infants. *J Pediatr.* 1981;98(2):281–287.

52. Delaney M, Mayock D, Knezevic A, et al. Postnatal cytomegalovirus infection: a pilot comparative effectiveness study of transfusion safety using leukoreduced-only transfusion strategy. *Transfusion.* 2016;56(8):1945–1950.

53. Yazer MH, Podlosky L, Clarke G, Nahirniak SM. The effect of prestorage WBC reduction on the rates of febrile nonhemolytic transfusion reactions to platelet concentrates and RBC. *Transfusion.* 2004;44(1):10–15.

54. Weisberg SP, Staley EM, Williams 3rd LA, et al. Survey on transfusion-transmitted cytomegalovirus and cytomegalovirus disease mitigation. *Arch Pathol Lab Med.* 2017;141(12):1705–1711.

55. Wu Y, Zou S, Cable R, et al. Direct assessment of cytomegalovirus transfusion-transmitted risks after universal leukoreduction. *Transfusion.* 2010;50(4):776–786.

56. Josephson CD, Caliendo AM, Easley KA, et al. Blood transfusion and breast milk transmission of cytomegalovirus in very-low-birth-weight infants: a prospective cohort study. *JAMA Pediatr.* 2014;168(11):1054–1062.

57. Mainou M, Alahdab F, Tobian AA, et al. Reducing the risk of transfusion-transmitted cytomegalovirus infection: a systematic review and meta-analysis. *Transfusion.* 2016;56(6 Pt 2):1569–1580.

58. Heddle NM, Boeckh M, Grossman B, et al. AABB Committee Report: reducing transfusion-transmitted cytomegalovirus infections. *Transfusion.* 2016;56(6 Pt 2): 1581–1587.

59. Olson J, Talekar M, Sachdev M, et al. Potassium changes associated with blood transfusion in pediatric patients. *Am J Clin Pathol.* 2013;139(6):800–805.

60. Lee AC, Reduque LL, Luban NL, Ness PM, Anton B, Heitmiller ES. Transfusion-associated hyperkalemic cardiac arrest in pediatric patients receiving massive transfusion. *Transfusion.* 2014;54(1):244–254.

61. Camazine MN, Karam O, Colvin R, et al. Outcomes related to the use of frozen plasma or pooled solvent/detergent-treated plasma in critically ill children. *Pediatr Crit Care Med.* 2017;18(5): e215–e223.

62. Vendramin C, McGuckin S, Alwan F, Westwood JP, Thomas M, Scully M. A single-center prospective study on the safety of plasma exchange procedures using a double-viral-inactivated and prion-reduced solvent/detergent fresh-frozen plasma as the replacement fluid in the treatment of thrombotic microangiopathy. *Transfusion.* 2017;57(1):131–136.

63. Vamvakas EC. Meta-analysis of the randomized controlled trials of the hemostatic efficacy and capacity of pathogen-reduced platelets. *Transfusion.* 2011;51(5):1058–1071.

64. Rebulla P, Vaglio S, Beccaria F, et al. Clinical effectiveness of platelets in additive solution treated with two commercial pathogen-reduction technologies. *Transfusion.* 2017;57(5):1171–1183.

65. Butler C, Doree C, Estcourt LJ, et al. Pathogen-reduced platelets for the prevention of bleeding. *Cochrane Database Syst Rev.* 2013;(3):CD009072.

66. Goodrich RP, Segatchian J. Special considerations for the use of pathogen reduced blood components in pediatric patients: an overview. *Transfus Apher Sci.* 2018.

67. *PMA BP140143: FDA Summary of Safety and Effectiveness Data.* December 18, 2014.

68. McCullough J, Vesole DH, Benjamin RJ, et al. Therapeutic efficacy and safety of platelets treated with a photochemical process for pathogen inactivation: the SPRINT Trial. *Blood.* 2004;104(5):1534–1541.

69. Stramer SA. *Prospective, Open Label, Treatment Use Study of Patient Safety Following Transfusion of INTERCEPT Platelet Components (TRUE).* American National Red Cross Cerus Corporation; 2016.

70. Snyder E, Raife T, Lin L, et al. Recovery and life span of 111indium-radiolabeled platelets treated with pathogen inactivation with amotosalen HCl (S-59) and ultraviolet A light. *Transfusion.* 2004;44(12):1732–1740.

71. Murphy S, Snyder E, Cable R, et al. Platelet dose consistency and its effect on the number of platelet transfusions for support of thrombocytopenia: an analysis of the SPRINT trial of platelets photochemically treated with amotosalen HCl and ultraviolet A light. *Transfusion.* 2006;46(1):24–33.

72. Slichter SJ, Kaufman RM, Assmann SF, et al. Dose of prophylactic platelet transfusions and prevention of hemorrhage. *N Engl J Med.* 2010;362(7): 600–613.

73. Corash L, Lin JS, Sherman CD, Eiden J. Determination of acute lung injury after repeated platelet transfusions. *Blood.* 2011;117(3):1014–1020.

74. Snyder E, McCullough J, Slichter SJ, et al. Clinical safety of platelets photochemically treated with amotosalen HCl and ultraviolet A light for pathogen inactivation: the SPRINT trial. *Transfusion.* 2005;45(12):1864–1875.

75. Janetzko K, Cazenave JP, Kluter H, et al. Therapeutic efficacy and safety of photochemically treated apheresis platelets processed with an optimized integrated set. *Transfusion.* 2005;45(9):1443–1452.

76. INTERCEPT® Blood System for Platelets –Small Volume (SV) Processing Set. Concord, CA: Cerus Corporation; 2016. [package insert].

77. INTERCEPT® Blood System for Platelets-Large Volume (LV) Processing Set. Concord, CA: Cerus Corporation; 2016. [package insert].

78. Knutson F, Osselaer J, Pierelli L, et al. A prospective, active haemovigilance study with combined cohort analysis of 19,175 transfusions of platelet components prepared with amotosalen-UVA photochemical treatment. *Vox Sang.* 2015;109(4):343–352.

79. A randomized controlled clinical trial evaluating the performance and safety of platelets treated with MIRASOL pathogen reduction technology. *Transfusion.* 2010;50(11):2362–2375.

80. Strauss RG, Burmeister LF, Johnson K, Cress G, Cordle D. Feasibility and safety of AS-3 red blood cells for neonatal transfusions. *J Pediatr.* 2000;136(2):215–219.

81. Fernandes da Cunha DH, Nunes Dos Santos AM, Kopelman BI, et al. Transfusions of CPDA-1 red blood cells stored for up to 28 days decrease donor exposures in very low-birth-weight premature infants. *Transfus Med.* 2005;15(6):467–473.

82. Weisberg SP, Shaz BH, Tumer G, Silliman CC, Kelher MR, Cohn CS. PAS-C platelets contain less plasma protein, lower anti-A and anti-B titers, and decreased HLA antibody specificities compared to plasma platelets. *Transfusion.* 2018;58(4):891–895.

83. Surowiecka M, Zantek N, Morgan S, Cohn CS, Dangerfield R. Anti-A and anti-B titers in group O platelet units are reduced in PAS C versus conventional plasma units. *Transfusion.* 2014;54(1):255–256.

84. Cohn CS, Stubbs J, Schwartz J, et al. A comparison of adverse reaction rates for PAS C versus plasma platelet units. *Transfusion.* 2014;54(8):1927–1934.

85. Tobian AA, Fuller AK, Uglik K, et al. The impact of platelet additive solution apheresis platelets on allergic transfusion reactions and corrected count increment (CME). *Transfusion.* 2014;54(6):1523–1529; quiz 1522.

86. Kerkhoffs JL, Eikenboom JC, Schipperus MS, et al. A multicenter randomized study of the efficacy of transfusions with platelets stored in platelet additive solution II versus plasma. *Blood.* 2006;108(9):3210–3215.

87. Kerkhoffs JL, van Putten WL, Novotny VM, et al. Clinical effectiveness of leucoreduced, pooled donor platelet concentrates, stored in plasma or additive solution with and without pathogen reduction. *Br J Haematol.* 2010;150(2):209–217.

88. Jay S, Epstein MD. Approval Letter - InterSol. In: *Research OoBRaRCfBEa.* 2009.

89. Poles D, et al. In: Bolton-Maggs P, ed. *The 2016 Annual SHOT Report.* London, UK: Royal College of Pathologists; 2017.

90. van der Meer PF. PAS or plasma for storage of platelets? A concise review. *Transfus Med.* 2016;26(5):339–342.

91. Garratty G. Problems associated with passively transfused blood group alloantibodies. *Am J Clin Pathol.* 1998;109(6):769–777.

92. Harris SB, Josephson CD, Kost CB, Hillyer CD. Nonfatal intravascular hemolysis in a pediatric patient after transfusion of a platelet unit with high-titer anti-A. *Transfusion.* 2007;47(8):1412–1417.

93. Fontaine MJ, Mills AM, Weiss S, Hong WJ, Viele M, Goodnough LT. How we treat: risk mitigation for ABO-incompatible plasma in plateletpheresis products. *Transfusion.* 2012;52(10):2081–2085.

94. Quillen K. Hemolysis from platelet transfusion: call to action for an underreported reaction. *Transfusion.* 2012;52(10):2072–2074.

95. Bercovitz RS, Josephson CD. Transfusion considerations in pediatric hematology and oncology patients. *Hematol Oncol Clin North Am.* 2016;30(3):695–709.

96. Nikolajeva O, Mijovic A, Hess D, et al. Single-donor granulocyte transfusions for improving the outcome of high-risk pediatric patients with known bacterial and fungal infections undergoing stem cell transplantation: a 10-year single-center experience. *Bone Marrow Transplant.* 2015;50(6):846–849.

97. Weingarten C, Pliez S, Tschiedel E, Grasemann C, Kreissig C, Schundeln MM. Granulocyte transfusions in critically ill children with prolonged neutropenia: side effects and survival rates from a single-center analysis. *Eur J Pediatr.* 2016;175(10):1361–1369.

98. Cugno C, Deola S, Filippini P, Stroncek DF, Rutella S. Granulocyte transfusions in children and adults with hematological malignancies: benefits and controversies. *J Transl Med.* 2015;13:362.

99. Lehrnbecher T, Sung L. Anti-infective prophylaxis in pediatric patients with acute myeloid leukemia. *Expert Rev Hematol.* 2014;7(6):819–830.

100. Gurlek Gokcebay D, Akpinar Tekgunduz S. Granulocyte transfusions in the management of neutropenic fever: a pediatric perspective. *Transfus Apher Sci.* 2018;57(1):16–19.

101. Dorsey KA, Moritz ED, Steele WR, Eder AF, Stramer SL. A comparison of human immunodeficiency virus, hepatitis C virus, hepatitis B virus, and human T-lymphotropic virus marker rates for directed versus volunteer blood donations to the American Red Cross during 2005 to 2010. *Transfusion.* 2013;53(6):1250–1256.

102. Mahmood I. Pharmacokinetic considerations in designing pediatric studies of proteins, antibodies, and plasma-derived products. *Am J Ther.* 2016;23(4):e1043–1056.

103. Kearns GL, Abdel-Rahman SM, Alander SW, Blowey DL, Leeder JS, Kauffman RE. Developmental pharmacology–drug disposition, action, and therapy in infants and children. *N Engl J Med.* 2003;349(12):1157–1167.

104. Bailey D, Bevilacqua V, Colantonio DA, et al. Pediatric within-day biological variation and quality specifications for 38 biochemical markers in the CALIPER cohort. *Clin Chem.* 2014;60(3):518–529.

105. Karbasy K, Ariadne P, Gaglione S, Nieuwesteeg M, Adeli K. Advances in pediatric reference intervals for biochemical markers: establishment of the Caliper database in healthy children and adolescents. *J Med Biochem.* 2015;34(1):23–30.

106. Wiegmann TL, Mintz PD. The growing role of AABB clinical practice guidelines in improving patient care. *Transfusion.* 2015;55(5):935–936.

107. Schiffer CA, Bohlke K, Delaney M, et al. Platelet transfusion for patients with cancer: American society of clinical oncology clinical practice guideline update. *J Clin Oncol.* 2018;36(3):283–299.

108. Kaufman RM, Djulbegovic B, Gernsheimer T, et al. Platelet transfusion: a clinical practice guideline from the AABB. *Ann Intern Med.* 2015;162(3):205–213.

109. Childs BR, Nahm NJ, Dolenc AJ, Vallier HA. Obesity is associated with more complications and longer hospital stays after orthopaedic trauma. *J Orthop Trauma.* 2015;29(11):504–509.

110. Blomberg M. Maternal obesity and risk of postpartum hemorrhage. *Obstet Gynecol.* 2011;118(3):561–568.

111. Mustain WC, Davenport DL, Hourigan JS, Vargas HD. Obesity and laparoscopic colectomy: outcomes from the ACS-NSQIP database. *Dis Colon Rectum.* 2012;55(4):429–435.

112. Murphy ME, McCutcheon BA, Kerezoudis P, et al. Morbid obesity increases risk of morbidity and reoperation in resection of benign cranial nerve neoplasms. *Clin Neurol Neurosurg.* 2016;148:105–109.

113. Frisch N, Wessell NM, Charters M, et al. Effect of body mass index on blood transfusion in total hip and knee arthroplasty. *Orthopedics.* 2016;39(5):e844–849.

114. Richards JE, Morris BJ, Guillamondegui OD, et al. The effect of body mass index on posttraumatic transfusion after pelvic trauma. *Am Surg.* 2015;81(3):239–244.

115. De Jong A, Deras P, Martinez O, et al. Relationship between obesity and massive transfusion needs in trauma patients, and validation of TASH score in obese population: a retrospective study on 910 trauma patients. *PLoS One.* 2016;11(3):e0152109.

116. Shaikh MG, Crabtree N, Kirk JM, Shaw NJ. The relationship between bone mass and body composition in children with hypothalamic and simple obesity. *Clin Endocrinol.* 2014;80(1):85–91.

117. Kowal M, Kryst L, Woronkowicz A, Sobiecki J. Long-term changes in body composition and prevalence of overweight and obesity in girls (aged 3–18 years) from Krakow (Poland) from 1983, 2000 and 2010. *Ann Hum Biol.* 2014;41(5):415–427.

118. Carasco CF, Fletcher P, Maconochie I. Review of commonly used age-based weight estimates for paediatric drug dosing in relation to the pharmacokinetic properties of resuscitation drugs. *Br J Clin Pharmacol.* 2016;81(5):849–856.

119. Palmieri TL. Children are not little adults: blood transfusion in children with burn injury. *Burns Trauma.* 2017;5:24.

120. Stanley HM, Friedman DF, Webb J, Kwiatkowski JL. Transfusional iron overload in a cohort of children with sickle cell disease: impact of magnetic resonance imaging, transfusion method, and chelation. *Pediatr Blood Cancer.* 2016;63(8):1414–1418.

121. Zalpuri S, Zwaginga JJ, le Cessie S, Elshuis J, Schonewille H, van der Bom JG. Red-blood-cell alloimmunization and number of red-blood-cell transfusions. *Vox Sang.* 2012;102(2):144–149.

122. Treml A, King KE. Red blood cell alloimmunization: lessons from sickle cell disease. *Transfusion.* 2013;53(4):692–695.

123. de Montalembert M, Dumont MD, Heilbronner C, et al. Delayed hemolytic transfusion reaction in children with sickle cell disease. *Haematologica.* 2011;96(6):801–807.

124. Talano JA, Hillery CA, Gottschall JL, Baylerian DM, Scott JP. Delayed hemolytic transfusion reaction/hyperhemolysis syndrome in children with sickle cell disease. *Pediatrics.* 2003;111(6 Pt 1):e661–e665.

125. Tahhan HR, Holbrook CT, Braddy LR, Brewer LD, Christie JD. Antigen-matched donor blood in the transfusion management of patients with sickle cell disease. *Transfusion.* 1994;34(7):562–569.

126. Lasalle-Williams M, Nuss R, Le T, et al. Extended red blood cell antigen matching for transfusions in sickle cell disease: a review of a 14-year experience from a single center (CME). *Transfusion.* 2011;51(8):1732–1739.

127. Chou ST, Jackson T, Vege S, Smith-Whitley K, Friedman DF, Westhoff CM. High prevalence of red blood cell alloimmunization in sickle cell disease despite transfusion from Rh-matched minority donors. *Blood.* 2013;122(6):1062–1071.

128. Chou ST, Flanagan JM, Vege S, et al. Whole-exome sequencing for RH genotyping and alloimmunization risk in children with sickle cell anemia. *Blood Adv.* 2017;1(18):1414–1422.

129. Noizat-Pirenne F, Tournamille C. Relevance of RH variants in transfusion of sickle cell patients. *Transfus Clin Biol.* 2011;18(5–6):527–535.

130. Peltoniemi OM, Rautiainen P, Kataja J, Ala-Kokko T. Pediatric intensive care in PICUs and adult ICUs: a 2-year cohort study in Finland. *Pediatr Crit Care Med.* 2016;17(2):e43–e49.

131. Lehn RA, Gross JB, McIsaac JH, Gipson KE. Needleless connectors substantially reduce flow of crystalloid and red blood cells during rapid infusion. *Anesth Analg.* 2015;120(4):801–804.

132. Barcelona SL, Vilich F, Cote CJ. A comparison of flow rates and warming capabilities of the Level 1 and Rapid Infusion System with various-size intravenous catheters. *Anesth Analg.* 2003;97(2):358–363, table of contents.

133. Murdoch LJ, Cameron VL. Smart infusion technology: a minimum safety standard for intensive care? *Br J Nurs.* 2008;17(10):630–636.

134. Hatcher I, Sullivan M, Hutchinson J, Thurman S, Gaffney FA. An intravenous medication safety system: preventing high-risk medication errors at the point of care. *J Nurs Adm.* 2004;34(10):437–439.

135. Bloomquist A, Seiberlich L. Reducing intermittent infusion syringe pump errors via weight-based safety parameters. *Biomed Instrum Technol.* 2015;(suppl):31–36.

136. Ohashi K, Dalleur O, Dykes PC, Bates DW. Benefits and risks of using smart pumps to reduce medication error rates: a systematic review. *Drug Saf.* 2014;37(12):1011–1020.

137. Olgun H, Buyukavci M, Sepetcigil O, Yildirim ZK, Karacan M, Ceviz N. Comparison of safety and effectiveness of two different transfusion rates in children with severe anemia. *J Pediatr Hematol Oncol.* 2009;31(11):843–846.

138. Barcelona SL, Thompson AA, Cote CJ. Intraoperative pediatric blood transfusion therapy: a review of common issues. Part I: hematologic and physiologic differences from adults; metabolic and infectious risks. *Paediatr Anaesth.* 2005;15(9):716–726.

139. Cooling L, Hoffmann S, Webb D, et al. Procedure-related complications and adverse events associated with pediatric autologous peripheral blood stem cell collection. *J Clin Apher.* 2017;32(1):35–48.

140. Gauvin F, Lacroix J, Robillard P, Lapointe H, Hume H. Acute transfusion reactions in the pediatric intensive care unit. *Transfusion.* 2006;46(11):1899–1908.

141. Ricci M, Goldman AP, de Leval MR, Cohen GA, Devaney F, Carthey J. Pitfalls of adverse event reporting in paediatric cardiac intensive care. *Arch Dis Child.* 2004;89(9):856–859.

142. Hendrickson JE, Roubinian NH, Chowdhury D, et al. Incidence of transfusion reactions: a multicenter study utilizing systematic active surveillance and expert adjudication. *Transfusion.* 2016;56(10):2587–2596.

143. Balamuth F, Alpern ER, Abbadessa MK, et al. Improving recognition of pediatric severe sepsis in the emergency department: contributions of a vital sign-based electronic alert and bedside clinician identification. *Ann Emerg Med.* 2017;70(6):759–768.e752.

144. Mulder HD, Augustijn QJ, van Woensel JB, Bos AP, Juffermans NP, Wosten-van Asperen RM. Incidence, risk factors, and outcome of transfusion-related acute lung injury in critically ill children: a retrospective study. *J Crit Care.* 2015;30(1):55–59.

145. Lieberman L, Petraszko T, Yi QL, Hannach B, Skeate R. Transfusion-related lung injury in children: a case series and review of the literature. *Transfusion.* 2014;54(1):57–64.

146. Win N, Chapman CE, Bowles KM, et al. How much residual plasma may cause TRALI? *Transfus Med.* 2008;18(5):276–280.

147. Derienzo C, Smith PB, Tanaka D, et al. Feeding practices and other risk factors for developing transfusion-associated necrotizing enterocolitis. *Early Hum Dev.* 2014;90(5):237–240.

148. Paul DA, Mackley A, Novitsky A, Zhao Y, Brooks A, Locke RG. Increased odds of necrotizing enterocolitis after transfusion of red blood cells in premature infants. *Pediatrics.* 2011;127(4):635–641.

149. Maheshwari A, Patel RM, Christensen RD. Anemia, red blood cell transfusions, and necrotizing enterocolitis. *Semin Pediatr Surg.* 2018;27(1):47–51.

150. Patel RM, Knezevic A, Shenvi N, et al. Association of red blood cell transfusion, anemia, and necrotizing enterocolitis in very low-birth-weight infants. *Jama.* 2016;315(9):889–897.

151. El-Dib M, Narang S, Lee E, Massaro AN, Aly H. Red blood cell transfusion, feeding and necrotizing enterocolitis in preterm infants. *J Perinatol.* 2011;31(3):183–187.

152. Talavera MM, Bixler G, Cozzi C, et al. Quality improvement initiative to reduce the necrotizing enterocolitis rate in premature infants. *Pediatrics.* 2016;137(5).

153. Rabe H, Diaz-Rossello JL, Duley L, Dowswell T. Effect of timing of umbilical cord clamping and other strategies to influence placental transfusion at preterm birth on maternal and infant outcomes. *Cochrane Database Syst Rev.* 2012;(8):CD003248.

CHAPTER 9

Informed Consent

J. MILLS BARBEAU, MD, JD

Informed consent is an essential feature of medical practice. If a physician treats a patient without obtaining consent, then the patient's autonomy—the right to control his or her own body—is violated. In 1914, Justice Benjamin Cardozo laid out the fundamental rule that every patient has the right to decide what shall be done with his or her own body. If a physician performs a procedure without the patient's consent, that action is considered to be assault and battery—or medical malpractice, depending on the jurisdiction (Fig. 9.1).[1]

Consent is a central concept of medical jurisprudence. In a routine primary care setting, a patient is deemed to have given *implied* consent to medical care by entering the doctor's office. At the same moment, by providing a medical consultation, the physician agrees to enter into a doctor-patient relationship with the patient.[2] Once implied consent and the initiation of the doctor-patient relationship have occurred, routine medical care activities such as obtaining detailed medical histories, performing physical examinations, prescribing medications, and even giving intramuscular injections and vaccinations do not require explicit written consent—although in the case of vaccinations, there has in recent years been a decided trend toward obtaining written consent. However, for significant medical procedures such as elective surgery, physicians and patients must go through a formal consent process in advance of the surgery, during which the physician provides disclosure of the risks and benefits of the proposed procedure, and offers an ample opportunity for the patient to ask questions.

Emergencies such as acute trauma are exceptional situations, and the law has carved out legal exceptions to the consent requirement, often in the form of Good Samaritan laws that render patient consent unnecessary. If an incapacitated person is unable to provide informed consent as a result of a medical emergency, Good Samaritan laws permit physicians (and typically helpful onlookers) to come to the person's aid. As long as physicians make their best efforts, they may provide assistance without fear of reprisal when the crisis has passed and the person is no longer incapacitated.

Similarly, in the emergency room, if the patient is incapacitated and a surrogate decision maker is not available to provide informed consent–as often happens in hospital trauma bays–physicians are exempt from the usual obligation to obtain informed consent. This exemption is particularly relevant for transfusion services, since blood products are often dispensed during trauma resuscitation, and members of the transfusion service are often directly involved in clinical decision making.

Surrogate decision makers are individuals such as family members or others who have been granted responsibility for the patient and are authorized to make medical decisions on behalf of the patient. If a patient is conscious, competent, and has reached the age at which the law of the jurisdiction permits medical decision making, then there is no need for a surrogate decision maker. If the patient is not capable of giving consent, and time permits, the medical team will seek a surrogate. Court-appointed guardians and individuals identified in advance care directives take priority as surrogates. Thereafter, default rules are typically based on kinship. The majority of states have statutes explicitly listing the priority in which family members are authorized to act as surrogates. The order is typically spouse, adult children, parents, then adult siblings. In practice, families often make decisions by consensus.[3] Providers tend to accommodate family dynamics if they are healthy and functional. As to the patient's wishes, some states specify that surrogates should base their decisions on what the incapacitated patient would have wanted, rather than what the surrogate thinks is in the patient's best interests. Advance directives can be very helpful when the patient's preferences would otherwise have been uncertain.

In our discussion of consent to medical treatments, we have touched on several ways patients and physicians may enter into doctor-patient relationships, including explicit consent to undergo major medical procedures, implied consent to routine medical care, Good Samaritan laws that permit emergency treatment, and surrogate decision makers who not only give consent on behalf of the patient, but also largely step into the doctor-patient

Risk Management in Transfusion Medicine. https://doi.org/10.1016/B978-0-323-54837-3.00009-2

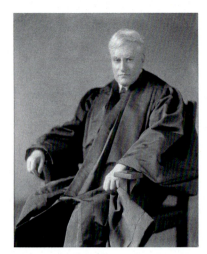

FIG. 9.1 Judge (and later Supreme Court Justice) Benjamin Cardoza.

- To give meaningful consent, the patient must understand the issues (be "informed"):
    - Why the procedure is being recommended
    - Available alternatives
    - The risks and benefits
        - Cannot omit important information
        - Must include the option of declining treatment, and the risks entailed
- Consent should/must be documented
- Information tailored to patient's aptitudes, emotional state, and desire to know details
- Allow ample opportunity for the patient to ask questions

FIG. 9.2 The elements of informed consent in clinical practice.

relationship on the patient's behalf. In all cases, whenever a doctor-patient relationship is formed, the physician binds herself professionally to a relationship based on trust, entering into a fiduciary relationship in which the physician puts the patient's interests ahead of her own. The doctor-patient relationship also commits the physician to a bond of absolute confidentiality that is deemed by society to be so socially valuable that the law will not permit even a judge to require the physician to breach the patient's privilege.

If informed consent to medical treatment is implied simply by walking into a doctor's office, when might it become necessary to obtain a more formally expressed consent to medical treatment? This is a key question. The answer is that the patient must give expressed informed consent for any medical procedure or treatment above minimal risk, as well as any circumstances that change the risk inherent in the patient's current course of treatment. Not only should the patient be informed of changes in risk, but the discussion should at the very least be documented in the patient's chart. For consent to medical procedures, written informed consent signed by the physician and the patient, whenever possible, is the standard of care. If written informed consent is not practicable under the circumstances, the informed consent discussion between the patient and physician should be memorialized in the chart.

To achieve truly informed consent to a proposed medical intervention, the patient must be provided with sufficient information to independently judge the advisability of the medical plan. The patient must understand the key issues involved in the decision, the options that are available to the patient, the advantages and disadvantages of each option, and the risks of each option, including the risk of doing nothing. All important information must be shared with the patient, and the patient must have ample opportunity to ask questions (Fig. 9.2).[4]

THE ETHICAL BASIS OF INFORMED CONSENT

The necessity of obtaining the patient's informed consent prior to performing a medical procedure is grounded in ethics, specifically the ethical principal of autonomy. Autonomy is the right of self-determination, that is, the right to make decisions for oneself. In the context of medical treatment, patient autonomy means that the patient decides what may be done to his or her body. It would be difficult to imagine a more fundamental right than the right to determine what may or may not be done to one's own body.

Autonomy, beneficence, and justice are the three core ethical principles, and the pillars upon which medical ethics are built.

- Autonomy: the patient's right of self-determination.
- Beneficence: maximizing benefits for the patient.
- Justice: maximizing healthcare resources for all, sharing duties and privileges equitably.

In the medical context, autonomy is achieved by respecting the patient's right to decide what may be done to his or her body. This is accomplished by ensuring that all medical decisions are made according to the patient's informed consent. Beneficence is seen in physicians' fiduciary duty to put their patients' interests ahead of her own, as well as in primum non nocere, "first do no harm". Justice is the equitable distribution of public health resources and the stewardship of those resources by providing quality care.

AUTONOMY AND CONSENT—A FALSE EQUIVALENCE?

As we have seen, autonomy is the right to decide one's own bodily integrity, the moral authority to decide how one's own physical embodiment may be treated. This chapter has examined how patient autonomy is safeguarded in clinical practice, and found that clinical practice relies heavily on informed consent to ensure that the patient's autonomy is protected.

To gain a more profound sense of how patient autonomy actually fares in daily medical practice, we may need to push the boundaries a bit. One way to test the boundaries is to ask how diligently the informed consent requirement is enforced in practice. At a fundamental level, we may start by asking how well we provide our patients with a chance to give *genuinely* informed consent. Intuitively we know that practices will vary considerably in different clinical settings. Informed consent will inevitably be more patient-centered in a fertility clinic than in a radiology department. Nevertheless, it may be informative for readers to consult their experience in familiar settings such as a medium sized medical-surgical hospital.

Many of us have experience with being on rounds when the chief resident tells the intern to "be sure to consent Mrs. X for surgery". First, "to consent" really should not be a transitive verb, as though consent is something we are doing to poor Mrs. X. We should be facilitating a decision-making process for Mrs. X, helping her to understand her options so that she can make the best possible decision for her own individual needs and objectives.

So "consenting" poor Mrs. X is a bit brutal. Perhaps the intern and chief resident simply need to be reminded of the importance of informed consent in practicing patient-centered medicine. Unfortunately, there are still hurdles to cross. Our overworked intern is now "consenting" the patient for a blood transfusion, "tanking her up" for surgery. Why is the transfusion being recommended? What are the indicia for transfusing blood, given her hemoglobin level and comorbidities? What are the possible complications that might arise from a blood transfusion? Mrs. X wants to know how likely it is that she will get HIV from the transfusion. Hepatitis? Ebola? The intern may not be able to contribute much information to this informed consent.

Now, we will push the boundaries a little further. Does the court system promote patient autonomy when Mrs. X sues her physician for failure to provide adequate information to allow her to give informed consent?[1] One may recall that Judge Cardoza's pronouncement in 1914, in the case of *Schloendorff v.*

Society of New York Hospital,[1] emphasized consent per se, using the language of assault and battery. By 1957, *Salgo v. Leland Stanford Jr. Univ. Bd. of Trs.*[5] shifted the focus from whether the procedure was authorized, to asking whether the patient's consent was adequately informed. *Salgo* thus places the emphasis on the information that was needed to allow the patient to provide adequately informed consent.

In the wake of the *Salgo* decision, courts across the country adopted the principle that patient autonomy relies on the adequacy of information provided to the patient. At this point, however, the story takes an unexpected twist. Many courts continued to give significant discretion to *physicians* to decide the amount of information that was sufficient for patients to make informed decisions. This was referred to as the "professional" or "physician" standard, in which the adequacy of disclosure was that which would be provided by a reasonable medical practitioner.[6]

Physicians, on the whole, may not always provide much information to patients, yet the physician standard of practice asked what the majority of physicians in the community would do. For jurisdictions that adopted the physician standard, expert medical testimony was required to establish what would be considered customary disclosure in the medical community. With the emphasis being placed on what physicians would do rather than the information that consenting patients would need, the physician standard arguably constituted a step away from patient autonomy.

In 1972, the influential D.C. Federal Circuit announced in the case of *Canterbury v. Spence*, that "it is the prerogative of the patient, not the physician, to determine for himself the direction in which his interests seem to lie."[7] The patient was the one who should determine the adequacy of the information being provided. *Canterbury*'s patient-oriented standard asked what a reasonable person in the patient's position would consider important. As a result, expert testimony was not relevant, since juries were better suited to determining what a reasonable patient would consider important. This new "patient-centered" approach created an alternative standard for judging the adequacy of the information provided to the patient.

In 2007, David Studdert and colleagues[8] performed an empirical study examining whether jurisdictions across the United States apply the physician standard (disclosure that a reasonable physician would make; based on expert medical testimony); the patient-centered standard (disclosure a reasonable patient would require; no expert testimony needed); or an alternative standard. Studdert and colleagues found that 25 states had adopted the patient-centered standard: 23 states followed the physician standard, and the remaining 2 states, Georgia and Colorado, used a hybrid standard. Thus, as of 2007, the nation is evenly split between the physician standard and the patient-based standard.

Returning to our question: When lawsuits allege that the treating physician provided inadequate information to allow the patient to give informed consent, do courts protect patient autonomy? We are now in a position to make several interesting conclusions. In the United States, state courts follow essentially two standards:

25 states:
- "Patient-centered" standard
  - Disclosure a reasonable patient would require to permit informed consent
  - No expert testimony needed
  - An OBJECTIVE standard

23 states:
- "Physician" standard
  - Disclosure a reasonable physician would make
  - Requires expert medical testimony
  - An OBJECTIVE standard

2 states:
- A hybrid

The patient-centered standard seeks the perspective of patients, whereas the physician standard seeks the perspective of doctors. This seemingly brings the patient-centered standard closer to protecting a patients' autonomy, which is the goal of informed consent. By contrast, the physician standard asks what physicians think is important. In fairness, it must be pointed out that physicians have more experience than the lay public with complications and risks attendant to procedures they perform. Physicians may arguably be better able to address the risks and benefits of a procedure. Nevertheless, juries may arguably be a step closer to a patient's actual worries.

Another important point is lurking in the background, and has yet to be addressed. In the law, there are two important burdens of proof for determining a defendant's fault or culpability. They are the objective standard and the subjective standard. The distinction comes up most often when comparing criminal law to civil law. In criminal law, we often hear that the state must prove "intent," meaning that the defendant

intended to do the illegal actions that he or she is accused of. In criminal law, the defendant must have mens rea, or "guilty mind," to be found guilty of a crime. This is referred to as a subjective standard, meaning that the defendant must actually have intended to perform the illegal acts.

In civil law, on the other hand, negligence cases involve one party claiming that another breached a duty of care, and that breach resulted in an injury. These are not criminal trials, and are instead referred to as "civil" cases. In civil cases, the injured party is not required to prove that the defendant intended to commit harm, which would be a subjective standard. Instead, the question is whether the defendant breached the "standard of care" that ordinarily prudent people would exercise in the same situation. This is an objective standard since the individual's mind is not at issue. The question is, objectively, would an ordinarily prudent person have behaved more carefully than the defendant did? If so, the defendant was negligent.

Now to the point. When determining the information that a physician must provide in order for the patient to make informed decisions, the court asks the jury to assess the adequacy of disclosure according to either the patient-centered standard or the physician standard. However, both the patient-centered standard and the physician standard of disclosure are objective standards. The patient-centered standard asks for the level of disclosure a *reasonable patient would require* to ensure informed consent; The physician standard asks for the level of disclosure a *reasonable physician would make* to ensure informed consent. Neither standard is subjective. Neither standard asks what thoughts were in the patient's own mind while she was deciding what to allow the doctors do to her body. If the legal standard genuinely seeks to enforce an individual patient's autonomy, it should seek to know her own concerns, rather than asking a group of jurors or a group of doctors what they would have done. Autonomy is about the very personal decisions a single individual makes regarding her own body. Personal autonomy, by definition, means having the right to have one's preferences respected, even if they are eccentric. Anything else is just a group decision.

As a practical matter, it would admittedly be difficult for juries to inquire into the mind of the plaintiff at the time of the informed consent discussion. It would also be very difficult to reconstruct the discussion sufficiently well to assess whether the physician was negligent. Nevertheless, juries have been entrusted to be fact finders for centuries. And perhaps, if autonomy is to be respected, we need to think about improving the

---

[1] Of course, failure to provide adequate information is not in itself sufficient to sustain a malpractice lawsuit. The failure must also have caused harm to the patient. All or the elements of a negligence action—duty, breach, causation, and harm—must be present for a plaintiff to prevail. For a more detailed discussion, see Chapter 10, *infra*, "Transfusion Medicine and the Law."

consent process in a manner that keeps patient autonomy at the forefront. Objective standards such as the patient-centered and physician standard are problematic. Imagine that the opinion of peer physicians is that, in thyroid surgery, the risk of injury to the recurrent laryngeal nerve is so remote that it would be unwise to include it in the informed consent conversation, lest the patient refuse the surgery out of excessive fear. Depending on how small the risk is, this approach may seem medically valid. Eventually, however, a physician will have a patient whose single greatest joy in life is singing in the church choir.

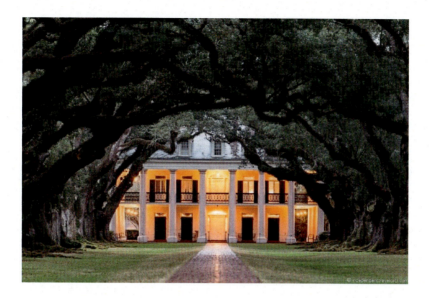

There have been many approaches to improving the informed consent process. Individual hospitals or hospital systems frequently design templates for specific procedures such as blood transfusions. Such templates can help ensure that the disclosures are complete, and they can be designed to include boxes to stimulate questions from the patient that can be noted on the form.

Some states have passed statutes designed to enhance the informed consent process. For example, the State of Louisiana passed the Uniform Consent Law,[9] which is designed for the purpose of improving faithful documentation of the informed consent process and clarifying proof issues should the informed consent be the subject of litigation. Under the Uniform Consent Law, if a patient sues a physician on the basis that the physician's disclosure of the risks was inadequate, the physician can only be liable for failure to disclose risks that could have influenced a reasonable person in deciding to give or withhold consent. In other words, the patient cannot argue that the consent did not address her own specific concerns, but only that a reasonable person would have considered the disclosure important. This is the "patient-based" standard discussed earlier.

The next important feature of Louisiana's Uniform Consent Law is that the Secretary of Health will prepare a list of procedures that require disclosure of risks, and specify the disclosure that is required for each such procedure. The statute then provides that, if a patient's consent to a procedure is documented on an approved form that contains the disclosures required by the Secretary of Health, the patient's consent is presumed. If a physician does not use the approved form, then the burden of proof shifts to the physician to demonstrate that the informed consent process was adequate. In short, if the physician uses the State's form, consent is presumed to be valid. Otherwise, the burden is on the physician to prove that the patient gave properly informed consent.

A TEST CASE: INCIDENTAL FINDINGS IN NEXT-GENERATION SEQUENCING[10]

In transfusion medicine, blood banking, and cellular therapy, as in virtually every field of medicine, next-generation genomic sequencing (NGS) is revolutionizing practice. Rapid genotyping of blood recipients and rapid donor sequencing is transforming personalized transfusion medicine. Human leukocyte antigen (HLA) typing can be performed using NGS, and rare blood group genotypes can be determined.

As genome-wide and exome-wide sequencing becomes more routine, an important question arises: How can we harness the information buried in the sequence data? There is presently a very active debate on that issue, which has significant implications for transfusion medicine, blood banking, and cellular therapy. Not surprisingly, issues of informed consent are at the center of the discussion. This chapter finishes with a "hot topic" in next-generation sequencing that involves many of the issues we have examined, and allows us to see them play out in a compelling context.

In 2013, the American College of Medical Genetics and Genomics (ACMG) published recommendations regarding "incidental findings" in NGS sequencing.[11] Incidental findings, as defined by ACMG, are genetic variants that are associated with disease, but were not targeted as part of the evaluation of the patient's current clinical condition. The document listed 56 genes that were associated with germline disorders and recommended that all 56 should be reviewed in every case in which exome or genome-wide NGS assays are performed.[11] The 56 genes are commonly referred to as the "minimum list". As proposed by ACMG, they are essentially a screening test to be performed in all cases of clinical NGS sequencing. ACMG modified their recommendations in 2017,[12] and at present, the ACMG gene panel has changed twice, with the addition of some genes and the removal of other genes.

The recommendations state that "constitutional mutations found in the genes on the minimum list should be reported by the laboratory to the ordering clinician, **regardless of the indication for which the clinical sequencing was ordered**" (emphasis added). The ACMG recommendations were highly controversial, for two reasons in particular: (1) ACMG recommended that everyone undergoing germline NGS must be tested for the minimum list with no ability to opt-out from the screening; and (2) positive findings from the minimum list must be reported to children, regardless of parental preferences such as waiting until the child is old enough to decide whether to receive the results.[13–17]

The ACMG recommendations are being raised in this context because the recommendations, as proposed, would apply to NGS germline sequencing in transfusion medicine, blood banking, and cellular therapy; and the recommendations raise important questions about informed consent, particularly the lack of an opt-out option and the requirement that results must be returned to children.

A program such as the one ACMG proposes would reveal germline variants whose significance must be assessed and explained to the patient. Meaningful informed consent for NGS testing would have to address the kind of findings that might be revealed by the testing, and the potential implications to the patient and/or family members.

The genomics field is still remarkably new. The Human Genome Project was completed in 2003. Whole genome sequencing (WGS) and whole exome sequencing (WES) entered clinical practice around 2009.[18] By 2012, clinical whole genome and whole exome sequencing results could be returned within 2 months, and cost about $10,000.[19] During the first decade after the Human Genome Project was complete, it became clear that large-scale genomic testing would routinely reveal incidental findings, including normal variants, genes conferring increased disease risks, and genes that were immediately clinically actionable.

Genetics experts quickly recognized that medical science had to race to keep up with the genetic data being produced. Reporting findings without being sure of their significance had the potential to cause more harm than good. One approach might be to adopt a "look back" policy, since the significance of a variant may later be clarified. Immediately actionable diseases would also be identified, leading to the need to alert the patient's physician. During the period between the completion of the Human Genome Project in 2003 to the emergence of clinical availability of NGS around 2013, the question of how to handle incidental findings was an increasingly important concern. It must also be noted that, during the decade from 2003 to 2013, the overwhelming majority of large-scale genomic testing was being performed in the context of research. In 2011, NIH Director Francis Collins testified before Congress, reporting that the return of results was "a hot topic in every conversation about every genetic research protocol that I'm involved in."[20] Science magazine called incidental findings "arguably the most pressing issue in genetics today."[21]

Ethically, one might require research subjects to agree to receive incidental findings as a condition of participation in a study. It seems far less ethical to tell clinical patients that they will not be allowed access to NGS testing unless they agree to receive unrelated genetic information discovered as an incidental finding. Furthermore, in the research context, testing may be provided at no cost, but clinical testing is typically paid for by third-party payers who may only want to pay for clinically actionable findings.

As NGS became common clinical practice around 2013, Ayuso et al.[22] published the first major systematic review of the literature on informed consent in genomic testing. Ayuso identified all relevant guidelines published by scientific societies, ethical boards, and individual experts that addressed the proper content of informed consent in clinical genomics. Some studies specifically discussed content regarding incidental findings.[6] Based on their findings, Ayuso et al. provided recommendations regarding information to be included in all informed consent documents for WGS in the clinical setting.[6] Given the fact that the review was published in 2013, it is not surprising that the majority of the recommendations closely tracked contemporary NIH research informed consent guidelines for research found in the Common Rule.[23] One notable exception was the final recommendation, stating that "NGS consent documents should include information discussing how incidental findings would be handled, and the right not to know."

In 2017, Mackley et al. at Oxford University published a systematic review exploring stakeholder preferences regarding incidental findings in whole genome and whole exome sequencing.[24] Makeley's approach was essentially the opposite of Ayoso's: Instead of reviewing guidelines of professional societies and experts, Mackley and colleagues collected empirical primary data on the views of patients, parents, other relatives, primary and tertiary care physicians, geneticists, researchers, institutional review boards, and the public.

The great majority of stakeholders, including genetics health care providers, believed that incidental findings should be returned, but the content of the disclosure should be determined by decisions made during the consent process. Patients as well as providers agreed that patient autonomy should be the guiding principle for determining whether incidental results should be returned to the patient. Patients should have the right to refuse to accept incidental findings. All stakeholder groups indicated that genetic counseling is crucial when results are reported. Universally, participants indicated a strong sense that patients should have ownership of their personal genetic information. In the Mackley study, 44 studies met the inclusion criteria, representing the viewpoints of 11,566 unique stakeholders.

Jada Hamilton and coworkers at the Memorial Sloan Kettering Cancer Institute reported patient preferences in the context of tumor genome profiling.[25] Patients with advanced cancer agreed to participate in interviews exploring how the patients would approach hypothetical decisions about receiving germline findings. Regarding decisional autonomy, participants believed that the decision to receive findings was theirs to make. The patients considered their oncologists to be an invaluable resource for helping them work through the decision process. In terms of information needs, participants wanted to know whether the information would be clinically beneficial to themselves or family members, and conversely, whether such knowledge might have negative consequences. Participants wanted sufficient time to weigh the decision, reflect, consult with others, and investigate the issues on their own—demonstrating needs that would have to be factored into the logistics of a meaningful informed consent process.

The ACMG minimum list raises remarkable issues regarding informed consent. The requirement that clinical patients must agree to receive incidental findings before they would be granted access to diagnostic next-generation sequencing seems a tremendous broadside blow to patient autonomy, as does the requirement that children must receive their incidental findings without regard to parental preferences, and without the option to wait until the child is old enough to decide for him- or herself. Ayoso, Makeley, and Hamilton's studies make it clear that patients and healthcare practitioners value patient autonomy, and they expect their physicians to be their partners in the process.

Many aspects of the ACMG recommendations are of concern from an informed consent point of view. The minimum list is essentially an example of opportunistic screening. Given the gaps in our knowledge, at this time the ACMG recommendations can fairly be characterized as a research project. This is not without precedent. Indeed, healthcare is evolving into a "learning healthcare system" in which knowledge can be gleaned from the vast amount of scientific and clinical data that we generate every day. Nevertheless, we must acknowledge potential risks to individual autonomy.

The learning healthcare system blends clinical practice and research. One major federal administration has adopted a progressive practice: If a physician orders a medication in the electronic health record and there is another medication with clinical utility that is in equipoise with the one being ordered, a window appears asking whether the ordering physician agrees to randomize the patient to either of the two medications. The concept is ingenious, and highly attractive. Nevertheless, we must be sure to recognize when we are equating clinical equipoise with informed consent, or inserting "objective" jurors into the shoes of autonomous, "subjective" patients, or even statutes that prioritize state-authorized boilerplate consent forms above earnest bedside conversations.

REFERENCES

1. Schloendorff v. *Society of New York Hospital* 211 NY 125, 105 NE 92, 93(1914).
2. Blake V. When is a patient-physician relationship established? *AMA J Ethics*. 2012;14(5):403–406.
3. Hafemeister TL. *End of Life Decision Making, Therapeutic Jurisprudence, and Preventive Law: Hierarchal V. Consensus-based Decision-making Model* 41 ARIZ. L. REV. 329(1999).
4. *AMA Code of Medical Ethics, Informed Consent, CME Opinion 2.1.1.* ; 2018. https://www.ama-assn.org/delivering-care/informed-consent.
5. Salgo V. Leland Stanford Jr. Univ. Bd. of Trs., 317 P.2d 170 (Cal. Dist. Ct. App. 1957).
6. Stohl HE. When consent does not help: challenges to women's access to a vaginal birth after cesarean section and the limitations of the informed consent doctrine. *Am J Law Med*. 2017;43:388–425.
7. Canterbury v. Spence, 464 F.2d 772 (D.C. Cir. 1972).
8. Studdert, et al. Geographic variation in informed consent law: two standards for disclosure of treatment risks. *4 J Empir Leg Stud*. 2007;103.
9. LA Rev Stat 40 §1299.40.
10. This discussion draws heavily from my participation in a College of American Pathologists white paper on incidental findings in tumor genomics, currently under submission for publication.
11. Green RC, Berg JS, Grody WW, et al. ACMG recommendations for reporting of incidental findings in clinical exome and genome sequencing. *Genet Med*. 2013;15(7):565–574.
12. Kalia SS, Adelman K, Bale SJ, et al. Recommendations for reporting of secondary findings in clinical exome and genome sequencing, 2016 update (ACMG SF v2.0): a policy statement of the American College of Medical Genetics and Genomics. *Genet Med*. 2017;19(2):249–255.
13. Scheuner MT, Peredo J, Benkendorf J, et al. Reporting genomic secondary findings: ACMG members weigh in. *Genet Med*. 2015;17(1):27–35.
14. Townsend A, Adam S, Birch PH, Friedman JM. Paternalism and the ACMG recommendations on genomic incidental findings: patients seen but not heard. *Genet Med*. 2013;15(9):751–752.
15. Holtzman NA. ACMG recommendations on incidental findings are flawed scientifically and ethically. *Genet Med*. 2013;15(9):750–751.
16. Rosenblatt DS. Who's on first in exome and whole genome sequencing? Is it the patient or the incidental findings? *Mol Genet Metab*. 2013;110(1–2):1–2.
17. Johnson KJ, Gehlert S. Return of results from genomic sequencing: a policy discussion of secondary findings for cancer predisposition. *J Cancer Policy*. 2014;2(3):75–80.
18. Lunshof JE, Bobe J, Aach J, et al. Personal genomes in progress: from the human genome project to the personal genome project. *Dialogues Clin Neurosci*. 2010;12(1):47–60.
19. Biesecker LG. Opportunities and challenges for the integration of massively parallel genomic sequencing into clinical practice: lessons from the ClinSeq project. *Genet Med*. 2012;14(4):393–398.
20. Wolf SM. The past, present, and future of the debate over return of research results and incidental findings. *Genet Med*. 2012;14(4):355–357.
21. Couzin-Frankel J. Human genome 10th anniversary. What would you do? *Science*. 2011;331(6018):662–665.
22. Ayuso C, Millan JM, Mancheno M, Dal-Re R. Informed consent for whole-genome sequencing studies in the clinical setting. Proposed recommendations on essential content and process. *Eur J Hum Genet*. 2013;21(10):1054–1059.
23. Basic HHS Policy for Protection of Human Research Subjects. 45 C.F.R. 46.
24. Mackley MP, Fletcher B, Parker M, Watkins H, Ormondroyd E. Stakeholder views on secondary findings in whole-genome and whole-exome sequencing: a systematic review of quantitative and qualitative studies. *Genet Med*. 2017;19(3):283–293.
25. Hamilton J, Shuk E, Garzon M, et al. Decision-making preferences about secondary germline findings that arise from tumor genomic profiling among patients with advanced cancers. http://10.1200/PO.17.00182. JCO Precision Oncology - published online December 21, 2017.

CHAPTER 10

Transfusion Medicine and the Law

J. MILLS BARBEAU, MD, JD

INTRODUCTION

An understanding of the law is fundamental to effective risk management. Fortunately, studying the law is not only interesting, but also highly practical. In this chapter, we will examine basic legal concepts that are already familiar to the reader and "unpack" them, contextualizing them and making them accessible for use in daily medical practice.

When physicians and other healthcare professionals think about the law, particularly in the context of risk management, they tend to think in terms of medical malpractice lawsuits. That is entirely appropriate. Indeed, every chapter in this book can be viewed as an essay on best practices to avoid harming patients. In a chapter on the law, medical malpractice is a good place to start.

It can be difficult to get a sense of how often patients are injured as a result of medical care they receive. The Institute of Medicine (IOM) issued a seminal report in 1999 entitled "To Err is Human: Building a Safer Health System".[1] Defining medical error as the failure of a planned action to be completed as intended or the use of a wrong plan, the report estimated that 44,000–98,000 deaths occur each year as a result of medical errors. Such errors include diagnostic errors, treatment errors, and systems failures such as failures in communication.[2]

In the 20 years since "To Err Is Human" was published, several studies have refined the estimate.[3–7] In 2016, Makary and Daniel[8] at Johns Hopkins University reviewed the studies and estimated that the mean annual death rate due to medical errors is 251,454. According to the authors, if we began recording deaths due to medical error on US death certificates, medical error would be the third leading cause of death, after heart disease and cancer (**Fig. 10.1**).

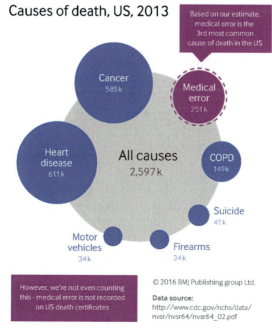

FIG. 10.1 According to a study by Makary and Daniel, if deaths due to medical error were recorded on U.S. death certificates, medical error would be the third leading cause of death, after heart disease and cancer.

Risk Management in Transfusion Medicine. https://doi.org/10.1016/B978-0-323-54837-3.00010-9

That is only counting deaths. The overall number of injuries due to medical errors would be considerably larger. The IOM estimated total costs of $17–29 billion per year. By definition, each of these events is a potential lawsuit. In terms of patient pain and suffering, loss of trust, and lost worker productivity, as well as healthcare workforce stress, morale, and reputational damage, the cost of medical errors is staggering.

How many medical malpractice suits are filed each year? Which specialties are sued the most? Which specialties are most likely to have to pay compensation, either in a settlement or due to a jury award? Data like that is hard to come by since private insurers have no obligation to disclose such information. Claims that are settled out of court are almost always subject to confidentiality agreements. A rare and fortuitous glimpse was provided to Jena and coworkers[9] at Harvard University when they were given access to more than 10,000 claims closed during 2002–05 by one of the largest national medical liability insurers in the United States. The data were released on condition of anonymity.

Results from Jena's study are summarized below:

Outcomes of Medical Malpractice Litigation Against US Physicians

(Jena, Arch Intern Med 2012;172:892-4)

- Examined > 10,000 claims closed 2002-05 by an unnamed national medical liability insurer
- 6% of pathologists are sued/year
  - 7.4% of all physicians
  - 19% of neurosurgeons
- Pathology had lowest percentage of cases dismissed (36.5%)
- Highest percentage of claims that went to trial (7.4%)
- Pathology was the specialty most likely to lose in trial
  - Mean payout for pathology: $384K (#2)
    - #1 is pediatrics ($520K)
    - #3 is neurosurgery ($345K)
    - Ob/Gyn is a close 4th
  - Note: Most were <u>surgical</u> pathology (not CP) cases, involving failure to diagnose

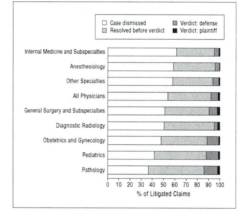

Figure. Outcomes of medical malpractice litigation according to physician specialty.

Among all physicians, 7.4% are sued each year.[10] Pathologists are slightly below that rate, at 6% per year. A stunning 19% of neurosurgeons are sued each year. When internal medicine specialists are sued, they do better than all other specialties in terms of dismissed cases (61.5%), settlements (33.3%), and favorable verdicts. Pathology may be sued infrequently, but when they are sued, they do not do well. Pathology has the lowest percentage of cases dismissed (36.5%) and the highest percentage of claims that go to trial (7.4%). When pathologists go to trial, they are the specialty most likely to lose—although the rate of plaintiff verdicts is less than 5% for all specialties. When pathologists lose, they lose badly. The mean payout for pediatrics is $520,000; pathology is next at $384,000; and neurosurgery is third, at $345,000; and Ob-Gyn is just behind neurosurgery.

Anatomy of a Lawsuit

Before addressing medical malpractice per se, it is useful to review some key legal concepts that apply to all civil lawsuits, and to highlight some important differences between criminal and civil cases. First, it is important to note that the state is not a party in civil cases. Civil actions are suits between private parties. It is a remarkable fact that, in civil law countries such as the United States and Great Britain, every citizen with a grievance against another citizen has the power to file a complaint, which institutes a court hearing and an order requiring the other citizen to appear before a judge to respond to the aggrieved party's complaint. Of course, the judge will promptly dismiss the complaint if it is not "actionable", that is, if it is not the type of wrong that a court will address, but plaintiffs still get their day in court, as well as a fair hearing. The party with the grievance–the party that files the "complaint"—is the "plaintiff", and the party being sued is the "defendant".

Differences between civil and criminal cases are summarized in **Fig. 10.2**. In criminal actions, the case is brought by the State. The State is, in essence, the plaintiff in a criminal case. Private citizens do not have the right to file criminal actions against other parties. Furthermore, the State cannot file criminal charges against a defendant unless the defendant's acts are specifically prohibited by a statute.

In civil cases, injured parties file lawsuits on their own behalf rather than depending on the State to do so. There is no requirement that the defendant's behavior be specifically prohibited by statute. Injuries in civil suits only need to be of the sort that have been recognized as compensable by prior courts over the years. For example, if a party creates a dangerous situation by behaving carelessly in a public place, and someone is hurt as a result, the injury may be compensable. The injured party is not required to identify a statute that addresses the particular behavior in which the defendant was engaged.

In criminal cases, the potential punishments, such as prison terms or payment of fines, are defined by statute. In civil suits, the injury must be compensable by monetary damages, meaning payment of money to "make the plaintiff whole". Monetary payment may not be capable of making the injured party whole, as for example, in a wrongful death case, but money is the only recourse in a civil suit.

Two final differences between criminal and civil suits are particularly important: the *mental standard* (subjective vs. objective) and the *burden of proof* (reasonable doubt vs. preponderance of the evidence). In criminal cases, the State must prove that the defendant intended to commit the criminal act. In other words, the prosecutor must prove mens rea (Latin for "guilty mind"). Pulling a lever expecting to turn on a light is quite different from pulling a lever expecting to detonate a bomb. In a criminal case, the State must demonstrate that the accused intended to perform the illegal acts. This is referred to as a "subjective"

standard, because it requires proof of the defendant's subjective intent.

In civil lawsuits, the plaintiff alleges that the defendant's negligence caused harm to the plaintiff. Here, guilt or innocence is not relevant. The question is whether the defendant exercised reasonable care in carrying out the activity. It is therefore up to the fact finders (usually a jury) to decide how carefully a reasonable person would have behaved when carrying out that activity. If the defendant did not exercise that degree of care, then the defendant was negligent. In a civil case for negligence, then, the defendant's liability is judged according to an "objective" standard—objective, since it asks how a reasonably prudent person would have behaved, rather than asking subjectively, what the defendant was thinking.

Finally, and crucially, the burden of proof differs between criminal and civil cases. In criminal trials, the defendant's guilt is in question, raising the stigma of personal culpability and the specter of punishment. In such cases, the State is required to prove guilt beyond a "reasonable doubt." This standard does not require the jury to be absolutely certain that the defendant is guilty. The jury is allowed to bring its common sense into the jury room. However, it does mean that the jury is confident that the defendant is guilty. In a civil trial for negligence, there is no reason at the outset to hold one party to a higher level of proof than the other. Maybe the defendant was negligent, or maybe not. For this reason, the burden of proof required for the plaintiff to win the case is a "preponderance of the evidence." The plaintiff must show that it is more probable than not that the defendant's behavior was below the standard of care, meaning that the defendant was less careful than an ordinarily prudent person would have been in the same circumstances.

Criminal versus Civil Lawsuits.

- Criminal:
  - Act is prohibited by statute
  - The plaintiff is the state
  - Requires *mens rea* ("guilty mind" –intent)
    - Subjective standard (what this person thought)
  - Punishment is defined by statute (prison, fine)
  - Burden of proof: Beyond a reasonable doubt

- Civil:
  - Plaintiff is the injured party
  - Classically based on negligence
    - Objective standard
      - How carefully would a reasonable person behave
  - Compensation is by $$$
  - Burden of proof: Preponderance of the evidence

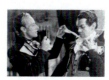

FIG. 10.2 Differences between civil and criminal lawsuits.

A medical malpractice lawsuit is a specialized type of negligence suit, in which the plaintiff alleges that a medical practitioner did not meet the profession's duty of care, causing injury to the patient. It is very useful to understand the elements of a civil suit for negligence before we discuss the nuances of actions alleging medical malpractice. The elements of a civil suit for negligence are as follows:

Civil Lawsuits for Negligence

Elements of a negligence claim:

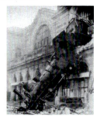

- Duty (duty of care)
- Breach
- Causation
  - Proximate cause
- Harm

For a plaintiff to have a "cause of action" (grounds for filing a suit) against a defendant, the defendant must owe a duty of care to the plaintiff. It is easy to overlook this element of a negligence claim. Imagine a person is driving a car. Drivers on a public roadway, availing themselves of the local byways, owe a duty of care to pedestrians, property owners, and other drivers. They must drive carefully and obey the laws of the road. Driving recklessly would constitute a breach of that duty.

Referring to the elements of a negligence claim, if the driver's recklessness caused a plaintiff to be injured, the elements are all satisfied: *duty* (established by availing oneself of a public roadway), *breach* (driving recklessly breached the duty), *harm* (the plaintiff was injured), and *causation* (the driver's recklessness caused the harm). On the other hand, if the driver was on her own property, and the property was fenced in by a 10-foot wall with "Beware Reckless Driver!" signs posted around the perimeter, then the driver may not have owed a duty of care to the plaintiff. This is not a trivial point. Many medical malpractice cases hinge on whether a doctor-patient relationship has been established. If there is no

such relationship, then the physician does not have a duty of care toward the plaintiff. When considering the merits of potential negligence suits, it is wise to start by evaluating each element of a claim.

Once a duty of care is established, what constitutes a breach of that duty? This is where the "ordinary person" standard comes in. The standard of care appropriate for a given activity is the degree of care an ordinary person would exercise while engaged in that activity. This is the "reasonable person" or "ordinary person" standard of care–the due care that a reasonable person would exercise in the same situation. Thus, if a pedestrian sues a railroad company for negligently striking him while he was walking along the rail, the jury would be required to determine the standard of care the train engineer should have followed, then determine whether the engineer breached that duty (of course, in this example the jury would also have to decide whether the plaintiff's negligence was to blame).

So, what is the standard of care for a physician? The answer is that a medical practitioner must provide the level of care that an "ordinary practitioner" would provide, that is, the care that a reasonably prudent, careful, knowledgeable, and competent physician would provide in the same circumstances. As an evidentiary matter, a jury would rely on the testimony of expert physicians to explain what the standard of practice would have been in the case in question. The jury would then have to decide whether the defendant physician breached the standard of care.

Of course, there is something special about the medical duty of care. Unlike automobile drivers navigating the roadways, physicians have a fiduciary duty to their patients, a duty of loyalty, an obligation to put the patient's interests ahead of their own. If an automobile driver is expected to stop for pedestrians, physicians are expected (figuratively) to get out of the car and help their patient across the street. Healthcare providers are expected to treat the patient as they would treat their own child or grandparent. Their duty is an ethics-based duty, grounded in beneficence. There is no Code of Ethics for automobile drivers.

Ordinary duty of care:

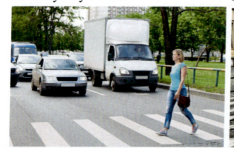

Medical duty of care:

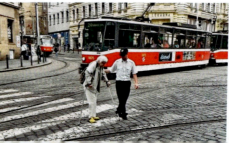

To summarize the elements of a civil suit for medical malpractice:

- Duty: A "doctor-patient" relationship must exist
- Breach: Medical care was not provided in a reasonably skilled, careful, and competent manner
  - The care did not meet the "medical standard of care"
- Causation: "Proximate cause"—the negligence directly caused the injury
- Harm: The patient suffered an actual injury
  - An injury that can be compensated with a monetary damage award

An excellent way to demonstrate that a blood service's transfusion practices meet the standard of care is by achieving laboratory certification and adhering to policies and procedures that are in accord with the requirements of the certifying organization. Consensus guidelines and medical practice guidelines such as Standards for Blood Banks and Transfusion Services and the AABB Technical Manual are also representative of best practices in the field. Adopting and adhering to standard operating procedures (SOPs) that reflect those practices is strong evidence that the service's practices meet the standard of care.

Despite all best efforts, one cannot fully protect oneself from being sued. In transfusion practice, certain types of claims are characteristic, for example, those in which it is alleged that:

- The transfusion was not necessary (did not need the blood) and harm occurred
- The transfusion was necessary but not provided (did not get blood) and harm occurred
- Reasonable and prudent alternatives to transfusion were not offered
  - Informed consent was inadequate
- Blood was improperly administered
  - Wrong blood (not compatible with patient)
  - Nerve damage by needle
- Blood was improperly tested
  - By transfusion service or blood supplier
- Antibody screen not performed properly
- Donor history questionnaire, infectious disease testing not performed properly

An Illustrative Example

It will be useful to see how these legal concepts play out in practice. The following scenario is based on real events, with occasional adjustments made for illustrative purposes. The reader may find it interesting to watch for the negligence elements of duty-breach-causation-harm as the case unfolds.

A 40-year old woman is scheduled for a hysterectomy to treat severely bleeding uterine fibroids. Her preoperative blood bank workup reveals an anti-Js^b antibody.

Patient History

- 40 y/o female scheduled for abdominal surgery

- Pre-operative blood bank workup: Anti-Js^b
  - Js^b is a high-incidence antigen in the Kell blood group

Phenotype	Whites	Blacks
Js (a-b+)	100	80
Js (a+b+)	Rare	19
Js (a+b-)	0	1

Fung, AABB Technical Manual, 19th ed.

Js^b is a high-incidence antigen in the Kell blood group.[11] As shown above, 99% of blacks in the United States are Js(b+), and whites are universally Js(b+). Indeed, Js(a+b–) has never been found in persons of non-African ancestry.[12] According to the United States Census Bureau, blacks comprise 13.4% of US citizens and whites 76.6%.[13] This means that, when pulling RBC units off the shelves to find Js(b-) negative blood, only (0.134) (0.01), or 0.134% of units, will be negative for Js^b.

Unfortunately, anti-Js^b acts very much like anti-K clinically.[14] One would expect Js(b+) donor blood to be cleared very quickly, and there would be the possibility of brisk hemolysis. The blood bank immediately called the blood bank medical director to communicate the information that there was a preoperative patient, scheduled for surgery that afternoon, who was found to have an anti-Js^b antibody.

The blood bank director promptly paged the surgical team, and the Ob-Gyn resident returned the page. The director explained that neither the blood bank nor the blood supplier would be able to locate Js(b-) RBC units, and locating compatible blood would require a national search. The search would take days, rather than hours. The director explained that Js^b is in the Kell blood group. If Js(b+) blood is transfused, the result would likely be an IgG-mediated extravascular ("delayed") hemolytic transfusion reaction. It would probably be severe, analogous to an anti-Kell reaction, possibly even fatal (stating for emphasis: "I can't guarantee that the patient wouldn't die on the table"). The resident replied that the patient's fibroids were bleeding very briskly and the need for surgical intervention was urgent. The resident promised to discuss the decision with the team and get back to the transfusion director. The director finished the conversation by saying "please be sure to contact me with any questions you might have."

The transfusion medicine director received an urgent call from the blood bank at 10:00 p.m. that evening. The Ob-Gyn team had decided that the operation could not be delayed. They were planning a laparoscopic hysterectomy and did not expect significant bleeding. Indeed, there was very little blood loss during surgery, only about 100 cc. Unfortunately, 10 h postoperatively, the patient suffered severe intraabdominal hemorrhage from a vessel that had been ligated during the procedure. The patient was urgently rushed back to the O.R. to control the bleeding. By the time the bleeding was brought under control, the patient had received 11 Js^b-positive RBC units.

The patient's transfusion-related laboratory values and transfusion course are charted:

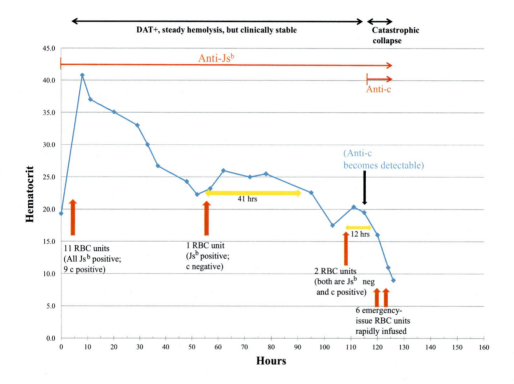

During the first 5 days after the patient's massive blood resuscitation, she experienced a brisk but stable delayed hemolytic transfusion reaction. The direct antiglobulin test (DAT) was 1+, indicating that the patient's red cells were coated with IgG immunoglobulin due to the presence of anti-Js^b antibodies opsonizing the Js^b antigen on the surface of the foreign red blood cells. There was steady hemolysis, but the patient was clinically stable.

On postsurgical day #6, however, an anti-c antibody became detectable. For the patient, it was like a gunshot. She rapidly decompensated. The DAT became 3+ and bilirubin shot up to 36.1 mg/dL. This rendered the samples too icteric to be able to report hemoglobin. The nucleated RBC count, which had been running at 2 per 100, skyrocketed up to 22 per 100, revealing the body's effort to replace the red cells being lost to hemolysis. The patient developed severe hypotension, hypoxia, rapid cardiovascular collapse, and death within 6 h of the time the anti-c was detected.

The attending surgeon's conclusion was "The little-c killed her."

At autopsy, the spleen revealed massive phagocytosis of the opsonized red blood cells by the splenic macrophages:

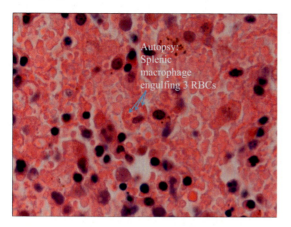

Autopsy: Splenic macrophage engulfing 3 RBCs

This case scenario raises several legally relevant questions to consider. First, was the blood banker's call to the Ob-Gyn team sufficiently informative? The discussion identified the antibody, explained its clinical significance, and provided an understanding of the logistics and timeframe involved in obtaining compatible blood. If the substance of the discussion was appropriate, was it acceptable to communicate with a resident rather than talking directly with the attending physician? There is probably no clear standard of practice on that issue. In teaching hospitals, the traditional practice has always been to rely on residents. The attending surgeon's responsibility is to lead the team, ensure that the workup is complete and the proper information has been gathered, and make the final decision regarding the care of the patient. Others would say that the world seldom lives up to such ideals, and if the information is highly important, the communication should be attending-to-attending. Of course, it is not clear in this case whether speaking directly with the attending Ob-Gyn physician would have changed the outcome.

Should the conversation between the transfusion specialist and the Ob-Gyn attending physician have been memorialized? The answer is certainly yes. If there is no record of the conversation, it will be very difficult to reconstruct at a later date what was said. No matter how certain the parties may be, their memories may differ substantially. Even more importantly, patient care, planning, and decision-making "speak through the chart". The chart has long been designated as the definitive source for ascertaining the patient's progress, defining the clinical plan, and communicating among caregivers. Particularly, in the era of the electronic health record, there is no excuse for failing to document important events in the course of the patient's treatment. To put it in risk management terms, one fails to document important events at one's peril–and at the patient's.

Was the decision to go forward with the hysterectomy reasonable? What would the "standard of care" be in this clinical setting? The answer to that question is considerably a matter of clinical judgment, and thus likely to be the hardest to assess. The obstetric surgeons believed that a laparoscopic approach was safe. Other obstetricians may differ on that point. If the case went to court, there would no doubt be a "battle of the experts" regarding whether it was appropriate to proceed with the surgery. A similar battle would probably be waged on the issue of whether it would have been best to have used an open or a laparoscopic approach.

Would the outcome have been different if surgery had been delayed long enough to obtain Js^b-negative blood? This is a powerful question. Once asked, the answer turns out to be rather unexpected. No, it probably would not have made a difference. The patient required 11 units of blood–an entire blood volume—to keep her alive while the hemorrhage was brought under control. Using a national search, it took four and a half days to obtain two units of Js^b-negative blood. The blood bank would not have accumulated enough blood to handle a massive transfusion before the surgeons went ahead with the procedure. Thus, failure to wait for Js(b−) units could not be said to have caused the patient's death.

Was the attending surgeon correct in concluding that the little-c killed her? A close look at the graph suggests that he may be right. During the first 55 h after the massive transfusion, the patient's hematocrit slowly decreased from about 42 to about 22. She was clinically fairly stable. At 55 h, at midnight, a cross-covering intern ordered transfusion of a single unit of Js(b+), c-negative blood. The hematocrit had a significant bump before returning to baseline 41 h later. Thus, the hemolysis of Js^b-positive red cells was not especially brisk. Two units of Js^b-negative–and *c-positive*–red blood cells arrived just before the c became detectable, and they were transfused immediately. The patient went into profound shock and was dead within the day.

One final question: Was a new informed consent obtained when the obstetric surgeons learned of the anti-Js^b antibody? This could have been dispositive of the whole case. When new information is learned that materially increases the risk of a procedure, the treating physicians must obtain new informed consent. The patient was not asked to reconsent in light of the new risk, so her consent for the procedure was no longer informed. The surgeons may have won the day up until this last question, but they may ultimately have lost the battle due to their failure to update the patient's consent in light of the increased risk posed by the anti-Js^b antibody.

Strict Product Liability

Strict liability is so named because, in the context of manufactured products, the law may hold a manufacturer liable for harm caused by a product, without requiring the injured party to prove that the manufacturer was negligent.[15] The manufacturer is therefore "strictly liable" for injuries caused by defects in the product.

Strict product liability for defective products makes parties who manufacture, sell, or distribute a defective product "strictly liable" (liable without negligence) for any defect in the product. Each product comes with an "implied warranty" that every product is safe for its intended use. Everyone in the chain of design, sale, and distribution is strictly liable for harm caused by a dangerous product.

One might wonder whether strict product liability is fair. The concept behind the doctrine is that a consumer is not in a position to inspect and evaluate every mechanical, electrical, or other product. Therefore, if a purchaser uses a product as intended, there should be an implied warranty of fitness for its intended use. One cannot use a lawn mower to trim the hedges. However, for cutting the lawn, the mower must be safe for its intended use. To hold otherwise would be barbaric. There are many other nuances to product liability law. For example, the doctrine recognizes that manufacturers are in a better position to defray the cost of injuries than are individual consumers. In addition, in the chain of distribution it is sometimes impossible to identify where the defect occurred, so shared liability shifts the burden of proof from the injured party to the manufacturer. Imagine a biological product such as a vaccine. If the vaccine is contaminated with bacteria, it may not be possible for the consumer to determine the source of contamination in the chain of distribution.

Strict liability is an important concept in transfusion medicine and blood banking. In 1954, in the case

of Perlmutter v. Beth David Hospital, a patient sued a hospital after having contracted hepatitis from a blood transfusion on the theory of strict liability for an unsafe product.[16] After all, we pay for the blood and refer to RBCs, plasma, and platelets as "blood products." It is a blood banking "industry." The blood banking community across the United States breathed a sigh of relief when the Court of Appeals of the State of New York held that the blood bank did not sell a product. Rather, it provided a medical service, so liability could rest only on a finding of negligence on the part of the providers.

The "industry" remained sanguine for 16 years until, in the case of Cunningham v. MacNeil Memorial Hospital (1970),[17] the Supreme Court of Illinois disagreed with Perlmutter and held that blood is a product. Almost every state in the country hurriedly passed "blood shield laws" declaring blood to be a service. This was highly fortuitous for avoiding a public health crisis when Hepatitis C and HIV entered the blood supply. The laws were in place and ready.

Even if blood shield laws did not exist, the blood industry would have some fall back. For example, some products avoid strict liability by being considered "unavoidably unsafe." These products are *inherently* unsafe products that cannot be made to be safe, but have a high degree of public utility and social benefit. They are therefore exempt from strict liability. Blood and blood products cannot be made completely safe, but they have very high public utility. They can therefore be exempt from strict liability.

Criminal Liability

Any intentional act that places a patient in danger may be criminal, just as it would be outside the realm of healthcare. Wanton recklessness, on the part of individual employees or the institution, can also be criminal if it creates a high enough level of risk to be unconscionable. There are also a wide variety of statutes, both federal and state, that bear upon healthcare and can result in criminal liability for the institution or its employees, such as the Occupational Safety and Health Act (OSHA), environmental statutes, and employment laws. A few federal laws that can be a source of criminal punishment in the healthcare realm are noted here for illustrative purposes:
a. Fraud and abuse
   The federal government pays billions of dollars each year to healthcare providers,[18] so is not surprising that criminal statutes have been put into place to discourage self-dealing by providers. The Office of the Inspector General (OIG), the Centers for Medicare & Medicaid Services (CMS), and the Department of Justice (DOJ) pay a great deal of attention

to identifying healthcare fraud (misrepresentation) and abuse (overbilling). Fraud and abuse can trigger stiff financial penalties, disqualification from CMS services, and criminal prosecution.

The Anti-Kickback Statute[19] makes it a crime to knowingly pay someone remuneration in order to induce them to refer services that are reimbursable by the federal government, or conversely, to receive payments in exchange for making referrals. It thus targets inducements, or "quid-pro-quo" arrangements. Payment includes any sort of remuneration, such as providing office space below fair market value. Imagine, for example, an orthopedic surgeon who pays reduced rent, in exchange for referring his patients to the physical rehabilitation clinic that owns the building. The anti-kickback law thus targets payments in exchange for referrals.

The Physician Self-Referral Law (Stark Law) prohibits physicians from referring health services to an entity in which the physician or an immediate family member has a financial relationship, such as ownership or investment interest. For example, a physician cannot refer a CMS beneficiary to a company that provides home health services and supplies if the physician has an interest in the company. The Stark self-referral law thus targets referring CMS-covered health services to oneself.

b. HIPAA

The Health Insurance Portability and Accountability Act of 1996 (HIPAA)[20] is undoubtedly familiar to all readers of this book, at least in terms of the statute's privacy rules. The essence of HIPAA's privacy rules is that protected health information (PHI) may not be disclosed unless authorized by the patient or specifically permitted by the statute. HIPAA allows PHI to be used without the patient's permission for treatment, payment, or healthcare operations, including for quality purposes. Users must limit the disclosures to the "minimum necessary" unless the disclosure is made for treatment purposes, in which case full disclosure is permitted for the patient's safety and care.

For improper disclosures of protected health information, severe breaches demonstrating careless disregard for the patient's interests can result in criminal punishment. If systematic mishandling of PHI occurs at the level of the institution, penalties can be severe. Civil and criminal penalties for privacy and security violations include fines up to $50,000 per violation to a maximum $1.5 million per year. Offenses committed with the intent to sell, transfer, or use individually identifiable health information for commercial advantage, personal gain, or malicious harm are punishable by fines up to $250,000 and imprisonment up to 10 years.

c. CLIA

Interestingly, the Clinical Laboratory Improvement Act of 1988 (CLIA) contain criminal provisions. The Act provides for criminal penalties for violating CLIA regulations, including a year's imprisonment, **civil** monetary penalties of $10,000 per day, and exclusion from federal programs.

REFERENCES

1. Kohn LT, Corrigan JM, Donaldson MS. *To Err Is Human: Building a Safer Health System*. Washington DC: National Academies Press; 2000.
2. Leape L, Lawthers AG, Brennan TA, et al. Preventing medical injury. *Qual Rev Bull*. 1993;19:144–149.
3. *HealthGrades Quality Study: Patient Safety in American Hospitals*; 2004. http://www.providersedge.com/ehdocs/ehr_articles/Patient_Safety_in_American_Hospitals-2004.pdf.
4. Department of Health and Human Services. *Adverse Events in Hospitals: National Incidence Among Medicare Beneficiaries*; 2010. https://oig.hhs.gov/oei/reports/oei-06-09-00090.pdf.
5. Classen D, Resar R, Griffin F, et al. Global "trigger tool" shows that adverse events in hospitals may be ten times greater than previously measured. *Health Aff*. 2011;30:581–589.
6. Landrigan CP, Parry GJ, Bones CB, et al. Temporal trends in rates of patient harm resulting from medical care. *N Engl J Med*. 2010;363:2124–2134.
7. James JTA. A new, evidence-based estimate of patient harms associated with hospital care. *J Patient Saf*. 2013;9:122–128.
8. Makary MA, Daniel M. Medical error – the third leading cause of death in the US. *BMJ*. 2016;353:i2139.
9. Jena AB, Chandra A, Lakdawalla D, Seabury S. Outcomes of medical malpractice litigation against U.S. physicians. *Arch Intern Med*. 2012;172(11):892–894.
10. Jena AB, Seabury S, Lakdawalla D, Chandra A. Malpractice risk according to physician specialty. *N Engl J Med*. 2011;365:629–636.
11. Fung MK, Elder AF, Spitalnik SL, et al., eds. *AABB Technical Manual*. 19th ed. Bethesda: AABB Press; 2017.
12. Fung MK, Elder AF, Spitalnik SL, et al., eds. *AABB Technical Manual*. 19th ed. Bethesda: AABB Press; 2017:329.
13. United States Census Bureau. *Quick Facts*; 2018. https://www.census.gov/quickfacts/fact/table/US/PST045217.
14. Yuan S, Ewing NP, Bailey D, et al. Transfusion of multiple units of Js(b+) red blood cells in the presence of anti-Jsb in a patient with sickle beta-thalassemia disease and a review of the literature. *Immunohematology*. 2007;23:75–80.

15. Restatement (Third) of Torts: Products Liability. *Chap.1, Topic 1, § 2. Categories of Product Defect*; 2012.
16. Perlmutter v. *Beth David Hospital, 308 N.Y. 100, 123 N.E.2d 792*; 1954.
17. Cunningham v. *MacNeil Memorial Hospital, 47 Ill. 2d 443, 266 N.E.2d 897*; 1970.
18. Medicare Fraud & Abuse. *Prevention, Detection, and Reporting. CMS Medicare Learning Network. ICN 006827*;

September 2017. https://www.cms.gov/Outreach-and-Education/Medicare-Learning-Network-MLN/MLNProducts/Downloads/Fraud-and-AbuseTextOnly.pdf.
19. The 42 U.S.C. § 1320a-7b(b).
20. *Health Insurance Portability and Accountability Act of 1996, Pub. L. No. 104-191, 110 Stat. 1936*(1996).

CHAPTER 11

Treating Jehovah's Witness Patients

J. MILLS BARBEAU, MD, JD

An important aspect of the Jehovah's Witness faith is that believers must refuse blood transfusions, even at the risk of losing their life. Given that exigency, Jehovah's Witness patients can present healthcare providers with difficult but highly instructive risk management challenges, legally, ethically, and professionally.

The mandate to refuse blood transfusions is derived from scripture. Adherents believe that the Bible makes it clear that one may not receive blood, citing passages such as the following:

Therefore, I said unto the children of Israel, No soul of you shall eat blood, neither shall any stranger that sojourneth among you eat blood. Leviticus 17:11–14

Ye shall eat the blood of no manner of flesh: for the life of all flesh is the blood thereof: whosoever eateth it shall be cut off. Leviticus 17:11–14

But flesh with the life thereof, which is the blood thereof, shall ye not eat. Genesis 9:4

That you abstain from things sacrificed to idols, and blood. Acts 15:29

The prohibition against receiving blood might appear to be consistent with other examples of Old Testament dietary laws. Jehovah's Witnesses reject that interpretation, however, adhering strictly to the view that the passages on "eating" blood mean that it is sinful to consume or derive sustenance from blood, and to do so will result in being cut off from God.

To willingly receive a blood transfusion not only cuts the believer off from God, but also from one's community. The decision to receive a transfusion is an affirmative act, and therefore the believer is considered to have affirmatively broken his or her ties with God. The decision has placed that individual's soul in moral peril, and as a result, that person may have brought sin into the community's midst. For that reason, one who accepts a blood transfusion risks "disfellowship," a termination of membership in the community. Rejecting the faith by accepting a blood transfusion places an individual at risk for being shunned by the community, which potentially includes friends, family, and children.

A review of the religion's history sheds some light on the origins of the Jehovah's Witnesses' strict interpretation of scripture. Allen Rostron,[1] a Yale Law School graduate and Professor of Law at the University of Missouri–Kansas City School of Law, has noted that in 1916, during the formative years of the faith, "Judge" Joseph Rutherford took over leadership of the Watch Tower Society and imposed a particularly legalistic stamp on the religion. Rutherford began his tenure by changing the Society's name to the Jehovah's Witnesses. He also brought to the faith a focus on the printed word. Active members of the faith were referred to as "publishers," and God was characterized in strict, law-and-order terms—God's mandates were spelled out in the bible and they were uncompromising. The faith's new-found legalistic bent also revealed itself in a propensity for litigation. Between 1938 and 1958, more than 50 cases involving Jehovah's Witnesses came before the United States Supreme Court. Remarkably, there has been only one since 1958.[2]

Through their court cases, the Jehovah's Witnesses won a reputation as champions of freedom of religion. Underlying their impact on First Amendment-based religious freedoms, the Witness' crusade seems also to have been motivated by a streak of sheer pugnaciousness. Their legal battles were fought over the right to refuse to salute the flag, celebrate Christmas or national holidays, or serve in the military, since the military, and indeed governments, are instruments of the devil.[3] Outside the courthouse, members actively shunned organized sports, Boy Scouts and Girl Scouts, and higher education. During the era of Judge Rutherford's influence, the Jehovah's Witnesses seemed eager to fight the world. Add in a mixture of strict biblical literalism and an apocalyptic, "end of days" world view, and the daring practice of refusing blood to save one's life was certain to capture attention, and perhaps even respect.

The Jehovah's Witness era of court battles ended 50 years ago. Joseph Rutherford himself died in 1942. Religions evolve, and so do the faithful. Today, one thing is certain: When a hemorrhaging Jehovah's Witness is

Risk Management in Transfusion Medicine. https://doi.org/10.1016/B978-0-323-54837-3.00011-0

rolled into the emergency room, we cannot learn everything about that person's beliefs by looking on the internet. We must inquire not only about Jehovah's Witness religious practices and principles today in the 21st century, but also about the individual patient's beliefs.

WHICH BLOOD PRODUCTS ARE FORBIDDEN?

One might expect that a Jehovah's Witness' refusal to accept blood products would simplify the patient's transfusion management. That is not the case. Transfusion medicine practitioners must be alert to nuances when caring for Jehovah's Witness patients, including the key decision points that must be navigated throughout the patient's course. Treatment pathways vary depending on each case. Each treatment decision has legal, ethical, and professional implications, and each decision represents a potential source of risk. The purpose of this chapter is to provide a general template for practitioners to negotiate the terrain with confidence.

If a Jehovah's Witness patient chooses to honor the prohibition against blood transfusions, it is probably safe to assume that the patient will refuse red blood cells. However, it is important to be cognizant of the fact that interpretation regarding other blood components, such as plasma and platelets, is left largely to the individual's conscience. It is therefore important to inquire into the patient's feelings about blood alternatives, recalling that the treating physician's responsibility is not to enforce the religion's doctrine, but rather to discover and honor the individual's personal values. Indeed, a physician who also happens to be a Jehovah's Witness should be particularly careful about making doctrinal assumptions about a patient's beliefs. Patient autonomy and patient-centered care requires us to respect the patient's personal religious beliefs, not to enforce the tenets of the church.

In addition to discussing the acceptability of specific blood components, one should also explore alternate transfusion techniques that might contribute to a successful outcome. Would autologous blood be acceptable? What about intraoperative blood salvage and/or normovolemic hemodilution? If a patient needs heart surgery, is cardiac bypass acceptable? If so, perhaps a system for minimalized extracorporeal bypass volume should be arranged.

To be sure of understanding the patient's preferences regarding transfusion options, it is important to have a candid conversation with the patient alone in a private setting. If family members, clergy, or others are present, the patient may not be able to speak freely. It is crucial to assure the patient of absolute confidentiality, and to explain that the patient's interests are the highest priority.

A surgeon from New Orleans relates an instructive story about a patient he encountered in his practice.[4] The patient came for a preoperative visit accompanied by his son. During the visit, the son informed the doctor that they were Jehovah's Witnesses, so his father must not receive blood. The patient confirmed that this was the case. The surgeon prepared a consent form that carefully documented the patient's refusal to receive blood or blood products. The consent form also waived any malpractice claims for withholding blood should it be needed.

The doctor rounded on the patient the night before the surgery. The patient was alone, and he took the opportunity to confide the fact that he was not averse to receiving blood should it be indicated. He simply had not wanted to admit that fact in front of his son. The surgeon understood, and he and his patient updated the consent accordingly.

As it turned out, the patient lost an unexpected amount of blood during the procedure, and he required a red cell transfusion. After the surgery was successfully completed, the doctor went out to meet with the family. Unbeknownst to the doctor, a hospital representative had already approached the family to ask if they wished to donate blood, since the patient had required a transfusion. Naturally, the first thing the son asked the surgeon when he arrived was whether it was true that his father had received blood. The surgeon was utterly taken aback. When he learned why the son had asked, he was confronted with an acute quandary: should he lie to the family, risking his own reputation for honesty, or should he protect his patient's secret? Maintaining his composure, the doctor told the family that their father had not been transfused, and the hospital representative was mistaken.

Ethics and professionalism are sometimes challenged when one least expects it. In that moment, the surgeon decided whether to place his patient's relationship with his family ahead of his own reputation for honesty. If he told the family that the patient had changed his mind about receiving blood, the patient's relationship within his own family and possibly his peers may have been severely disrupted. The doctor could not be sure of this, but under the circumstances he had to assume the worst, which meant placing his own personal integrity at risk, rather than betraying his patient's trust.

The foundation of a physician's ethical compass is the doctor-patient relationship. It is a fiduciary relationship, meaning that the physician places the patient's interests ahead of his or her own. In daily practice, the sanctity of the physician-patient relationship can have literally life-and-death importance, as we saw in the New Orleans surgeon's experience. If the patient had not trusted his doctor's confidentiality, he may have died on the table. Patients routinely disclose their most private concerns to their doctors, knowing that the disclosures will remain confidential. The sanctity of the doctor-patient relationship is such that even a judge in a court of law cannot compel a physician to disclose a patient's private medical information. All physicians should take this responsibility very seriously.

PATIENT AUTONOMY

In the previous section, we discussed the importance of building trust and maintaining open communication with Jehovah's Witnesses who decline blood products. Interestingly, that trust begins at a societal level. Physicians as a profession must adhere to the highest level of professionalism and responsibility toward their patients. From a risk management perspective, the foundation upon which optimal physician-patient decision making is built on this level of trust.

The prior section focused on the Jehovah's Witness patient's right to determine the metes and bounds of his or her transfusion restrictions, specifying permissible blood products or, conversely, confiding a willingness to accept blood if a transfusion becomes necessary. This section will discuss the other side of the same coin: The patient's right to refuse blood.

Every adult has a fundamental right to decide what may be done to his or her body.[5] Indeed, it would be difficult to imagine a human right that is more fundamental. Respect for the patient's autonomy imposes a mandate to obtain consent for any medical procedure being recommended to the patient. Respect for patient autonomy—the right to control one's own body—finds its fullest expression in the requirement to obtain informed consent. For that reason, if a patient refuses to consent to a blood transfusion, the transfusion cannot be performed.

Legally and ethically, caregivers are required to respect a patient's autonomy, meaning that personal autonomy is a restraint placed on caregivers, preventing them from performing acts on the patient—even healing acts—without the patient's permission. A caregiver cannot decide what is best for the patient, even if the patient is refusing lifesaving treatment.

There is a problem, however. Medical providers also operate under another compelling ethical imperative: beneficence. Different from patient autonomy, which places limitations on caregivers' actions, the ethical principle of beneficence focuses on how caregivers must act. Beneficence means caring for the patient, demonstrating the caregiver's fiduciary duty, putting the patient's interests ahead of one's own. Beneficence is expressed by medicine's well-known first principle, primum non nocere ("first do no harm"). Unfortunately, beneficence and autonomy are in perfect conflict when a Jehovah's Witness refuses blood.

When beneficence and autonomy collide, probably the most compelling pathway out of the dilemma is to focus on patient-centered care. People who are not Jehovah's Witnesses may perceive a lifesaving transfusion to be a necessary beneficent act. A patient-centered view, however, may recognize that the life-affirming, faith-based course of action for a Jehovah's Witness may be to refuse transfusion and trust in God. In this light, the Jehovah's Witness' decision might be seen as akin to an elderly patient foregoing chemotherapy to spend her remaining "good days" with her grandchildren. In both cases, the patient is electing to refuse treatment in order to have a preferred, life-affirming benefit. In both cases, the decision is a patient-centered, value-based choice.

Answers are not always easy, however. Consider a Jehovah's Witness patient with severe postpartum hemorrhage. Blood is urgently needed to keep the patient alive until the bleeding can be brought under control, after which the patient would be expected to have a full recovery. Instead, the mother bleeds to death while her newborn cries for her in the nursery.

Anyone on the mother's treatment team would likely feel profoundly resentful about having to participate in such an outcome. Here, beneficence would begin to feel more like a right than an obligation. One may ask whether the patient's autonomy must always trump beneficence. Does a caregiver ever have the right to save the life of a competent, adult patient over the patient's objections? The short answer, legally, is no. Interestingly, the sense of injustice does seem to have some theoretical basis. Older academic literature in the social sciences suggested that, in the relationship between patient and caregiver, there is a certain element of quid pro quo, supported by an underlying societal understanding that the relationship between beneficence and autonomy involves a mutual obligation between caregiver and patient. Consent to treatment relinquishes some of the patient's autonomy. In exchange, the patient receives the full measure of the caregiver's beneficence. A Jehovah's Witness who refuses a lifesaving transfusion may thus violate an unspoken social norm, even if not a legal norm, hence the caregiver's sense of injustice.[6]

A PATIENT'S RIGHT TO DIE

The law in the United States dealing with a patient's "right to die" holds that the degree of respect accorded to patient autonomy depends on an assessment of the patient's judgment. In the case of Curzan v. Director, Missouri Department of Health,[7] the United States Supreme Court held that a competent person who understands the consequences of his or her actions has a constitutional right to refuse lifesaving medical treatment, in this case nutrition and hydration. Accordingly, an adult Jehovah's Witness may refuse a lifesaving transfusion if he or she possesses decision-making capacity and understands the consequences of refusing treatment. In short, if the Jehovah's Witness has a clear mind, autonomy prevails and the patient has the right to refuse blood.

Cases involving Jehovah's Witnesses who refuse blood can be viewed as demonstrating that autonomy trumps beneficence: The patient's right to withhold consent trumps the caregiver's right to heal. But does it? Curzan can lead to some aberrant results.

Imagine that a Jehovah's Witness is brought to the emergency room hemorrhaging to death. Her heart racing, she implores the emergency room physicians, "Please save my life! I have everything to live for and I do not want to die. Do everything you can for me, but you may not under any circumstances give me blood–even if I bleed to death." We are obligated to respect the patient's wishes even if it means she dies.

Ten minutes later, a patient comes into the emergency room having slit his wrists in a suicide attempt. He screams: "Do NOT save my life! I have nothing to live for and I want to die. You may not under any circumstances give me blood–I want to bleed to death." In this case, the ER team does not hesitate to override the patient's wishes. They start an urgent blood transfusion and pull the patient back from the brink of a nearly successful suicide attempt.

In the first instance, respect for the patient's autonomy prevails. In the second, beneficence wins. How do we reconcile the two? The salient difference between the two cases appears to be the fact that the Jehovah's Witness is operating from a religious conviction, whereas the person attempting suicide is presumed to be suffering from a pathologic suicidal ideation that is clouding his judgment. If the patient poses a threat to himself or others, interventions such as sedation or physical restraints are considered to be justified.[8] In the case of a suicide attempt, once we stabilize the patient we anticipate being able to cure what we have identified as a pathologic medical condition. If the suicidal patient can be saved and brought back to mental health, perhaps treated for depression, he will be glad to be alive. Of course, there are instances of Jehovah's Witnesses being saved and later being grateful to be alive, just as there are cases of Jehovah's Witnesses who let their children bleed to death and later regret that decision.[9] In terms of mental capacity, however, we "medicalize" suicide attempts, which are deemed to imply pathology, while religious convictions are presumed to be the result of a clear mind. Thus, medical beneficence is not always subordinate to patient autonomy. Physicians are allowed to override severely depressed patients, but not religious ones. The result is that the patient who wants to live is allowed to bleed to death and the one who wants to die is saved.

ADVANCE DIRECTIVES

Many Jehovah's Witnesses carry advance directive cards, living wills, or Medical Alert badges explaining that, in case of an emergency, they do not wish to receive blood. Such directives can be problematic. By definition, the directives are intended to be used precisely when the patient lacks the ability to communicate his or her wish not to receive blood, that is, when the patient lacks decision-making capacity due to trauma. Canada seems to have examined the legal aspects of Jehovah's Witnesses' advanced directives more thoroughly than the United States. In one case, a severely injured patient arrived unconscious in the emergency room with a Medical Alert card in her purse stating that she was a Jehovah's Witness and instructing caregivers not to transfuse blood or blood products under any circumstances. The patient had signed the card, but it was not witnessed or dated. The patient was in shock on arrival and the treating physician elected to ignore the card and give the patient a lifesaving blood transfusion. The patient survived, sued for damages, and won. The Ontario Court of Appeals found that the treating physician had violated the patient's right to control her own body.[10]

Jehovah's Witnesses frequently carry cards instructing caregivers not to transfuse blood. Indeed, it is expected in some communities. One may well ask whether such cards are sufficiently reliable evidence of a patient's beliefs to justify permitting her to die on the strength of a card found in a purse. She may have changed her mind since signing the card, or she may have signed under pressure from her family. She may not have been mentally competent when she signed the card. The card may not even be hers. It may have been dropped into her purse by a deranged prankster. Even if a close friend or family member is available to attest to the patient's beliefs, would this be sufficient evidence to construe the card as a binding commitment to refuse blood to save the patient's life?

Decisions have varied among jurisdictions, but generally the United States has not gone as far as Canada in honoring Medical Alert cards or even advanced directives. In Werth v. Taylor,[11] a pregnant Jehovah's Witness who was being admitted to a Michigan hospital signed a hospital preregistration form in which she stated that she would not permit transfusions. She delivered twins and had severe postpartum hemorrhage. Her physicians transfused her despite the directive she had signed during the admission process. The patient then sued for battery and lost. The court found that the patient's:

> refusals were made when she was contemplating merely routine elective surgery and not when life-threatening circumstances were present. . . It could not be said that she made the decision to refuse a blood transfusion. . . while fully aware that death would result from such refusal. The record reflects the unexpected development of a medical emergency requiring blood transfusion to prevent death or serious compromise of the patient's well-being.

The court held that a refusal to consent to lifesaving transfusions must be "contemporaneous and informed" to be enforced.

Case law varies among jurisdictions, however. Not all states have adopted Michigan's "contemporaneous and informed" rule. When caregivers are confronted with such situations, an emergency consultation with the institution's attorney is strongly advised. Generally, in the United States, if it is an emergency and the patient is incapacitated, courts and juries tend to defer to the physician's judgment in ignoring a written, noncontemporaneous refusal to permit transfusions. By contrast, if a patient consciously refuses blood during an emergency and there is no reason to doubt her mental capacity or her ability to understand the consequences of refusal, then according to the United States Supreme Court in *Curzan*, the physician is obligated to follow the patient's wishes.

CHILDREN

Where children are involved, courts and health care providers must always err on the side of protecting a child's health and safety. Questions of parental rights are deferred until the child's safety is assured. Ideally, the providers who are treating the child will be able to be supportive of the parents' concerns, even if the parents' wishes cannot be accommodated. Parents who are Jehovah's Witnesses may feel that it is in their child's best interests to save the child's soul rather than the child's body, but it is universally accepted that physicians should protect the minor's health and safety by transfusing if necessary.

In the case of Prince v. Massachusetts,[12] the United States Supreme Court held that religious freedom does not authorize parents to place their children at risk, nor does religion impose a limit on the State's right to intervene in the child's best interests. This rule was enunciated in 1944, in a case involving parents who were Jehovah's Witnesses. U.S. Supreme Court Justice Rutledge articulated the principle memorably: "Parents may be free to become martyrs themselves. But it does not follow that they are free, in identical circumstances, to make martyrs of their children."

The State has an interest in protecting children, and it has the authority to intercede when parental decisions place a child at risk. States invariably have child protection laws that authorize physicians to take action–often in the form of assuming custody of the child–if parents are putting a child's health at significant risk by withholding consent for standard-of-care treatment. If circumstances permit, physicians should contact the healthcare facility's attorney and responsible administrator prior to acting. The attorney will likely inform the court about the case to be ready to move quickly should a hearing and a court order become necessary.

If the child's physical condition places the child in danger of death or permanent bodily harm, the physician is ethically bound to treat the child immediately, and can do so with confidence that he or she is authorized by law to take the necessary action. As a practical matter, it is highly advisable to obtain at least one other physician's opinion that the medical intervention is necessary, and to document the second opinion in the patient's chart. Some states have statutes that specifically list the steps that must be taken, including a second or even third physician's signature, but where time is of the essence such documentation can be deferred until the patient is stable. Ideal risk management and compassionate care for the family unit can best be achieved by treating the parents with respect, and it is highly advisable to provide a full, honest disclosure of the steps being taken and the reasons why they are being taken, as well as reassurance and recognition of the parents' distress. The healthcare team must endeavor to maintain open, respectful communication with the parents, and be honest about the course of action one plans to take, even when that plan is contrary to the parents' wishes.

ADOLESCENTS

The need for medical consent by minors becomes more complicated when children reach adolescence. When children are young, they lack the capacity to provide or withhold informed consent for medical treatment because they do not have sufficient intellectual capacity to understand the implications of their decisions. Simply put, their consent cannot qualify as "informed." Adolescents, on the other hand, often have the ability to understand the risks and benefits of proposed medical interventions. They may reach maturity before they reach the age of majority. States that follow the "mature minor" rule allow adolescents to give valid consent if they are judged to be capable of providing such consent, at least for less serious medical procedures. Many states follow the mature minor rule, but the rule is problematic to apply because it is left to the physician to assess the minor's capacity. In addition, depending on the jurisdiction, the mature minor rule may not authorize minors to make more serious decisions, including decisions regarding medically necessary blood transfusions.

One should also be aware that some states have very specific laws governing medical consent by minors for particular treatments. Such laws typically authorize minors who have reached a specified age, usually in the teens, to obtain medical treatment without parental consent in circumstances such as pregnancy care, treatment for sexually transmitted diseases, and treating drug addiction. Such statutes vary widely by jurisdiction, and each is subject to amendment, so this discussion can only address the topic in general terms. The healthcare facility's attorney will be aware of the relevant statutes in the relevant jurisdiction that pertain to treating minors. It is highly advisable to consult the attorney early in the care of an adolescent Jehovah's Witness.

ALTERNATIVES TO TRANSFUSION

The foregoing discussions have taken a traditional approach to exploring the ethical and legal considerations raised by a Jehovah's Witness' refusal to accept blood transfusions, in the sense that the illustrative examples tend to involve uncontrollably hemorrhaging patients dying before our eyes. These scenarios are helpful for exploring the rules, but in practice, unless you are an emergency physician or a trauma surgeon, you are probably unlikely to treat a Jehovah's Witness in extremis. Instead, like the New Orleans surgical patient at the start of this chapter, issues of transfusing Jehovah's Witness patients are more likely to arise in the context of a planned operation or procedure that may involve blood loss. For that reason, it is fortuitous that transfusion practices and surgical techniques are currently undergoing a marked transition toward minimizing unnecessary transfusions for all patients.

Multiple studies have demonstrated clinical settings in which lowered hemoglobin transfusion thresholds have produced equal or improved outcomes.[13] Transfusion-free surgery using blood conservation techniques and lowered transfusion triggers are regularly demonstrating their worth. A commitment to avoiding surgical transfusion starts with preoperative planning that includes a careful medical history, medication history, physical examination, and when indicated, laboratory evaluation to identify clotting deficiencies. Preoperative anemia may be treated, as appropriate, with vitamin B12, folic acid, iron therapy, or possibly an erythropoietin analog. Surgery might involve intraoperative normovolemic hemodilution, which advantageously lowers viscosity during the surgery. Blood is drawn off early in surgery and volume is maintained with fluids. The blood is then replaced at the end of the surgery. Intraoperative blood salvage is another useful technique for avoiding transfusions, especially for procedures associated with highly anticipated blood loss.

Developing a patient blood management program to guide transfusion practices throughout the hospital can itself be viewed as an ethical obligation. Blood is a scarce resource, so the principle of distributive justice argues in favor of a carefully planned blood stewardship program. Lowering transfusion thresholds minimizes exposure to infectious risks, thus exemplifying the beneficence–or more properly, the nonmaleficence—embodied in "first, do no harm." Developing best transfusion practices at one's institution is therefore the right thing to do, and fortuitously, it goes a long way toward being able to offer strategies of providing care to Jehovah's Witnesses refusing blood. Optimal risk management occurs when best clinical practices, quality, and efficiency unite.

Brezina and Moskop[14] share an illustrative example of compassionate and ethical care provided to an adolescent Jehovah's Witness and her family in North Carolina. The patient was a 15-year-old girl whose parents brought her to the emergency department with a distended, tense abdomen. The parents immediately announced that they were Jehovah's Witnesses, and under no circumstances would their daughter receive a transfusion, even if it meant her death. The daughter concurred. The parents also insisted on remaining at their daughter's bedside at all times. The hospital ethics team was consulted and hospital administration was notified. A CT scan revealed a large ovarian mass and massive ascites. Draining the fluid produced a large amount of blood. The girl's hematocrit dropped from 32.5% to 20.9%, and she had worsening tachycardia. An urgent meeting was convened with the patient, her parents, the clinical team, several church elders, the ethics team, and the hospital attorney. The patient and parents were determined to refuse all blood products. The ethics consultants suggested locating a facility with a well-developed bloodless surgery program. Meanwhile, the hospital attorney made preliminary contact with a local judge in case a court hearing became necessary. The girl's low hematocrit remained relatively stable, and 2 days later she was transferred to a tertiary hospital in North Carolina that had a dedicated blood conservation program.

Both hospitals had at all times demonstrated respect for the family's faith and a willingness to avoid transfusing the daughter if possible. The family was included in all decision making, and church representatives were included as participants. The caregivers were also forthright in stating that the law permitted them to override the girl's and her parents' wishes, and they would do so if it became necessary to save her life. As a result of strengthened relationships and honest, ongoing communication, all three family members consented to the surgery and signed an "acknowledgment statement" affirming their understanding that blood would be given if needed. The surgeons removed a 10 cm ovarian mass and 5 L of bloody ascites, but no blood was transfused. The patient was ultimately discharged in stable condition.

CONCLUSIONS

Most Jehovah's Witnesses have very strongly held religious beliefs regarding blood transfusions. When treating Jehovah's Witness patients, it is important to understand precisely what the individual patient's personal religious requirements are. Under Curzan, and in keeping with the ethical concept of respect for patient autonomy, a competent adult who understands the consequences of refusing a blood transfusion has a constitutional right to do so, and the patient's decision cannot be overridden by a health care provider. It is a different matter with children. One must place a child's health and safety first and

transfuse if necessary, even if it means overriding the parents' wishes. The situation can be more complex when caring for adolescents. The laws vary from jurisdiction to jurisdiction, so it is important to contact the institution's attorney and administrator early in all such cases. Above all, when disagreements with Jehovah's Witnesses arise regarding blood transfusions, it is important to treat everyone involved with respect, to communicate openly and honestly, and to think creatively about how to address the problem. Finally, be sure to consider state-of-the-art blood management practices, which may offer a way to achieve both religious and clinical goals.

REFERENCES*

1. Rostron A. Demythologizing the legal history of the Jehovah's Witnesses and the first amendment. *Quinnipiac Law Rev.* 2004;22:493–522.
2. Watchtower Society v. *Village of Stratton, 536 U.S. 150;* 2002.
3. Koehne JA. *Witnesses on Trial: Judicial Intrusion Upon the Practices of Jehovah's Witness Parents;* 1993. 21 Fla. St. U. L. Rev. 205.
4. Baum N. *Transfusion a Jehovah's Witness During Surgery;* 2018. Available at: https://www.kevinmd.com/blog/2011/05/transfusing-jehovahs-witness-surgery.html.
5. Schloendorff v. *Society of New York Hospital* 211 N.Y. 125, 105 N.E. 92. 1914.
6. Burnham JC. Why sociologists abandoned the sick role concept. *Hist Hum Sci.* 2014;27:70–87.
7. Curzan v. *Director, Missouri Department of Health* 110 S. Ct. 2841, 111 L. ed. 2d 224. 1990.
8. Hirschfeld RMA, Russell JM. Assessment and treatment of suicidal patients. *N Engl J Med.* 1997;337(13):910–915.
9. Catlin A. The dilemma of Jehovah's Witness children who need blood to survive. *HEC Forum.* 1996;8:195–207.
10. Malette v. Shulman. *Ontario Court of Appeal, No 29–88;* 1990.
11. Werth v. Taylor. *475 N.W.2d. 426, 190 Mich. Ap. 444;* 1991.
12. Prince v. Massachusetts. *321 U.S. 158, 64 S. Ct. 438, 88 L. ed. 645;* 1944.
13. Carson JL, Hebert PC. Should we universally adopt a restrictive approach to blood transfusion? It's all about the number. *Am J Med.* 2014;127:103–104.
14. Brezina PR, Moscop JC. Urgent medical decision making regarding a Jehovah's Witness minor: a case report and discussion. *NC Med J.* 2007;68:312–316.

*The author wrote an earlier version of this chapter that appeared in Domen RE. Ethical Issues in Transfusion Medicine and Cellular Therapies. Bethesda, Maryland: AABB Press; 2015. AABB Press has kindly given the author permission to borrow freely from the earlier text.

CHAPTER 12

Risk Management in Massive Transfusion

JOHN R. HESS, MD, MPH, FACP, FAAAS

INTRODUCTION

Massive transfusion is a response to massive hemorrhage, and massive hemorrhage occurs in both emergent and planned medical situations. Unplanned massive hemorrhage can occur with severe or profound injury, rupture of abdominal aortic aneurisms, and gastrointestinal hemorrhage. Planned massive hemorrhage can occur during liver transplantation in severely cirrhotic patients, in complex cardiovascular surgery, and with the delivery of women with extensively invasive placentation. In each of these situations, the acuity and extent of the bleeding can vary widely.

As a result, there are multiple definitions of massive transfusion. The historic definition, the replacement of one blood volume in 24 h, has been used since the 1950s and most extensively explored in the review of 92,000 such episodes in the combined Swedish and Danish blood transfusion databases over a 27-year period.[1] The study pointed out that 61% of massive hemorrhage events occur in a surgical setting, usually cardiac or transplant, and that trauma and obstetrical hemorrhage represent only 15% and 2% of such episodes, respectively. Even larger bleeding episodes where more than 20 units of RBCs were given over a 2-day period have been described in a multinational study.[2] In this study, performed in 11 hospitals in six developed nations between 2009 and 2013, the most common use was in organ transplant, and in this group even those patients using 60 units of RBCs or more in 2 days had a 75% survival. In an effort to understand urgency, interest has centered on short and intense episodes of blood use and the Critical Administration Threshold of 3 units of any blood products given in 1 h (CAT-1). In a study of 316 transfused trauma patients, 51% of whom met CAT-1 criteria, mortality was twice as great among those who met this urgency criterion.[3]

Risk management of massive transfusion can be considered in terms of the World Health Organization mantra that "Safe blood is the right product to the right patient in a timely manner and for the right reason." In this chapter, we will discuss the roles of different products, patient identification rules, massive transfusion protocols, and patient blood management in the safety and effectiveness of massive blood transfusion.

THE RIGHT PRODUCT

The physiologic goals of resuscitation of massive hemorrhage are to restore cardiac output, replace and maintain oxygen carrying capacity, and repair and sustain hemostatic capacity. The latter two functions require blood products. As no blood product perfectly meets the needs of all patients, risk management in massive transfusion requires choices about the products to be made available. Those choices will impact the outcomes of specific patients as well as the blood supply and overall public health.

It may seem obvious that massively bleeding patients are losing whole blood and that whole blood is the best resuscitation fluid. Group O whole blood has a long history of lifesaving and safe use in World Wars I and II, Korea, and Vietnam, and its reemergence in military activity in the first Iraq invasion, Somalia, Bosnia, Kosovo, and again in Iraq and Afghanistan suggests that it is the product of choice for field medical use.[4]

However, the question arises of what is "universal donor" whole blood in the modern age. Need it be Rh(D) negative, leukoreduced, low titer for anti-A and anti-B, or risk mitigated for transfusion-related acute lung injury (TRALI)? When dealing with young male military populations the answer is probably no. The two cases of hepatitis C, the one case of TRALI, and even the fatal case of transfusion-associated graft versus host disease from the wars in central Asia seem a small price to have paid for the approximately 200 lives saved with whole blood transfusion.[5]

In the civilian setting in a developed country, the calculus may be different. Whole blood stored in citrate, phosphate, dextrose (CPD) has a shelf life of only 3 weeks and raises the specter of wasting a third of it, as occurred in the US national blood system before storage was finally lengthened to 5 weeks in 1979. It

Risk Management in Transfusion Medicine. https://doi.org/10.1016/B978-0-323-54837-3.00012-2

is still possible to store whole blood for 5 weeks in CPDA-1 but there are no good studies of the quality of the plasma and platelets late in that storage period. As group O RBCs are already scarce in the blood system, the idea of committing a significant fraction of them to a product that is intrinsically wasteful (as only a portion are used) is concerning.

The problem of wasting a limited resource becomes more critical in discussions of Rh(D)-negative whole blood. Only one Caucasian donor in seven is Rh(D) negative, less for other racial groups, so group O Rh(D)-negative RBCs are a scarce commodity available from only 6% of all donors and already frequently in short supply around the country. There is probably not enough group O Rh(D)-negative whole blood to support its wide use as universal donor whole blood for trauma, yet the alternative, using O Rh(D)-positive whole blood, has the risk of alloimmunizing young women of child-bearing potential. Notwithstanding the relative rarity of young Rh(D)-negative women in the trauma population, the reported reduced risk of alloimmunization following trauma, and the high rate of successful pregnancy in Rh(D) alloimmunized women, the potential social and legal consequences of alloimmunizing a young woman need to be considered as a risk management issue.[6]

Leukoreduction is difficult with whole blood. The only available whole blood leukoreduction filter is only 80% platelet sparing and is not available with the 5-week CPDA-1 anticoagulant/storage solution. The attempt to recover the RBCs from units of whole blood after 2 weeks in the emergency refrigerator will result in units with RBCs that are damaged by WBC metabolism and enzymes, plasma that is contaminated with cytokines, and white blood cells that leukoreduce poorly due to their age.

A potential concern about using group O whole blood as universal donor is the rare occurrence of units from donors with high titers of anti-A or anti-B. Hemolytic reactions and deaths have been reported.[7] RBCs in additive solution have 3/4s of their plasma removed, providing some protection, and units or donors can have their anti-A and anti-B levels titered to exclude units with high concentrations.

Risk mitigation for TRALI has been US national policy since 2007. It requires the exclusion of plasma components from women who have been pregnant or their testing for human leukocyte antigen (HLA) antibodies. It is one more pressure on the limited supply of group O Rh(D)-negative blood.

The alternative to whole blood is the use of conventional blood components in ratios that address the requirements to sustain concentrations of RBCs, platelets, and coagulation factors. Although exact ratios of currently available components necessary to do this are unknown, substantial experience suggests that they are close to 1:1:1 when expressed in the old whole blood-derived unit nomenclature.[8] However, in a country in which more than 90% of all platelets are collected and provided as apheresis units many providers find it difficult to remember what the real ratio of bags of components are. Thus, even if ratio driven resuscitation is a goal, it can be difficult to achieve without substantial training. Legal suits have been brought when doctors got the ratios wrong. The importance of massive transfusion protocols cannot be overemphasized.

Components are readily available because component therapy has been standard in US hospitals for 30 years. This means that low-plasma group O RhD positive and negative RBCs in additive solution are readily available, as are plasma from group AB or A donors. Group A plasma can be titered for anti-B or drawn from known low-titer donors to potentially improve its safety for group B or AB recipients.[9] High-quality apheresis platelets are also widely available in large centers.

Apart from the risks of complexity, the use of components means that patients ultimately get less concentrated products because of the addition of RBC additive storage solutions and the losses for RBCs, platelets, and plasma involved in leukoreduction. The total amount of extra crystalloid solution given with 10 rounds of 1:1:1 component resuscitation is 1 L more than with 10 units of whole blood. The clinical consequences are unknown, as excellent hemostatic resuscitation has been possible with both systems and reported mortality is about half of the historic 40% associated with massive crystalloid resuscitation at the turn of the millennium.[10] The level of restraint in crystalloid use may be more important for the degree of hemostatic resuscitation and morbidity and mortality outcomes than the actual blood components used. The massive transfusion protocol is part of a larger resuscitation protocol, and the transfusion service only has control over the latter. It must collaborate responsively to influence the wider aspects of resuscitation.[11]

Blood for transfusion must be available, safe, effective, and cheap. Risk management of massive transfusion must take all these factors into account. Specialty products such as group A low-titer anti-B liquid plasma, which carries a 26-day outdate, can both improve plasma availability and serve multiple functions. At Harborview Medical Center in Seattle, we use about 25 units of this product each week. In their first week, they are deployed at air ambulance bases around the Pacific Northwest and used as universal donor plasma, but when returned they are used as A plasma in general inpatient care. We mitigate the potential risk of bacterial overgrowth in these cold-stored components by trying to use them by 19 days of storage as cold-stored RBCs rarely exhibit bacterial contamination consequences before 20 days of storage.

The Right Patient

The problems with identifying unknown trauma patients for purposes of transfusion are well known. Such patients are frequently unable to identify themselves, and sometimes they are carrying false identification. Systems for surrogate naming or arm-banding unknown patients are widely used, but each has potential pitfalls. All seven deaths from hemolytic transfusion reactions among US soldiers in Vietnam occurred in patients receiving supposedly crossmatched blood despite dogtags, armbands, and having their names sewed or stenciled on their shirts.

Surrogate naming systems are widely used in trauma centers. An unknown patient arriving at Harborview Medical Center will receive a gender-specific "Doe" name such as Doe Bobby that serves as a temporary name for purposes of admission and record keeping. In the transfusion service, such a name in conjunction with a hospital number allows original and second sample typing and the issuing of type compatible or fully crossmatched blood. However, the hospital policy is to change the name of record of the patient when the true identify is discovered, so the transfusion service can be dealing with patients whose blood is crossmatched under one name and for whom products are requested under another with no time to request two more samples. In a recent mass casualty situation, a new system of Disaster names appeared: Disaster Jack, Disaster Jill, etc. When the two most seriously injured patients arrived and were named Disaster Akiro and Disaster Alexa, with sequential hospital numbers, the potential for confusion was high.

Armbands are a critical part of many aspects of hospital care, including blood drawing and blood administration. However, patients can remove them unconsciously or purposefully, they can become soiled or unreadable, and staff can remove them due to injury or for vascular access. They can be covered by drapes in surgery.

Massive transfusions present unique problems of their own just because of the large amount of blood products present and the pressure of events. Early in the author's career as a transfusion service medical director, I offered to carry several units of group A RBCs down to the Trauma Receiving Unit while on my way to observe a critically injured massive transfusion recipient. I handed the units to the Head Nurse and then in a series of mistakes they were given to the group O massive transfusion patient. Although the patient survived and the group A RBCs circulated for 2 days, this kind of circumstance can lead to fatal ABO transfusion reactions. Moreover, this taught me as a medical director not to interfere with standard operating procedures except to protect a patient.

In a related kind of situation in a multiple casualty event, an anesthesiologist grabbed a unit of RBCs out of a massive transfusion container and hung them on another casualty, failing to realize the first casualty had been typed and the uncrossmatched group O RBCs had been replaced with type specific group A red cells. In this case, the second patient died of an acute hemolytic transfusion reaction. Situations around massive transfusion, in which large amounts of blood products are present, are risky both for the patients and the products. In these situations, having blood safety officers present can occasionally be lifesaving.

In a Timely Manner

Patients with uncontrolled hemorrhage die quickly. In a series of 68,000 direct admissions to the Cowley Shock Trauma Center at the University of Maryland in Baltimore between 1996 and 2008, just over 700 died of uncontrolled bleeding after arriving alive and surviving at least 15 min. Time to death in this group was short, with 30% of those who would die dead in 1 h, 43% dead at 90 min, 50% dead by 2 h, and 63% dead by 3 h. Eighty percent of those who would die of bleeding were dead by 6 h and 90% by 12 h. If a transfusion service is going to make a difference in the outcome of the massively bleeding patient, it must act quickly.

In the Prospective Observational Multicenter Massive Transfusion Study (PROMMTT), time to the delivery of balanced resuscitation was observed. This study performed in 2008 and 2009 in 10 academic trauma centers confirmed that times to get hemostatic blood products, plasma, platelets, and cryoprecipitate, to severely and profoundly injured trauma patients were long. Essentially no one received a balanced resuscitation in the first hour, and only 50% of survivors had received a balance of plasma and RBCs by 3 h. For platelets, it was 30%. Death rates in patients who did not receive balanced resuscitation were twice as high as in those who did, but it was not clear whether patients died because they did not receive plasma or they did not get plasma because they died.

In the subsequent Pragmatic Randomized Optimal Plasma and Platelet Ratio (PROPPR) trial, the demonstrated ability to get 6 units of RBCs, 6 units of thawed plasma, and 1 unit of apheresis platelets to the bedside within 10 min of a blood bank call was a requirement for trauma centers to participate in the study. During the study, 11 of the 12 centers met that goal. In a retrospective review of PROPPR blood delivery, every minute of delay in administering blood was associated with a 5% increase in mortality. There was also a pattern observed in the behavior of the surgeons in the PROPPR study based on their transfusion service support. In trauma centers in which the response time of their transfusion service in delivering blood to the bedside was less than 5 min, the surgeons took time to evaluate the patient before calling the blood bank, whereas in the centers where blood service was slower the doctors called the blood bank when the patients arrived resulting in more calls and more unnecessary urgent activations. It appeared that both the fact and the perception of service mattered.

Harborview has maintained the basic form of the 1:1:1 arm of the PROPPR trial as its massive transfusion protocol (MTP). We send a blood bank certified laboratory technician with a refrigerator containing 6 units of uncrossmatched group O RBCs, Rh(D) negative for women of potentially child-bearing age and for children, and 6 units of thawed or liquid plasma to every adult MTP activation. A unit of apheresis platelets is also sent in a room temperature box. Blood products are issued at the bedside. In the PROPPR trial, our mean response time, telephone activation to emergency room bedside, was 3 min.

In 2016, we audited all 309 MTP activations in the hospital. Again, our time to bedside for patients in the physically close emergency room and operating rooms was 3 min. It took longer to reach many of the wards because of waiting times for elevators. Our ratio of transfused products was 1:0.98:1:12 when a unit of apheresis platelets was counted as equivalent to six whole blood-derived platelets. The mean injury severity score (ISS) of the 237 treated trauma patients was 32, unchanged from PROPPR and well above the severe-profound injury boundary of ISS scores greater than 25, so there has not been an increase in activations for patients not needing blood where the rate remains at 5%. Hospital mortality in the trauma patients was 15%, well below the 40% typical of 20 years ago and predicted by the level of injury severity. The average number of RBC units transfused on an MTP activation was 6.8 units, again supporting the recognition in the Damage Control Resuscitation literature that balanced resuscitation reduces blood use and changes the epidemiology of massive resuscitation.

We have also placed a blood refrigerator in the emergency department (ED). The refrigerator is small, locked with a simple electronic code known to all the ED nurses, and contains 2 units of group O Rh(D)-positive RBCs on the top shelf, 2 units of group AB thawed plasma or group A low-titer anti-B liquid plasma on the middle shelf, and 2 units of group O Rh(D)-negative RBCs on the bottom shelf. The shelves are labeled with what they contain and who the products are indicated for. There is also a sign on the door to call the Transfusion Service if a baby needs blood emergently. The ER blood refrigerator was used 135 times the first year and 245 times the second year it was in place. Usage was audited in the middle of the second year by a pathology resident and a junior faculty member and found to be overwhelming appropriate. The door of the ED refrigerator is monitored and rings in the Transfusion Service if it is open. When the door monitor rings, a transfusion service technician or clinical laboratory scientist goes up to the ED to confirm removal of blood, determine where it went, and initiate replacement of the removed units. A transfusion safety nurse, laboratory medicine resident, or faculty member may go as well as these events are often interesting and teachable moments.

For the Right Reason

Risk management in an age of evidence-based patient blood management starts with the question, do the patients need the blood at all. In situations of massive hemorrhage and transfusion, unlike the well-studied situations surrounding RBC transfusion triggers of 7 versus 10 g of hemoglobin or prophylactic platelet transfusion triggers of 10 or $20 \times 10^3/\mu L$ in nonbleeding oncology patients, it is unlikely that the patients would do just as well without the blood. It is also unlikely that we will have level 1 evidence for the utility of massive transfusion better than the PROPPR trial any time soon. From the patient's point of view, the most important thing we can do is make blood for hemostatically balanced massive transfusion available, safe, effective, and cheap.

Availability of blood products for massive transfusion is a constant, multifaceted, and constantly changing challenge. Harborview Medical Center uses about 8000 units of RBCs a year, 22 units a day, down from 15,000 units in 2003. This means that we keep 104 units of group O Rh(D)-positive RBCs and 36 units of group O Rh(D)-negative units in house as our basic emergency inventory at any time. This is enough to treat one or several massive transfusion patients at a time but would fail quickly in a large mass shooter incident or earthquake. Regional and national blood system backup for major disasters in the physically isolated population centers of the Pacific Northwest is uncharted territory.

Keeping group O Rh(D)-negative RBC units available for 10 widely disbursed air ambulances means that our usage of such units is 12% of our total RBC usage. This is twice the fraction in the donor population and puts a significant strain on our blood suppliers. We manage these units closely and wasted 0.3% of them in the second year of operation.

We have met the challenge of the limited donor base and supply of AB universal donor plasma by working with our major regional blood supplier to build capacity for producing group A low-titer anti-B liquid plasma as A donors are 10 times as common as AB donors, 40 versus 4% of the population. This has had the secondary benefit that they are now providing anti-A and anti-B titers for our group O apheresis platelets as well, helping us determine the units that might be best to give out of type to meet day-to-day demand. The failure of the country to support the development of a universal freeze-dried plasma product for use in military, field, and remote care remains a limiting problem in delivering resuscitation across the sparsely populated parts of the Washington, Wyoming, Alaska, Montana, and Idaho (WWAMI) region that the University of Washington hospitals supports.

Maintaining a platelet inventory in a hospital that uses only 1400 units of apheresis platelets a year but may use 10 or more units on a single patient going through 10 or more cycles of a 6:6:1 MTP in several hours requires hard choices about inventory size. We use 4 ± 2 U of apheresis platelets a day in a random pattern. We are lucky that our major regional blood supplier is six blocks down the street and our restocking time can be as short as an hour. We have chosen to keep 5 units of apheresis platelets on hand. Increasing outpatient oncology patients and longer platelet storage offer potential ways to allow a larger inventory without wasting a valuable resource.

Cryoprecipitate, the fourth component often used in massive transfusion, is easily maintained in inventory because it has a 1-year storage outdate. We give it only in response to a measured low plasma fibrinogen and use about 300 pools of 5 units each year.

The air ambulance blood system, which we developed slowly over a period of several years, is based on small eutectic coolers holding 2 units of group O Rh(D)-negative RBCs and 2 units of group A low-titer anti-B liquid plasma. The boxes are sealed with a breakaway plastic lock and validated to maintain temperature for

a week if the box itself is not out of the refrigerator for more than 24 h during that time. Small, continuously reading electronic temperature monitors are in each box, and as a back up to the temperature monitoring system, high precision measuring of the temperature of the units is performed at the time the box is unpacked. Once a box is opened for use, it is to be returned immediately thereafter to protect the unused units, and the whole box is replaced. With 10 boxes out at any time, four components in each box, and 52 weeks in a year, we cycled more than 2000 components through the system in 2017, using 207 units in the field and providing blood products to 102 patients. We wasted a dozen units through storage failures. With intensive training of the flight nurses, we have instituted the practice of providing plasma as the first unit given. As a result, 70% of all the units we give are plasma with a concomitant savings of the rare O Rh(D)-negative RBCs.

It is important to note that our approach to massive transfusion is integral to our service's overall risk management strategy. The safest blood product remains the one not given. As a highly academic hospital that took up some of the pieces of patient blood management early, Harborview has seen its blood use decline by almost 65% since 2003. This represents a 50% decrease in RBCs, a 70% decrease in plasma units, a 75% decrease in platelet units, and a 90% decrease in cryoprecipitate pools. The 23,000 blood products a year that are no longer given have saved the hospital more than $2 million a year in blood costs, 46,000 h per year of nursing time, and probably prevented 200 transfusion reactions each year.

We have a robust quality system for a small transfusion service. Our Quality Manager is a Certified Quality Accountant and Certified Quality Manager by the American Society for Quality. We conduct continuous and spot audits constantly. Our Transfusion Service Manager is a Blood Bank Inspector who serves on the AABB Inspections Committee, and our Training Lead is on the AABB Standards Committee. Our Medical Directors contributed 40 papers and book chapters to the literature last year while serving on AABB committees in leadership roles. We maintain a culture of continuing education and evidence-based excellence as was noted on our last AABB inspection, which was observed by the Washington State Department of Health and Center for Medicare & Medicaid Services. They found no deficiencies.

It takes time to build a system like this one. We are blessed with good leadership and good governance. Our workers struggle to improve their skills and we are training our sixth Specialist in Blood Banking in

7 years. The attention to education and quality has paid off as higher grades in the national certifying exams of our undergraduate Clinical Laboratory Scientist students and our Clinical Pathology Residents. In turn, our students and residents help with our quality audits.

The effectiveness of blood products and blood usage is hard to measure. In the PROPPR trial, Harborview had better than average mortality in both arms of the study and delivered RBC units that were younger than any other study site. We participated in the BEST Collaborative STAT study comparing the safety and effectiveness of A plasma in trauma but chose to locally shorten the outdate on the product to improve the function of coagulation factors known to have short effective half-lives. Specifically, we have not taken up pathogen reduction technologies for individual clinical blood components because we believe that the trade-offs between substantial loss of potency and minimal gains in safety represent a net loss in utility for our massively transfused patients.[12] Similarly, we are trying to maintain full supplies of apheresis platelets in plasma rather than move to probably minimally safer platelet additive solutions because the loss of 200 mL of plasma per unit represents a potential loss of hemostatic effectiveness during massive transfusion which, using estimates from the PROPPR study, might cost hundreds of lives each year in the country and so outweighs the risk of TRALI and other plasma transfusion risks.

As mentioned in the section on availability earlier, there is a need for a broader range and higher effectiveness of blood products. The need for better and longer lasting platelet storage needs no comment. As we try to develop new freeze-dried plasma products, efforts should be made to remove the antibodies to reduce reactions, and remove some of the albumin to increase the effective concentrations of the coagulation factors while maintaining the volume expanding properties of a unit. Finally, better storage of RBCs with a lower acid load and better 2,3-DPG preservation have already been developed and licensed.

And finally, cost. The high cost of medical care is a risk to the health of us all. Any of us may eventually need the healthcare services we try to provide for everyone, so if we price those services out of range they will not be there when we need them. The cost of a 10-unit hemostatic massive transfusion is about $4000 in basic blood components and perhaps four times that much when the cost of the transfusion service and the associated clinical care are added. In other words, it is about half the cost of a cardiac pacemaker.[13]

Cost is a risk because, as my administrator says, "no margin, no mission". In a situation of declining resources, administrators look for places to cut expenses. Blood bank quality programs and education programs like our transfusion safety officer's "Blood School" are vulnerable despite demonstrably saving more money than they cost, simply because they are not viewed as direct care. A simple way to think about the problem is that a Transfusion Medicine physician can pay for themself just by talking another physician out of giving a unit of platelets each day.

Risk management in massive transfusion is a sophisticated science and art. On the science side, it needs to deliver the right products to the right patient in a timely manner and for the right reason. On the art side, it needs to be available, safe, effective, and cheap. Other doctors, nurses, and administrators need to think of massive transfusion as not a disaster, but as a protocol that in their hands and hospital runs smoothly and effectively. We want them to be proud of taking part in a lifesaving protocol while showing appropriate stewardship for an expensive and rare regional resource. We want our patients to do well in a situation where speed and accuracy count. Risk is all around us. Management is a science and an art.

REFERENCES

1. Halmin M, Chiesa F, Vasan SK, et al. Epidemiology of massive transfusion: a binational study from Sweden and Denmark. *Crit Care Med.* 2016;44(3):468–477.
2. Dzik WS, Ziman A, Cohn C, et al. Biomedical excellence for safer transfusion collaborative. Survival after ultra-massive transfusion: a review of 1360 cases. *Transfusion.* 2016;56(3):558–563.
3. Savage SA, Sumislawski JJ, Zarzaur BL, Dutton WP, Croce MA, Fabian TC. The new metric to define large-volume hemorrhage: results of a prospective study of the critical administration threshold. *J Trauma Acute Care Surg.* 2015;78(2):224–229.
4. Hess JR, Thomas MJG. Blood use in war and disaster: lessons from the last century. *Transfusion.* 2003;43:1622–1633.
5. Spinella PC, Perkins JG, Grathwohl KW, Beekley AC, Holcomb JB. Warm fresh whole blood is independently associated with improved survival for patients with combat-related traumatic injuries. *J Trauma.* 2009;66(4 Suppl): S69–S76.
6. Moise Jr KJ, Argoti PS. Management and prevention of red cell alloimmunization in pregnancy: a systematic review. *Obstet Gynecol.* 2012;120(5):1132–1139.
7. Daniel-Johnson J1, Leitman S, Klein H, et al. Quillen K Probiotic-associated high-titer anti-B in a group A platelet donor as a cause of severe hemolytic transfusion reactions. *Transfusion.* 2009;49(9):1845–1849.

8. Malone DL, Hess JR, Fingerhut A. Massive transfusion practices around the globe and a suggestion for a common massive transfusion protocol. *J Trauma*. 2006;60(suppl 6): S91–S96.

9. Dunbar NM, Yazer MH. Biomedical excellence for safer transfusion (BEST) collaborative and the STAT study investigators. Safety of the use of group A plasma in trauma: the STAT study. *Transfusion*. 2017;57(8):1879–1884.

10. Como JJ, Dutton RP, Scalea TJ, Edelman BB, Hess JR. Blood transfusion rates in the care of acute trauma. *Transfusion*. 2004;44:809–813.

11. Hess JR, Ramos PJ, Sen NE, et al. Quality management of a massive transfusion protocol. *Transfusion*. 2018;58: 480–484.

12. Hess JR, Pagano MB, Barbeau JM, Johannson PI. Will pathogen reduction of blood components harm more people than it helps in developed countries? *Transfusion*. 2016;56(5):1236–1241.

13. Shander A, Hofmann A, Ozawa S, Theusinger OM, Gombotz H, Spahn DR. Activity-based costs of blood transfusions in surgical patients at four hospitals. *Transfusion*. 2010;50(4):753–765.

CHAPTER 13

Clinical Risk in Apheresis-Derived Cellular Therapy

CAROLINE R. ALQUIST, MD, PHD, D(ABHI)

INTRODUCTION

Risk management programs require active engagement with, and understanding of, process points encountered regularly by hospital services. The process by which Transfusion Medicine Services, in collaboration with clinical colleagues, obtain, store, and utilize apheresis-derived cellular therapy products is fraught with clinical risk at each step. This chapter aims to lay bare these inherent and residual risks, while exploring potential controls and requirements, many of which are mandated by accrediting body standards. The authors hope this information will facilitate controlled self-assessment processes in your own institutions.

APHERESIS-DERIVED CELLULAR PRODUCTS

Cellular immunotherapy is a rapidly growing field that harnesses the immunologic potential of autologous and allogeneic cellular products. These products are divided into subcategories, based upon the following:

1. the product composition at collection and
2. the product's target cell population after enumeration, manufacturing, or processing steps.[1]

In the first category, cellular therapy products obtained by apheresis include hematopoietic progenitor cells (HPC(A)) and mononuclear cells (MNC(A)). If these products are to be used for direct infusion, they maintain their original nomenclature. If manipulated, these products are placed in the second subcategory of nomenclature and renamed accordingly as follows: dendritic cells (DC(A)), malignant cells (MALIG(A)), natural killer cells (NK(A)), or T lymphocytes (T CELLS(A)). In an important exception, HPC(A) may retain their name despite manipulation if they are used as a source for hematopoietic progenitor cells.[1] Nomenclature is summarized in Table 13.1.

HPC(A) products contain mobilized autologous or allogenic CD34+ cell-rich peripheral blood mononuclear cells. It is worth noting that while hematopoietic progenitor cells for stem cell transplant are invariably mobilized for apheresis collection, other collections for cellular immunotherapy using hematopoietic progenitors, lymphocytes, and monocytes are assumed not to have been mobilized unless otherwise indicated. HPC(A) products have been increasingly used to replace the hematologic system in patients with hematologic disease, following varied preparative conditioning regimens of chemotherapy and radiation. Autologous HPC transplant use is optimized for curative treatment of non-Hodgkin and Hodgkin lymphomas and to promote disease-free survival in patients with multiple myeloma. Lack of graft versus host disease (GVHD), and therefore decreased mortality, in autologous transplant renders them more amenable to use in older patients.[2] By comparison, allogeneic HPC products are potentially curative in acute and chronic leukemia, myelodysplastic syndrome, and aplastic anemia. Advances in human leukocyte antigen (HLA) matching, pretransplant conditioning regimens, and earlier interventions continue to improve allogeneic transplant outcomes.[2]

Allogeneic minimally manipulated MNC product, MNC(A), is frequently collected in tandem with mobilized allogeneic HPC(A) for donor lymphocyte infusion (DLI), but mobilization is not required. CD3+ cell counts are used as surrogate markers for immunotherapeutic potency of the product, as higher initial CD3+ cell doses correlate with increased antitumor properties and GVHD risk.[3,4] Although no standard treatment exists for relapse following allogenic hematopoietic stem cell transplant, DLI with deescalated immune suppression is a common therapy.[4] DLI effectiveness has been highlighted in the treatment of relapsing chronic myeloid leukemia (CML) after transplant, but responses in other hematologic malignancies posttransplant remain poorly defined.[4]

Autologous peripheral blood MNC(A) may be collected for adoptive cell transfer therapy. Peripheral blood MNC source product is required for lymphocyte isolation and creation of T CELL(A). Amplified memory T lymphocytes of T CELL(A) can be used to create stimulated naïve T lymphocytes and engineered (transfected or transduced) T lymphocytes capable of

Risk Management in Transfusion Medicine. https://doi.org/10.1016/B978-0-323-54837-3.00013-4

TABLE 13.1
Apheresis-Derived Cellular Therapy Products

Subcategory 1: Product Composition at Collection	Subcategory 2: Product Target Cell Population after Manipulation
HPC(A): hematopoietic progenitor cells	HPC(A): hematopoietic progenitor cells[a]
MNC(A): mononuclear cells	T CELLS(A): T lymphocytes
	DC(A): dendritic cells
	NK(A): natural killer cells
	MALIG(A): malignant cells

[a]HPC(A) do not technically fall under subcategory 2, but are placed there to graphically demonstrate that these cells may retain their nomenclature despite manipulation.

highly targeted behaviors. Autologous cells T CELL(A) exposed in vivo to tumoral antigens can be cocultured with antigen presenting cells (APCs), then expanded in the presence of IL-2, stimulatory antibodies, and irradiated accessory cells or antigen-coated beads.[5] T cells exposed to viruses require only repeated exposure to viral antigen-exposed APCs and IL-2. After in vitro expansion, clonal reactivity to antigen of interest is confirmed and then the cells are ready for recipient infusion or cryopreservation. Conversely, naïve T-cell conversion to antigen-specific T cells requires ex vivo exposure to dendritic cells that have been primed with tumoral or viral antigens of interest, followed by clonal T-cell expansion, as discussed earlier. Once infused, these cells have been shown to home to tumoral sites but do not typically persist in the circulation beyond 3 weeks.[5] Because less differentiated effector cells have been shown to persist longer than more differentiated effector cells, culture methods to enrich for less differentiated CD8+ memory T cells are being optimized.

Autologous T cells from T CELL(A) can also be engineered to express specific cloned T-cell receptors (TCRs) or artificial chimeric antigen receptors (CARs). TCRs known to recognize specific tumoral antigens in cloned populations can be induced in autologous cells via transduction with a viral vector encoding TCRα and β chain genes. This methodology is limited by the existing library of conserved tumor-specific proteins. Roughly 40% of transduced cells will express the TCR of interest, which can be expanded and infused into the patient.[5] In CAR T-cell engineering, however, autologous T cells are transduced to express artificial antibody variable regions that do not require major histocompatibility complex antigen

presentation and can recognize cell surface protein and nonprotein targets. Primed or engineered, expanded T cells will secrete cytokines, proliferate, and trigger cell death when they encounter their targets. Successful application of CAR T-cell therapy has been reported in both hematologic malignancies and solid tumors. The ability of CAR T cells to recognize any surface antigen, protein or otherwise, make them particularly adept at recognizing poorly immunogenic or immunoevasive tumoral cells.[6,7]

Autologous MNC(A) or HPC(A) may also be used as source products for dendritic cells (DC(A)). Dendritic cells can be directly isolated or differentiated ex vivo, and then matured in culture with inflammatory cytokines, and exposed to target antigens.[8,9] These antigens may be introduced in the form of peptides, proteins, immune complexes, whole cells, cell lysates, microbial vectors, or nucleic acids.[5,8] This process arms the dendritic cells with relevant surface antigens that will induce and guide cytotoxic T-cell behavior in vivo. After preparation, dendritic cells may be infused fresh or stored frozen without compromising activity.[10] Utilization capitalizes on their antigen-presentation and T-cell stimulating properties. Essentially, infusion of tumor or viral antigen-exposed dendritic cells serves as an antitumor "vaccine", activating highly specific cytotoxic and memory T-cell activities. Active Phase III clinical trials continue to explore this immunotherapy in prostate cancer, colorectal malignancies, glioblastoma, and melanoma.

Enriched for cells expressing CD56 and not CD3, NK(A) may also be derived from either autologous or allogeneic MNC(A) or HPC(A) and show a strong potential for clinical use in DLI or for CAR-engineering purposes. Allogeneic NK-DLI, unstimulated or primed in vitro with IL-2, may exert a promising graft versus leukemia or tumor effect when administered following stem cell transplantation.[11-13] CAR-engineered cells may also be generated from NK(A) using the aforementioned techniques, but experience has been primarily limited to preclinical trials and often utilizes NK cell lines rather than NK(A) source material.[14]

MALIG(A) isolation may be helpful in a variety of situations, such as in research requiring the investigation of the tumoral antigens or mechanisms or for target antigen priming of effector cells.

DONOR SELECTION AND EVALUATION

The process of donor appraisal prior to acceptance for apheresis collection addresses three main areas of inherent risk: infectious disease transmission; injury to the donor or recipient; and ensuring that all involved parties understand the procedure. The latter concern is no less important than the others. Complete understanding and endorsement of the procedure empowers the participants and assures fully informed consent.

Infectious disease transmission risk is inherent to any procedure in which an allogeneic product is transferred to another individual. Steps must be taken to address risks posed by any products that could potentially cross-contaminate other units in storage. Infectious risk is addressed early in the process via donor eligibility screening. Potential donors are asked to complete a donor health history questionnaire (DHQ), undergo a limited physical exam. They also undergo a battery of infectious disease testing, and have their available medical records reviewed for high-risk exposures or behaviors.

The DHQ is a standardized guide for those performing donor history evaluations to identify infectious disease risk due to medical history or behavioral factors. This questionnaire addresses risk for hepatitis, HIV, HTLV, West Nile virus, transmissible spongiform encephalopathy, parasites (e.g., malaria, Chagas, babesiosis), bacterial contamination, xenotransplantation, or recent vaccination. The limited physical exam assesses viral risk via identification of tattoos, body piercings, or recent vaccinations. FDA-mandated laboratory evaluation for blood-borne pathogens includes testing for HIV-1, HIV-2, Hepatitis B, Hepatitis C, syphilis, HTLV-1, HTLV-2, West Nile, and cytomegalovirus. Additional testing may also include tests for Chagas disease, *Toxoplasma gondii*, varicella zoster virus, herpes simplex virus, and Epstein-Barr virus. Additionally, testing for microbial contamination of all cellular therapy products is required by the FDA to further ensure its safety. This will be addressed in the storage and manufacturing section of this chapter.

Based on the results of the aforementioned screening, the donor can be designated as "eligible" or "noneligible" and the product labeled accordingly. A "noneligible" designation does not preclude the ability to donate cellular product if the donor is found to be medically suitable and urgent medical need exists (and is documented). Medical suitability is addressed later.

To mitigate the risk of injuring the donor or harming the recipient, separate physicians from the clinical team take responsibility for determining donor and recipient medical suitability, respectively. For the donor, this evaluation includes a history and physical exam to assess overall health, a chest X-ray, an electrocardiogram, and laboratory tests to rule out hematologic and metabolic disorders. The general health assessment, similar to any standard history and physical exam, must include a health history, review of medications and allergies, and a review of family and social histories. The laboratory evaluation for medical suitability typically includes a complete blood count with differential, complete metabolic panel, urinalysis, ABO/Rh typing, and albumin or protein electrophoresis. Additionally, serum pregnancy tests and hemoglobin S screening are required, as applicable. Donor testing is designed to evaluate for hematologic and metabolic disorders, as well as conditions that may put the donor at risk during the collection process. For example, pregnancy is typically a contraindication for donation and sickle hemoglobinopathies can place a donor at risk for splenic rupture if given filgrastim for HPC(A) mobilization.

The physical exam process assesses overall health and identifies issues that may impact the safety and efficacy of donated cellular product, as well as the safety of the collection process. Beyond the detection of factors that would render a cellular product undesirable, such as genetic diseases of the hematopoietic system, focus is placed on candidacy for donation modality. Direct marrow extraction versus HPC(A) collection require separate health considerations, as these procedures are not without potential danger. Given the risk of mechanical injury or surgical complications, the ability to donate marrow may be hindered by a history of previous surgeries or anticipated difficulty accessing the iliac crest areas, unfavorable experiences with anesthesia, presence of neurologic, cardiovascular, respiratory, or musculoskeletal issues, or presence of acute or chronic pain of the back or lower extremities. Conversely, patients are generally excluded from HPC(A) donations if they are found to have an autoimmune disease, sickle cell disease or trait, splenic disorders, thrombocytopenia, thrombotic disorders, iritis or episcleritis, sensitivity to *E. coli* derived recombinant protein products, or are currently breastfeeding or taking lithium. Presence of these factors may jeopardize the health and well-being of the donor. The process of medical suitability or deferral may steer a donor toward one collection methodology or another, or may eliminate collection candidacy all together.

The clinical team must also take care to confirm that the patient has adequately comprehended and considered the presented information. Donors with limited English proficiency are common and the value of interpreter services cannot be underestimated. Care must be taken to use interpreters with medical procedure and consenting familiarity, rather than family members alone. Easy access to these services has been shown not only to improve patient satisfaction, but also to improve quality of care and outcomes.[15]

Other situations may also confound the consenting process, such as situations involving related or minor donors. Transplant teams must take care to avoid conflicts of interest in the evaluation process and explore feelings of obligation in these cases to protect the donor and recipient adequately. Ethical and legal issues surrounding appropriate consent and assent to collection must also be addressed and documented in pediatric donor candidate workups. Both autologous and allogeneic cellular therapy regimens require intense interdisciplinary coordination to ensure a safe treatment regimen. Avoidable delays or cancellations in donation due to misunderstandings or incomplete donor evaluation can have devastating consequences for the potential recipient.

APHERESIS COLLECTION

Beyond donor eligibility and medical suitability, the donor must be adequately briefed on the procedure and potential complications and consent to the procedure early in the planning process. Potential donors must be adequately prepared, physically and mentally, prior to initiation of collection. Donor consent must include the explanation of why the cellular product is needed, why they have been selected as a candidate, and the clinical process of mobilization, collection, and potential side effects. The consent for collection is typically obtained by the Transfusion Medicine apheresis physician.

Hematopoietic progenitor cell (HPC) collection once relied solely upon direct marrow harvest, but advances in mobilization strategies now permit peripheral blood collections by apheresis. Circulating HPC numbers can be augmented via cytoreductive chemotherapy (e.g., cyclophosphamide, etoposide, ifosfamide, and paclitaxel) and chemokine administration (e.g., G-CSF, GM-CSF, and plerixafor).[2] Mobilization and collection processes are not without risk. Filgrastim, a recombinant form of G-CSF, is commonly used for HPC(A) mobilization and is associated with mild splenomegaly for up to 10 days following collection. Splenic rupture and lung injury have been reported as rare but potential complications of G-CSF dosages.[16] Counseling patients to avoid activities that may result in splenic trauma is advised. Additionally, filgrastim may cause increased alanine aminotransferase, alkaline phosphatase, and lactate dehydrogenase levels; transient thrombocytopenia and neutropenia; bone pain; and flu-like symptoms. Other rare serious adverse events include capillary leak syndrome, retinal hemorrhage, acute iritis, gouty arthritis, and thrombotic events.[17]

Given these risks, filgrastim should not be administered if leukocytes counts are greater than 60 K/μL. The long-term risks of filgrastim administration are unknown, but none have been conclusively identified to date. Additionally, HPC(A) donors may also receive plerixafor to augment their circulating hematopoietic progenitor counts. Nausea, diarrhea, injection site reactions, bone pain, paresthesias, headache, and dizziness have all been reported as side effects, which must be discussed with the potential donor.[17,18]

Reliable venous access is requisite to adequate apheresis collections and options must be discussed with the donor. Peripheral access is typically preferred, although the positional requirements, potential venospasm, and anticipated duration of collection must be discussed with the donor. Discomfort due to venospasm, hematoma, or infection at the site of the needle, which will be in place for several hours, may occur. Central venous access is available for those with tenuous venous access, positional limitations, or preference, but is accompanied by other concerns. These include anesthesia requirements for placement, procedural complications at insertion, sepsis risk, thrombus formation, and catheter fracture or embolization.

The basics of HPC(A) and MNC(A) collections involve drawing whole blood into a system in which it is separated by centrifugal forces. The buffy coat is diverted into a separate chamber where opposing centrifugal and inlet blood flow forces retain the mononuclear cells of interest while pushing platelet and red blood cell content back to the donor's return line. These procedures require large volume processing and are typically quite time intensive. The most common risks to discuss with a donor involve the effects of citrate anticoagulant. Lowered calcium levels may cause tingling sensations around the mouth, hands and body or muscle cramps, nausea, and vomiting. Symptoms may progress to tetany and seizures if calcium levels continue to fall.[19] In addition to calcium, citrate also binds magnesium. Symptoms of hypomagnesemia include muscle spasms, muscle weakness, decreased vascular tone, and impaired cardiac contractility.[19] To combat these citrate effects, apheresis donors may be proactively repleted with calcium and postprocedural serum chemistries are routinely ordered to identify and treat any potential deficiencies prior to discharge.

Platelet and red blood cell loss with collection may occur as a result of the centrifugal separation method. To combat this possibility, it is routine to obtain a post-collection complete blood count to assess for iatrogenic anemia and thrombocytopenia. Platelet or red blood cell transfusions are routinely offered in these cases and the consenting process should address the relative risks of reaction and infectious disease transmission.

Regardless of access type, a small risk of air bubble formation is present given the use of a circuit in continuous flow with the central venous system. Death or brain damage due to air embolism is exceedingly rare. Risk is mitigated for this unlikely occurrence by the multiple sensors and alarms present on the machine and nurse presence during the procedure, but the patient must be briefed on this theoretical danger. Should an air embolus be suspected, the patient should be placed in Trendelenburg positioning on their left side, while evaluating and assessing the event. If the concern for a large air embolus is high, surgical intervention may be required.[19]

Additionally, hypotension, lightheadedness, and syncope may occur during routine apheresis procedures due to a combination of vasovagal, fluid shift, and citrate reactions. Lastly, shock, irregular heartbeats, and death have been reported in association with this procedure, but are attributed to underlying illnesses rather than the cellular therapy collection per se.[17]

Overall apheresis collections are typically uneventful except for the stress of central venous line placement or peripheral venous access, which may require sustained uncomfortable arm placement. In contrast, bone marrow donors of HPC or other cellular products require anesthesia, with its associated rare complications, along with potential mechanical injury to the bone and soft tissue of the pelvic region. After the completion of either apheresis or marrow collection, the most common reported symptoms are skeletal pain, fatigue, and insomnia. The median time to resolution of these complaints is 3 weeks for marrow donation and 1 week for HPC(A) donation.[17] Transfusion Services or apheresis teams routinely perform these time-intensive procedures without incident, but care must be taken to explain the anticipated and remote risks associated with each collection method so that they do not come as surprise. All cellular therapy programs must maintain a process to detect, report, evaluate, and manage donor adverse events in accordance with the facility's policies, applicable laws, and accrediting agency standards, and regulations.[20]

STORAGE AND MANUFACTURING OF THE CELLULAR THERAPY PRODUCT

Following a successful apheresis collection, the product must be transferred to storage and/or manufacturing facilities. As the cells move from bedside to lab to storage location, chain of custody remains an important concept to prevent errors in storage and delivery to the correct patient with appropriate viability. Seamless communication and training between all clinical entities is key. In addition, transport times and temperature impact viability. Accrediting agencies have issued guidance to standardize these processes, including temperature and transport requirements, and require facility agreements that address these rules and responsibilities.[20]

Once the product has arrived at the lab, it must be enumerated and evaluated for contamination and viability. Enumeration of HPC(A) requires a CD34 positive cell count. CD34 is a surface protein expressed by many primitive progenitor cells, including HPCs, and serves as a surrogate marker for hematopoietic regenerative potency and is typically measured by flow cytometry. Typical dosages for HPC transplant require CD34+ cell numbers $>2 \times 10^6$ CD34+ cells/kg. MNC(A) enumeration may utilize a simple hemocytometer or more sophisticated surface protein staining to characterize the product's target cell population. The product would then be renamed as DC(A), MALIG(A), NK(A), or T CELLS(A), as appropriate. Further manipulation may occur to stimulate, amplify, differentiate, or engineer cellular products for the intended therapeutic effect. The products may be infused fresh to the recipient, or stored, typically in liquid nitrogen, until needed.

The cryopreservation process utilizes a cryoprotectant known as dimethyl sulfoxide (DMSO) to preserve cells. DMSO concentrations are not standardized. Facilities report using 5%, 7.5%, or 10% DMSO concentrations. Lab-specific freezing parameters may also employ hydroxyethyl starch (HES), dextran, albumin, plasma, saline, normosol, and plasmalyte. The long-term effectiveness of these different freezing solutions are still being evaluated. Additionally the cryopreservation protocols differ by institution and may use controlled rate or dump method freezing procedures. All methods must balance viability concerns of intracellular ice crystal formation seen when freezing rates are too rapid, with cellular crenation seen when freezing rates are too slow and water moves out of the cells. Additionally, procedures must be in place to evaluate white blood cell counts and assess contamination.

Bacterial contamination remains a concern throughout collection and processing. It has been reported that approximately 3% of peripheral blood HPCs are bacterially contaminated.[21] Microbial contamination testing is required on all products, but the ability to confirm sterility may be superseded by the required timely infusion of the product. Sources of contamination for cellular products include chronic persistent donor infection, indwelling catheters, endemic hospital flora, or, in the case of cord blood or fetal cell sources, vaginal and fecal bacteria. Conventional sterilization mechanisms, such as filtration or heating, are not feasible with cellular therapy products. Importantly, contaminated products may still be used with appropriate antimicrobial treatment in concert with urgent medical need documentation and clinical physician approval.

Viral contamination must also be considered, as even units from negative donors may be vulnerable in storage. Hepatitis B product cross-contamination and spread has been reported in liquid phase nitrogen storage.[22] For this reason, most facilities not only store cryopreserved products in vapor phase liquid nitrogen, but also physically quarantine in separate freezers products that are untested or have positive infectious disease results.

Another risk management practice in cellular therapy storage is the requirement of facility-specific plans for internal and external disasters. Examples of internal disasters include fire, loss of utilities, worker strikes, workplace violence, smoke, fumes, release of chemicals or radiation, hostage situation, or bomb threats. External disasters include earthquakes, hurricanes, tornadoes, storms, floods, fire, riots, train derailment, plane crashes, power outages, and terrorist attacks. Required components of an emergency plan must address communication and notification procedures, assessment of required services, defined staffing needs and capabilities, decision-making trees, and service expectations. Additionally, facilities must consider priority transport of active patient products, as well as additional inventory relocation methods. Agreements with other facilities for housing must be in place to accommodate defined evacuation plans.

Another storage consideration must be the lengths of storage and terms of removal from inventory. No federally established maximum expiration date for cellular products has been established and no reimbursement code for storage of cellular therapy product exists. The exponential space requirements and cost of storage in a growing program is absorbed by lab. Clinical programs must proactively discuss storage limits and indications for disposal beyond patient demise.

CELLULAR THERAPY PRODUCT UTILIZATION

Risk is inherent in the product infusion phase of cellular therapy, as well. One of the most well-known cellular therapy infusion risks is due to the previously discussed cryopreservative DMSO. When used for cryopreservation, this agent may constitute 10% of HPC(A) product and has been associated with a lengthy list of adverse effects. During infusion a noxious garlic odor can be noted by anyone in the room, which may be accompanied by nausea and vomiting by the recipient. DMSO may also initiate histamine-associated symptoms, including pruritis, rash, flushing, wheezing, and low-grade fever. These symptoms may be impossible to distinguish from mild allergic reactions that may occur with any cellular therapy infusion, but, in either case, they are treated similarly. More serious reported sequelae include hypertension, tachycardia, and myocardial infarction, although the pathogenesis of these more severe reactions is unknown. DMSO toxicity is mitigated by limiting infusion volumes to 1 mL per kilogram of recipient weight per day, reducing the thaw to infusion timeline to prevent DMSO warming, and premedication with antihistamines and antiemetics. Alternatively, cellular products may be washed to remove cryopreservant, but potential for diminished yield is a concern.

When a patient receives allogeneic cellular therapy products, blood group and antibody incompatibility must be considered. Antibodies to ABO and other blood system antigens have the potential to cause acute intravascular hemolysis, which typically manifests as a fever with flank or lower back pain, tachycardia, and hypotension. Hemoglobinuria and hemoglobinemia may also occur. Acute renal failure, disseminated intravascular coagulation, shock, or death may occur secondary to the hemolysis. Treatment of this adverse event type is primarily supportive, aimed at preventing or treating shock and protecting the kidneys. To prevent such events, donors and recipients are ABO/Rh typed and screened for blood antibodies. If an incompatible ABO/Rh is necessary, red cell depletion or plasma reduction of the product can be performed, with similar concerns for product loss, as mentioned previously. Additionally, preinfusion therapeutic plasma exchange can facilitate recipient antibody removal.

As previously mentioned, bacterial contamination is not uncommon in cellular therapy products and is not an absolute contraindication to infusion. Cultures obtained following collection are typically sufficient to identify contaminating organisms so that appropriate antimicrobial therapy can be initiated prior to or during the relevant product infusion. Symptoms may include fever, tachycardia, hypotension, nausea, and vomiting. In cases where bacterial contamination of an infused product is suspected despite negative cultures, supportive care and broad spectrum antibiotics should be initiated until appropriate microbial identification and susceptibilities are completed. Decisions to stop product infusion must be relayed to the clinical team.

Volume overload remains a concern whenever any product is intravenously infused. Any volume may precipitate acute respiratory distress if it cannot be effectively processed by the recipient due to excessive infusion rate or underlying heart or lung pathology. Symptoms may include dyspnea, hypoxemia, tachycardia, hypertension, and jugular venous distension. If this occurs, the infusion rate should be slowed while the head of the patient's bed is elevated. Supportive care and diuresis may be necessary.

In the absence of volume overload, dyspnea, hypoxemia, tachycardia during cellular product infusion is likely to suggest acute lung injury. Granulocytes and plasma containing neutrophil antibodies or other proinflammatory cytokines, if present in a cellular therapy product, may contribute to acute lung injury via induced capillary leakage, similar to the pathogenesis of transfusion-related acute lung injury (TRALI). In case of oxygen saturation levels dipping below 90%, supplemental oxygen should be provided in additional to supportive care and consideration of stopping the infusion. Plasma reduction of allogeneic cellular products may reduce the incidence of this complication.

Acute febrile reactions without hemolysis are common cellular therapy infusion events given high granulocyte content and the inability to leukoreduce these products. These reactions are generally short-lived and consist of low grade fevers, rigors, chills, and mild dyspnea in the absence of hemolysis. They can be managed with or without antipyretic medication and supportive therapy, but should be considered a diagnosis of exclusion. TRALI, hemolysis, and sepsis must be ruled out.

Lastly, cytokine release syndrome is another potentially life-threatening condition that may occur in response to antibody therapy, certain cancer drugs, stem cell transplants, or T-cell engaging immunotherapy infusions.[23] Elevated levels of cytokines, such as IL-10, IL-6, and IFN-γ, are released by the host in response to the product's immune activation. Symptoms range in severity from fever, myalgia, and fatigue to cardiac dysfunction, adult respiratory distress syndrome, neurologic toxicity, renal failure, hepatic failure, and disseminated intravascular coagulation.[23,24] Corticosteroids may be used to control these responses, but may also dampen the desired immunologic effects of the therapy.[24]

Although cellular product infusions are generally well tolerated, closely monitoring vital signs throughout and following the infusion process is imperative to quickly recognize and appropriately treat any acute infusion-related adverse outcomes. All cellular therapy programs must have an active system for processes to detect, report, evaluate, and manage adverse events related to cellular therapy, including infusion, in accordance with the facility's policies, these CT Standards, and applicable laws and regulations. Reaction management is always specific to symptoms. As a last resort in each reaction, cessation of infusion is an option, though rarely employed given the grim outcomes without an alternative source of cells.

REFERENCES

1. *ISBT 128 STANDARD Standard Terminology for Medical Products of Human Origin, Version 7.7, 2017.*
2. Copelan EA. Hematopoietic stem-cell transplantation. *N Engl J Med.* 2006;354(17):1813–1826. https://doi.org/10.1056/NEJMra052638.
3. Chalandon Y, Passweg J, Schmid C, et al. Outcome of patients developing GVHD after DLI given to treat CML relapse: a study by the chronic leukemia working party of the EBMT. *Bone Marrow Transplant.* 2010;45(3):558–564.
4. Porter DL, Alyea EP, Antin JH, et al. NCI first international workshop on the biology, prevention, and treatment of relapse after allogeneic hematopoietic stem cell transplantation: report from the committee on treatment of relapse after allogeneic hematopoietic stem cell transplantation. *Biol Blood Marrow Transplant.* 2010;16(11):1467–1503.
5. McLeod BC, Szczepiorkowski Z, Weinstein R, Winters J. *Apheresis: Principles and Practice.* Karger, S; 2010.
6. Barrett DM, Singh N, Porter DL, Grupp SA, June CH. Chimeric antigen receptor therapy for cancer. *Annu Rev Med.* 2014;65:333–347. https://doi.org/10.1146/annurev-med-060512-150254.
7. Lee DW, Kochenderfer JN, Stetler-Stevenson M, et al. T cells expressing CD19 chimeric antigen receptors for acute lymphoblastic leukaemia in children and young adults: a phase 1 dose-escalation trial. *Lancet.* 2015;385(9967):517–528.
8. Thurner B, Röder C, Dieckmann D, et al. Generation of large numbers of fully mature and stable dendritic cells from leukapheresis products for clinical application. *J Immunol Methods.* 1999;223(1):1–15.
9. Yuan J, Kendle R, Ireland J, et al. Scalable expansion of potent genetically modified human langerhans cells in a closed system for clinical applications. *J Immunother.* 2007;30(6):634–643. https://doi.org/10.1097/CJI.0b013e31804efc8b.
10. Thumann P, Moc I, Humrich J, et al. Antigen loading of dendritic cells with whole tumor cell preparations. *J Immunol Methods.* 2003;277(1):1–16.
11. Rubnitz JE, et al. NKAML: a pilot study to determine the safety and feasibility of haploidentical natural killer cell transplantation in childhood acute myeloid leukemia. *J Clin Oncol.* 2010;28.6:955.

12. Ruggeri L, et al. Effectiveness of donor natural killer cell alloreactivity in mismatched hematopoietic transplants. *Science.* 2002;295(5562):2097–2100.

13. Passweg JR, et al. Natural-killer-cell-based treatment in haematopoietic stem-cell transplantation. *Best Practice Res Clin Haematol.* 2006;19.4:811–824.

14. Glienke W, et al. Advantages and applications of CAR-expressing natural killer cells. *Front Pharmacol.* 2015;6:21.

15. Flores G. The impact of medical interpreter services on the quality of health care: a systematic review. *Med Care Res Rev.* 2005;62.3:255–299.

16. Tigue CC, et al. Granulocyte-colony stimulating factor administration to healthy individuals and persons with chronic neutropenia or cancer: an overview of safety considerations from the Research on Adverse Drug Events and Reports project. *Bone Marrow Transplant.* 2007;40(3): 185–192.

17. Wingard JR, et al., ed. *Hematopoietic Stem Cell Transplantation: A Handbook for Clinicians.* AABB; 2015.

18. Dugan MJ, et al. Safety and preliminary efficacy of plerixafor (Mozobil) in combination with chemotherapy and G-CSF: an open-label, multicenter, exploratory trial in patients with multiple myeloma and non-Hodgkin's lymphoma undergoing stem cell mobilization. *Bone Marrow Transplant.* 2010;45(1):39.

19. Winters JL. Complications of donor apheresis. *J Clin Apher.* 2006;21(2):132–141.

20. *AABB Standards for Cellular Therapy Services.* 8th ed, September 2017.

21. Störmer M, et al. Bacterial safety of cell-based therapeutic preparations, focusing on haematopoietic progenitor cells. *Vox Sanguinis.* 2014;106(4):285–296.

22. Tedder RS, et al. Hepatitis B transmission from contaminated cryopreservation tank. *Lancet.* 1995;346(8968): 137–140.

23. Shimabukuro-Vornhagen A, et al. Cytokine release syndrome. *J Immunother Cancer.* 2018;6(1):56.

24. Maude SL, et al. Managing cytokine release syndrome associated with novel T cell-engaging therapies. *Cancer J.* 2014;20(2):119.

CHAPTER 14

Research Risks in Transfusion Medicine and Cellular Therapy

J. MILLS BARBEAU, MD, JD

Risk management and human subject research ethics intersect in fascinating ways in the context of transfusion medicine and cellular therapy research. In research involving human subjects, the study volunteer is paramount. The imperative to comply with ethical research requirements can potentially derail study protocols and limit data acquisition, in some cases restricting the amount of information that can be derived from a study. Important clinical questions must sometimes remain unanswered, even if the answers would improve patient outcomes or guide more rational therapy decisions. If the subject's autonomy or welfare is jeopardized, clinical progress must give way to the study subject's best interests. Unanswered questions must be sent back to the clinical arena.

Research on human subjects can raise important legal and compliance issues. If the research is federally funded, compliance with federally established principles and procedures is mandatory. Many institutions have also elected to adhere to federal standards voluntarily by executing a Federalwide Assurance[1] document, which is an election to follow federal standards for human subject research protections even for research that is not federally funded. Thus, human subject research standards, particularly those promulgated by federal regulations, establish a standard of care to which researchers are expected to adhere. Depending on the circumstances, a breach of that standard may give rise to lawsuits or sanctions.

Even research that is not specifically subject to federal regulations must take federal standards into account, since the standards are evidence of best practices in research. For federally regulated research, investigators and/or their institutions may be penalized for severe violations of human subject research protections with loss of eligibility for federal research funding. If private medical information is implicated in the negligence, privacy regulations such as HIPAA[2] establish causes of action for privacy breaches, as well as statutory civil and criminal penalties to the organizations conducting the research. In addition, individuals and organizations can suffer very significant reputational harm if they are guilty of ethical lapses that harm research subjects and/or disadvantaged populations.

Human subject research protections are not punitive, but protective. It is a tautology to state that adhering to the established ethical principles of human subject research is the right thing to do. The present, comprehensive framework of human subject research protections should be seen as a comprehensive risk management program: adherence to the protections is a highly reliable way to protect research subjects.

In this chapter, we will see how risk-based decisions in the research context have an impact on clinical practice. Thus, a focus of this chapter is the interplay between human subject research ethics and clinical decision making. We will start with a brief review of the core ethical principles governing human subjects research. The remaining sections will demonstrate how these ethical principles manifest themselves in familiar research settings in transfusion medicine and cellular therapy, and how research ethics impact clinical practice.

BACKGROUND: HUMAN SUBJECT RESEARCH ETHICS

The three ethical pillars of human subject research protections are autonomy, beneficence, and justice. How did this come to be? Prior to World War II, it was generally taken for granted that physicians and other scientists could be trusted to protect research volunteers. However, the war forced the international community to come to terms with horrific human experiments performed by Nazi physicians and scientists. The "Nazi Doctors Trial," was the second phase of the Nuremberg Trials. Twenty-three defendants were charged with atrocities relating to medical research. Prior to the Doctors Trial, it was unprecedented to try medical researchers criminally for abuses against humanity. Therefore, it was first necessary to set out universally accepted ethical principles of human subject research to use as a benchmark by which to judge the defendants' actions. The result was the

Risk Management in Transfusion Medicine. https://doi.org/10.1016/B978-0-323-54837-3.00014-6

Nuremberg Code. Two of the key protections set forth in the Nuremberg Code were the informed consent of research subjects (autonomy, also known as "respect for persons") and the avoidance of physical or mental suffering (beneficence, or more specifically, nonmalificence).

After World War II, there was a natural inclination, particularly in the United States, to see the Nazi doctors' atrocities as an aberration that could only have occurred in the unique context of Nazi Germany. Given the horrors that had been inflicted, such an assumption was perhaps understandable, although unfortunately not realistic. In fact, Nazi Germany was not the only axis country that performed reprehensible medical research on human beings during the Second World War.[3] Commentators, particularly in Europe, warned against complacency and suggested that the ethical principles guiding even routine clinical research needed to be clarified. In 1953, the World Medical Association (WMA) began developing an ethical framework for clinical research that incorporated and expanded upon the Nuremberg Code. In 1964, the WMA issued the Declaration of Helsinki, which among other things, reaffirmed the Nuremberg Code's principles of autonomy and beneficence. Later versions of the Declaration of Helsinki incorporated a third pillar, the ethical principle of justice, into the now-familiar triumvirate. Throughout this time period, a process of critical self-examination was taking place in the United States as well.[4] Ethical lapses were identified in several American research studies, and the lessons from those missteps ultimately contributed to the development of a highly refined system of federally mandated human subject research protections.

In the United States, the clinical trial that emphasized most clearly the importance of justice as a cornerstone of research ethics was the "Tuskegee Study of Untreated Syphilis in the Negro Male," which was carried out in Macon County, Alabama by the US Public Health Service beginning in 1932.[5] The purpose of the study was to observe the natural history of untreated syphilis. Subjects were recruited without being informed of the study's purpose, or in some cases, even being informed that they had syphilis. When the study began, there was no effective treatment for syphilis. The intent was to provide basic medical care to the subjects while studying the natural history of the disease. The observation period was initially planned to last only for a period of months. Incredibly, the project was extended several times, and was ultimately closed in 1972. Equally incredible was the fact that when penicillin was established in the late 1940s as an effective cure for syphilis, the Tuskegee subjects were not treated

with the drug. Tragically, several of the subjects' wives contracted syphilis during the study period (recall that the subjects were not aware of the diagnosis), and several children were born with congenital syphilis. The Tuskegee Study clearly violated the ethical obligation to respect subjects' *autonomy*, as evidenced by the lack of informed consent, and the duty of *beneficence* toward subjects, as evidenced by failing to inform them that they had syphilis and failing to treat them when penicillin became available. The Tuskegee Study also starkly illustrated the need to include *justice* as a pillar of human subject research protections. In human subject research, justice requires that one segment of society must not inequitably suffer the burdens of research for the benefit of other constituencies. Justice, the third ethical pillar, was clearly violated in the Tuskegee Study.

In the aftermath of Tuskegee and other cases, Congress passed the National Research Act in 1974.[6] The Act directed HHS to promulgate regulations for protecting human research subjects, and commissioned a report on the fundamental ethical principles that should guide those regulations. The Act also mandated Institutional Review Board (IRB) oversight at institutions performing federally funded human research. The commissioned report, known as the Belmont Report, was issued in 1979. It is the fundamental statement of ethical principles guiding human subject research in the United States. The core principles enunciated in the Belmont Report are autonomy, beneficence, and justice. In the regulations that were promulgated pursuant to the National Research Act, the primary expression of the Belmont Report is referred to as the "Common Rule" found in 45 CFR 46, Subpart A.[7]

The three ethical pillars of human subject research—autonomy, beneficence, and justice—can be considered pillars of clinical medical practice as well. The principle of autonomy, for example, requires informed consent prior to performing a procedure on a patient. Beneficence requires the utmost diligence in providing care, and placing the patient's interests before one's own. Nonmaleficence, the corollary of beneficence, is embodied in the preeminent clinical directive "first, do no harm". The concept of justice in an individual physician's clinical practice includes, for example, the distributive justice obligation to incorporate best practices into diagnostic and treatment decisions, to provide the most efficient, cost-effective medical care.

The three ethical principles also guide clinical research. However, because clinical research is largely controlled by federal regulations, the concepts of autonomy, beneficence, and justice have become more operationally defined in the research setting than they are in general medical practice. Autonomy (respect for persons) expresses itself in the requirement of informed consent. In the context of federally funded research, the content of consent forms is clearly delineated. In the case of vulnerable persons with limited autonomy, such as prisoners, children, or the intellectually impaired, respect for persons means identifying a surrogate decision maker who can provide consent on behalf of the subject, and who will protect the subject's best interests and withhold consent if appropriate. In the context of research, beneficence means that risks are minimized and reasonable in relation to the anticipated benefits expected to result from the research and the importance of the knowledge that will be generated. Justice means that selection of subjects is not disproportionate in terms of the allocation of burdens and benefits of the research, and research protocols must be designed to include as many subpopulations as is practicable so that all may share the benefits of the knowledge gained.

RESTRICTIONS IN TRAUMA RESEARCH AND WAIVERS OF INFORMED CONSENT

Research performed on trauma patients evokes concerns about patient autonomy because many research subjects will be in distress, under the influence of drugs or alcohol, or unconscious. Informed consent to treatment—let alone consent to participate in clinical research—may not be possible in many instances. For example, a randomized, controlled clinical trial protocol involving massive hemorrhage in trauma will inevitably involve patients who are unable to provide consent prior to being randomized to a treatment group. Surrogate decision makers cannot be a reliable option, since severely injured patients often arrive alone in an ambulance or life flight helicopter, often without reliable identification. One can randomize patients as they arrive, then approach them for consent after they have stabilized, deenrolling them if they refuse to give retroactive consent. However, these patients have already received treatment, which may or may not be the treatment they would have received had they not been randomized to one of the treatment arms. In short, they will have already participated in the trial, and the only available option is to suppress data, a solution that does not comport well with patient autonomy.

The US Department of Health and Human Services (DHHS) has developed a procedure for obtaining a waiver of consent for emergency research.[8] Although this might at first glance appear to be the solution to the problem of massive trauma research, the requirements for the waiver can be rigorous. To qualify for

the waiver, the following must be true: (1) subjects must be unable to provide informed consent due to the emergency; (2) it must be necessary to administer the intervention immediately, before it is feasible to obtain surrogate consent; (3) there can be no way to identify in advance the individuals likely to become eligible for participation in the study; (4) the subjects must be in a life-threatening situation; and (5) "available treatments are unproven or unsatisfactory." In fact, providing blood is a well-proven treatment for massive hemorrhage, nor could it be said to be "unsatisfactory." Indeed, as discussed in Chapter 12, several years of substantial experience derived from wartime[9] observations and followed by civilian practice,[10] have indicated that a close 1:1:1 ratio[11] of RBCs, plasma, and platelets is highly successful in improving outcomes in massive trauma. Close ratio resuscitation is responsible for saving countless lives, and at this point the close-ratio formula is well proven and satisfactory. However, can it be better? Close ratio resuscitation was discovered and validated almost entirely by retrospective reviews, and it has been so successful that it is now the standard of care for massive hemorrhage in trauma. Must we stop improving our protocols simply because the present approach is not "unproven or unsatisfactory"? The rule governing waivers of consent for emergency research suggest that further experimentation may not be permissible. At the very least, the rule suggests that there are risks associated with determining how to proceed.

Another source of risk must be considered when contemplating research involving trauma. The waiver of informed consent for emergency research is not available for research involving vulnerable populations, which includes prisoners. The line is grey as to whether some patients arriving in an emergency department might be considered prisoners. In trauma centers that care for patients suffering from penetrating trauma due to gun or knife injuries, or in emergency departments treating drunk drivers, some of whom may have killed or injured others in automobile accidents, or even in the case of individuals with outstanding bench warrants, the police may well be present and exercising a level of police custody, even if the patients themselves were rushed into the trauma bay on a stretcher. Such patients, if they qualify as prisoners, may not be acceptable subjects for waivers of informed consent for emergency research.

Another restriction placed on waivers of informed consent for emergency research is that the researchers must consult with representatives of the communities in which the research will be conducted, and from which the subjects will be drawn. The consultation must include descriptions of the research plan, the risks and expected benefits of the research, and the anticipated demographic characteristics of the study population. The notion behind the consultation is to explore community sensitivities and to achieve something akin to surrogate approval from individuals who share commonality with the as-yet unknown individuals who will be enrolled in the study.

RESEARCH ON THE RED BLOOD CELL STORAGE LESION

The issue of fresh versus old blood proved to be a context in which the principles of research ethics can be challenging. The red cell storage lesion consists of a constellation of changes that occur during red cell storage, such as alterations in the shape of the red blood cell, changes in the cell membrane, acidosis with concomitant changes in 2,3-diphosphoglycerate, decrease in nitric oxide binding to hemoglobin, and loss of ion compartmentalization.[12,13] These changes suggest that, with age, RBCs may become less effective in providing oxygen to tissues.

FDA did not consider clinical effectiveness when establishing storage requirements for red blood cells. The permitted shelf life of red blood cells was instead based on studies measuring in vitro hemolysis and in vivo recovery of radiolabeled red cells, rather than on clinical trials measuring effectiveness.[14] For licensure, the FDA requires evidence that at the end of the storage period, at least 75% of the transfused red cells remain in the circulation 24 h after infusion, and hemolysis must not exceed 1%.[15] Clinically, unanswered questions remained regarding the correlation, if any, between the red cell storage lesion and the clinical effectiveness of red blood cells. Many retrospective studies have been performed, but their findings are inconclusive, typically showing only slight differences or no differences at all in outcomes associated with red cell age.[16]

Large, prospective, randomized controlled trials were launched to try to resolve the issue of whether the age of stored red cells impacts their clinical effectiveness. The Age of Blood Evaluation (ABLE) trial, based in Canada, studied severely ill, adult ICU patients who were randomized into two groups, one receiving exclusively fresh RBCs ≤7 days old, and the other receiving standard-issue RBC units.[17] The Age of Red Blood Cells in Premature Infants (ARIPI) trial studied the clinical effect of fresh blood stored ≤7 days compared to standard issue red cells in very low birth weight infants in intensive care units.[18] The Red Cell Storage Duration Study (RECESS) study compared the effect of fresh RBCs of ≤10 days storage age versus units that were ≥21 days old in midsternotomy cardiac patients.[19]

The RECESS trial ran into ethical objections to its study design from the outset.[20] Most study designs, such as ABLE and ARIPI, compare fresh blood with standard practice, which means taking whatever is on the shelf in the order of "first in, first out" (FIFO). As stated by Flegel, Natanson, and Klein:

> Patients can be randomized to a fresh RBC group, which is commonly perceived as the improved treatment arm. Patients should not be treated with old RBC by design, and the control group is typically standard-issue RBC (oldest in inventory).... [S]tandard of care is "first in, first out" and the oldest available ABO identical RBC unit is transfused. This ethically imperative constraint restricts design options and can limit the power of any RCT.[11]

The RECESS study design compares outcomes of patients receiving red cells stored ≤10 days versus red cells stored ≥21 days. The first ethical concern raised by this approach is discussed above: older blood is believed to be inferior to fresh blood, so it may be unethical to assign patients "by design" to a treatment group that receives blood that is ≥21 days old, which is considered inferior. A second, more nuanced, ethical concern lies in the fact that the plan does not compare the investigational intervention (fresh red cells) to the standard of care (first in, first out). The proposed design is questionable because it does not compare the investigational intervention with standard practice as the benchmark. Instead, it compares two investigational interventions with each other (≤10 days old and ≥21 days old). In the worst-case scenario, it is possible that both interventions are harmful compared with the standard of care. Without a standard-of-care arm for comparison, potential harmful effects will not be detected.

The researchers in the RECESS trial justified the study design with the explanation that randomization to the ≤10 day or ≥21 day arms would take place only if the blood bank had sufficient units in the inventory to satisfy assignment into either arm, "hence, subjects randomized to the ≥21 day arm will receive RBC of the same storage time as they would have following the standard inventory practice of 'oldest units out first.'" The study proceeded accordingly. This approach may have addressed the first ethical concern, but not the second. Without question however, the study design sharpened the contrast between the fresh RBC and old RBC groups: the red cell storage times between groups had minimal overlap in storage duration and there was a 20-day difference in the mean durations of storage between the two arms.

The safest way to study the clinical effects of fresh versus old blood is to review data from past transfusions to see whether the age of the transfused red blood cells correlated with clinical outcomes such as death or increased hospital length of stay. Several retrospective reviews provided ambiguous results. A large meta-analysis published by Wang[21] et al. reported a 1.16 (1.07–1.24) odds ratio of death in patients treated with old blood. Does that mean the storage age of blood makes a difference? Perhaps not. In a busy hospital, patients receiving only a few units of blood may occasionally receive fresh units, but the more blood a patient receives, the more likely it is that the patient will receive a mixture of fresh and old blood. Fresher blood is therefore associated with smaller transfusion volumes and better outcomes, and older blood is associated with greater transfusion volumes and worse outcomes. Irrespective of storage age, larger volumes of blood are associated with increased odds of mortality. Only one of the studies in the meta-analysis attempted to correct for this confounder.[22] Thus, the small difference in outcomes observed in the meta-analysis could be explained by the correlation of volume transfused and increasing average storage age of blood.

Research addressing the clinical significance of the red blood cell storage lesion provides an illustration of how ethical limitations in human subject research can lead to challenging decision-making in clinical practice. Given the available retrospective data, clinicians must decide what to do for their patients. Does the sum of the in vitro evidence that points to a worrisome red cell storage lesion, combined with retrospective reviews hinting that fresh blood might be safer, mandate giving fresh blood to their patients? Beneficence may favor that approach. On the other hand, general adoption of that course would require costly, disruptive changes in the blood collection infrastructure. Even in the face of Wang et al.'s evidence presented in their meta-analysis, the authors themselves argued against instituting any changes in blood collection or utilization based on their findings. They noted that presently, fewer than 5% of red blood cells become outdated before being used and fewer than 5% of hospitals cancel surgeries due to lack of blood, and they concluded that the evidence did not yet support disrupting this hard-won success. To put the clinical decision into ethical terms, absent very compelling evidence, providing hypothetically "better" blood to some, at the expense of risking the adequacy of the blood supply for others who might have to do without, violates the principle of justice. Additionally, the cost of achieving an incremental improvement in blood potency due to the use of fresher blood may not be justified when compared to other potential uses for those health care dollars. Cognizant of those concerns, Wang et al. advocated further study using well-designed,

adequately powered, randomized controlled trials to determine whether it is imperative to institute major changes in blood collection and transfusion practice.

The ARIPI, RECESS, and ABLE trials are now complete. All three found no difference in clinical outcomes between patients who received fresh blood and those who received older blood. Given the potential disruption to the blood supply, these results were greeted with significant relief. Nevertheless, those studies did not settle all outstanding questions. Writing in the journal *Blood*, James Zimring[23] describes the results from ARIPI, RECESS, and ABLE as reassuring, but he notes that 5 million patients in the United States receive a red cell transfusion each year, so a mortality difference of only 1% would still translate into 50,000 patients annually. To put this number into perspective, the FDA reported that there were only 281 transfusion-related fatalities during the 4-year period from 2012 to 2016, due to such causes as TRALI, circulatory overload, incompatible blood, and infectious causes.[24] The loss of an additional 50,000 patients per year due to the age of blood being transfused would transform transfusion-related deaths into a staggering number. ABLE, RECESS, and ARIPI are not sufficiently powered to detect a 1% difference in mortality, so such a number of deaths could remain hidden from view. Zimring notes that animal studies are designed to maximize detection of clinical effects by transfusing large quantities of blood, and animal studies do in fact reveal substantial differences in mortality. ABLE, RECESS, and ARIPI all involved low transfusion volumes compared to the massive blood resuscitations seen in transplant, obstetric, and trauma settings. It would appear to be important to conduct trials evaluating fresh versus old blood in massive trauma resuscitation, for example, where the red cell storage lesion may have a much greater impact. If further large-scale trials are not practicable, then in light of the present evidence, can clinicians feel comfortable applying the results of ABLE, RECESS, and ARIPI to trauma resuscitation? These are important questions. However, as this discussion has emphasized, many practical, clinically relevant questions in blood safety are not definitively answered by research studies, for a variety of reasons. The questions therefore come back to clinicians who must use their best judgment, operating in the context incomplete information and scarce resources.

RISKS IN RESEARCH INVOLVING GENETICS AND HUMAN TISSUES

Transfusion medicine and cellular therapy research has by no means shunned molecular genetics. Techniques such as gene expression profiling and microRNA analysis are being used to study cellular responses to immunologic stimulation. The field of immunogenetics is being transformed by contemporary molecular techniques. In clinical practice, serology is being enhanced, and sometimes supplanted by, innovations in molecular testing. In the field of cellular therapy, the impact of donor and patient genetic heterogeneity is increasingly well understood due to newly available molecular techniques.

Clinical research involving human genetic analysis is subject to all of the complexities of other types of clinical research, while also bringing exceptional concerns of its own. For example, under the Federal Policy for the Protection of Human Subjects (most often referred to as the "Common Rule"),[25] human subject research is defined as research performed on a living individual, from whom an investigator obtains private, identifiable information through intervention or interaction with the individual. Thus, to be considered human subject research, the data relating to the subject must be identifiable, meaning that it can be traced to the research subject. If the information is not identifiable and cannot be traced to the subject, then the activity is not considered human subject research. This can be a very convenient state of affairs for researchers, because informed consent is not necessary if the activity is not human subject research. Contemporary tissue banks and biobanks are built on the understanding that nonidentifiable human tissues with accompanying clinical histories can be accessed without obtaining consent from the original subjects. Similarly, at the culmination of a research project, researchers often delete the personal information linking the tissue and clinical data to the research participants. The specimen and the accompanying clinical information have thus been "de-identified," meaning that the information can no longer be traced to the study subject who provided it, except perhaps through a responsible individual who maintains a key to link the information back to the subject if necessary. In such cases, investigators may obtain a waiver of informed consent to interrogate the biomaterial and its clinical data for use in additional research. An even stronger protection is achieved when the information is "anonymized," meaning that the link to the individual is irreversibly severed, and the subject can never be reidentified. In these cases, the research is exempt from oversight, and neither informed consent nor a waiver of informed consent is necessary.

We have entered into the genomic era, so samples containing genetic material, for example, any material containing nucleated cells, can never really be completely deidentified or anonymized because the DNA can always be unambiguously traced to the individual (barring cases such as identical twins). This causes a significant problem. Tissue banks are treasures of genetic material and accompanying clinical information that are carefully designed not to be traceable to the source. Consent is not required, so researchers can perform new research projects on the material without asking for the subject's permission. For example, to investigate whether a particular genetic mutation is associated with a particular tumor type, a researcher simply needs to pull the tissue off the shelf to find out, without having to locate the original subjects and obtain new informed consent.

On July 26, 2011, the United States Department of Health and Human Services (DHHS) announced an advance notice of proposed rulemaking (ANPRM), which proposed the first major revision of the Common Rule since it was adopted over 20 years previously.[26] The announcement observed that none of the prior statutes or rules governing human subjects research protections were "written with an eye toward the advances that have come in genetic and information technologies that make complete deidentification of biospecimens impossible and reidentification of sensitive health data easier." In its advance notice of proposed rulemaking, the Department of Health and Human Services proposed a significant number of changes to the Common Rule, but key among them was the proposed requirement that researchers must obtain a new informed consent for each future use of stored tissues. This requirement, if adopted, would impose a dramatic limitation in how banked tissues and other biobanks could be used. In the nascent era of genomic research, enormous data banks of genomic, biochemical, and clinical information were being built to enable bioinformatics techniques to reveal associations among clinical diseases, perturbations in physiology, and genetic variants. Databases of such magnitude—sometimes international in scope–would not lend themselves to reconsenting every subject for each new research project.

Four years later, on September 8, 2015, DHHS followed its advance notice of proposed rulemaking with publication of a Notice of Proposed Rulemaking (NPRM).[27] Similar to the Advanced Notice that preceded it, the NPRM advocated that new informed consent must be obtained from each research subject before additional research involving their nonidentified biospecimens could be conducted. During the comment period, Health and Human Services received more than 2100 comments on the proposed rules. Almost 50% of those comments addressed the proposal to require informed consent for nonidentified biospecimens, and 80% of those comments voiced opposition to the proposal. The dispositive resolution was announced in January, 2017, when the Final Rule was announced.[28] In the Final Rule, DHHS elected not to adopt the proposed change. No reconsent will be necessary for nonidentified biospecimens. The Final Rule goes into effect in 2018, as this book goes into print. The rules governing research use of nonidentified biospecimens will remain as they were in 2005.

As seen earlier, the use of tissue banks and genomic data repositories for research can raise significant issues involving privacy and personhood (i.e., autonomy) in the era of genomics and bioinformatics. These very concerns became even more acute in the case of Henrietta Lacks,[29] a mother of five young children. Lacks died of metastatic cervical cancer in 1951 at the young age of 31. Unbeknownst to Lacks or her family, tissue from her tumor had been removed and stored, and ultimately provided the cells that became the immortalized HeLa cell line. During the ensuing six decades, HeLa cells have been instrumental in incalculable numbers of scientific experiments and medical breakthroughs. They have also been commercialized, generating considerable revenue from research labs. Every aspect of the cell line, including its genome, has been thoroughly characterized, making HeLa cells a very valuable commodity.

The Lacks family learned of Henrietta's immortalized cell line in the 1970s, when members were asked to submit samples of their own for genetic analysis. Lacks' five children, whose ages ranged from 11 months to 16 years old when she died, were astonished to learn that cells from their mother were still alive. They were also surprised to learn of the scientific importance of their mother's cell line and the revenue that had been generated without the knowledge or permission of their mother or anyone in her family. Many of the children expressed pride that their mother's cell line had made such a significant contribution to science, but they nevertheless had important privacy concerns, including concerns about published genetic information that could reveal aspects of their own genomes. It is now reasonably well established from a legal point of view that Henrietta Lacks' family does not have property rights in the cell line derived from their mother's discarded tumor tissue.[30] Nor were all family members particularly interested in financial compensation. However, from the children's perspective, the cells were still alive, and they were from their mother' body. Some aspect of the mother they had lost as young children was still alive and contributing to society. An element of their mother's personhood was being perpetuated and facilitating important scientific work in the world—and her family had not even been informed. Such sentiments may or may not demand financial compensation, but unquestionably they are worthy of respect.

Beyond questions of their mother's personhood, the privacy concern for Lacks' children was real and immediate. Simply sequencing HeLa cells could place anyone in possession of 50% of each child's genome. The National Institutes of Health (NIH) did not believe that it had any legal obligations per se toward Lacks' family. However, representatives met with the family members several times and eventually reached an agreement that placed two family members on a committee that would regulate access to the genetic code of their mother's cells. This sharing of control over access to the genomic information contained in the cells demonstrated respect for the family members' privacy and also made it possible for them to participate in the science that was their mother's legacy. There is no perfect solution, but ongoing efforts by Lacks' family and the scientific community have continued to this day.

The enormous importance of large-scale genetic research will inevitably lead to vexing ethical questions. For example, when sequencing research subjects' genes, one might discover variants that are associated with a high risk of acquiring a disease or producing children with a disease. Among other considerations, this raises the question of whether the investigator has a duty to "return" research findings to the subject.[31] A clinically actionable finding might be the subject of the research project or it may be an "incidental" finding, that is, not part of the study but potentially clinically significant. At one end of the spectrum, some argue that an investigator has a duty to perform an analysis of all genetic information generated by the study and inform the subject of every finding that may be clinically significant. This could be extremely challenging. For the foreseeable future, the vast majority of incidental genetic findings are likely to be of uncertain significance, perhaps being the subject of scientific investigation in the research literature, but likely not of established clinical significance.[32] Many investigators argue that, in the absence of a physician-patient relationship and a specific agreement to return findings to research subjects, they should not share any information with the subject at all. The argument is that a doctor-patient relationship does not exist and the test was not performed as part of medical care, so there is no duty to disclose findings. Perhaps this seems harsh in the abstract, but the practical reality is that the relationship between the investigator and the research subject may be tenuous, and a forum for meeting with the subject to discuss research findings may not exist. The key is to recognize that significant risk lies in uncertainty. The proper resolution of questions regarding an investigator's duty to return clinically significant findings will ultimately depend on the nature of the findings and on the parties' expectations, which in turn depend on factors such as the existence of a concurrent physician-patient relationship, the availability of the subject for follow-up, and above all, the expectations on each side that were established at the outset. Ideally, all expectations about incidental findings should be discussed and agreed upon at the time of consent.

A NOVEL RISK: MEDICAL INNOVATION AND THE THERAPEUTIC MISCONCEPTION

The field that was once called "blood banking" is now referred to as "transfusion medicine and cellular therapy". As discussed in detail in Chapter 13, cellular products are living human tissue intended for use in treating patients. The field encompasses the collection, processing, manipulation, and infusion of somatic and embryonic stem cells, the entrainment of dendritic and other immune cells, the cellular delivery of viral vectors, and an increasing variety of other cellular techniques involving harvesting, extracorporeal manipulation, product characterization, and reinfusion. The clinical laboratory's role in cellular therapy is unlikely to diminish. As cell-based therapies become integrated into clinical practice, FDA requirements will demand the field's expertise, to consistently achieve and document regulatory compliance, and ensure the safety, purity, potency, and effectiveness of cellular products.

Valerie Gutmann Koch[33] and her coauthors, in a chapter on *Contemporary Ethical Issues in Stem Cell Research*, explore a useful distinction between clinical research in the field of cellular therapy and clinical research in other fields. In more mature areas of research, the concept of clinical equipoise—that is, a genuine uncertainty about the superiority of standard treatment over the experimental therapy—is generally considered to be an ethical imperative. Randomized, controlled, blinded clinical trials are the gold standard for establishing best practices, and enrolling large numbers of subjects improves investigators' ability to distinguish which is the superior therapy.

Cellular therapy, on the other hand, is a new area of clinical science. Research in cellular therapy is appropriately characterized as "medical innovation research." Clinical trials are not the gold standard in medical innovation research because there is no standard of care

against which to compare the experimental therapy. Instead, such research must be justified by a compelling scientific rationale as well as preclinical experimental evidence that supports the decision to attempt a trial in human subjects. Cellular therapy research is generally less formulaic than clinical trials involving drugs or devices. It is imperative that investigators pay a great deal of attention to the procedural protocol, product preparation, treatment regimen, data collection, outcomes assessment, and safety monitoring.

Different from a randomized clinical trial using large numbers of subjects to detect small differences in outcome, medical innovation research focuses on one individual at a time. The relationship between patient and investigator is complex: The subject is also a patient, and the trial therapy is intended to treat the patient's condition. It is easy to see why the therapeutic misconception is of particular concern in medical innovation research. A medical innovation trial can easily be perceived as a genuine, albeit unproven, treatment to help one's patient. It is therefore easy for a patient to expect the elements of a doctor-patient relationship to be in full effect during a trial. The danger with the therapeutic misconception is that the patient may perceive the trial as the physician's best effort at treatment, especially if the innovation is intended to cure a disease for which there has been no cure. The use of treatment or therapy-related terms such as "experimental treatment" or "gene therapy" to describe the research can unintentionally reinforce the therapeutic misconception.

From a research ethics point of view, the key danger of the therapeutic misconception is that it engenders a diminished appreciation on the part of the research subject that the intervention is an experiment rather than a treatment. To the extent that this misconception occurs, it negatively impacts the informed consent process and undermines patient autonomy.

That being said, we must also guard against being excessively paternalistic toward research subjects who participate in medical innovation research. It is entirely reasonable for a patient to understand that an innovative therapy is experimental, but still hope for a benefit. It is also entirely rational for an individual who suffers from a disease to be willing to participate in laying the groundwork for developing a cure for future sufferers of the same disease. In such cases, simply being aware of the risk of the therapeutic misconception and being careful to speak in frank and factual terms about the nature and goals of the research may be the best way to protect the research subject while honoring that individual's autonomy.

REFERENCES*

1. *Federalwide Assurance (FWA) for the Protection of Human Subjects.* 2018. https://www.hhs.gov/ohrp/register-irbs-and-obtain-fwas/fwas/index.html.
2. *Health Insurance Portability and Accountability Act of 1996,* Pub. L. No. 104-191. 1996. 110 Stat. 1936.
3. Tsuchiya T. The imperial Japanese experiments in China. In: Emanuel EJ, Grady C, Crouch RA, et al., eds. *The Oxford Textbook of Clinical Research Ethics.* New York: Oxford University Press; 2008:31–45.
4. Beecher HK. Ethics and clinical research. *N Engl J Med.* 1966;274:1354–1360.
5. Jones JH. *Bad Blood: The Tuskegee Syphilis Experiment.* New York: The Free Press; 1993.
6. National Research Service Award Act of 1974. 88 Stat. 342.
7. Code of Federal Regulations. *Basic HHS Policy for Protection of Human Research Subjects. Title 45, CFR Part 46(A).* Washington, DC: US Government Printing Office; 2014. revised annually).
8. Department of Health, Human Services. Waiver of informed consent requirements in certain emergency research. *Fed Regist.* 1996;61:51531–51533.
9. Borgman MA, Spinella PC, Perkins JG, et al. The ratio of blood products transfused affects mortality in patients receiving massive transfusions at a combat support hospital. *J Trauma.* 2007;63(4):805–813.
10. Duchesne JC, Hunt JP, Wahl G, et al. Review of current blood transfusion strategies in a mature level I trauma center: were we wrong for the last 60 years? *J Trauma.* 2008;65(2):272–276.
11. Perkins JG, Cap AP, Spinella PC, Blackbourne LH, et al. An evaluation of the impact of apheresis platelets used in the setting of massively transfused trauma patients. *J Trauma.* 2009;66(suppl 4):S77–S84.
12. Liumbruno GM, AuBuchon JP. Old blood, new blood or better stored blood? *Blood Transfus.* 2010;8:217–219.
13. D'Alessandro A, Liumbruno GM, Grazzini G, et al. Red blood cell storage: the story so far. *Blood Transfus.* 2010;8:82–88.
14. Flegel WA, Natanson C, Klein HG. Does prolonged storage of red blood cells cause harm? *Br J Haematol.* 2014;165:3–16.
15. *FDA Workshop on Red Cells Stored in Additive Solution Systems.* Bethesda, MD: US Food and Drug Administration; 1985.
16. Duchesne JB, Barbeau JM, Islam TM, et al. Damage control resuscitation: from emergency department to the operating room. *Am Surg.* 2011;77:201–206.
17. Lacroix J, Hebert PC, Fergusson DA, et al. Age of transfused blood in critically ill adults. *N Engl J Med.* 2015;372:1410–1418.
18. Fergusson DA, Hebert P, Hogan DL, et al. Effect of fresh red blood cell transfusions on clinical outcomes in premature, very-low birth weight infants. *J Am Med Assoc.* 2012;308:1443–1451.
19. Steiner ME, Ness PM, Assmann SF, et al. Effects of red-cell storage duration on patients undergoing cardiac surgery. *N Engl J Med.* 2015;372:1419–1429.
20. Alliance for Human Research Protection. *An Ethically Dubious Experiment: RECESS;* 2018. Available at: http://ahrp.org/an-ethically-dubious-blood-experiment-recess/.
21. Wang D, Sun J, Solomon SB, et al. Transfusion of older stored blood and risk of death: a meta-analysis. *Transfusion.* 2012;52:1184–1195.
22. Weinberg JA, McGwin G, Vandromme MJ, Marques MB. Duration of red cell storage influences mortality after trauma. *J Trauma.* 2012;69:1427–1432.
23. Zimring JC. Established and theoretical factors to consider in assessing the red cell storage lesion. *Blood.* 2015;125:2185–2190.
24. Food, Drug Administration. *Fatalities Reported to FDA Following Blood Collection and Transfusion: Annual Summary for Fiscal Year 2016.* Silver Spring, MD: CBER Office of Communication, Outreach, and Development; 2016–2018. https://www.fda.gov/downloads/BiologicsBloodVaccines/SafetyAvailability/ReportaProblem/TransfusionDonationFatalities/UCM598243.pdf.
25. 45 CFR part 46, subpart A.
26. Department of Health, Human Services. Human-subject research protections: enhancing protections for research subjects and reducing burden, delay, and ambiguity for investigators. *Fed Regist.* 2011;76:44512–44513.
27. Department of Health, Human Services. *Federal Policy for the Protection of Human Subjects. 80 Fed Reg 53931;* September 8, 2015. https://www.federalregister.gov/documents/2015/09/08/2015-21756/federal-policy-for-the-protection-of-human-subjects.
28. Department of Health, Human Services. *Common Rule Final Rule. 82 Fed Reg 7149, at 7164;* January 19, 2017. https://www.hhs.gov/ohrp/regulations-and-policy/regulations/finalized-revisions-common-rule/index.html.
29. Skloot R. *The Immortal Life of Henrietta Lacks.* New York: Crown Publishers; 2010.
30. Moore v. *Reagents of the University of California. 51 Cal. 3d 120; 271 Cal. Rptr. 146; 793 P.2d 479;* 1990.
31. Wolf SM. The past, present, and future of the debate over return of research results and incidental findings. *Genet Med.* 2012;14:355–357.
32. Couzin-Frankel J. What would you do? *Science.* 2011;331:662–665.
33. Koch VG, Roxland BE, Pohl B, Keech SK. Contemporary ethical issues in stem cell research. In: Sell S, ed. *Stem Cells Handbook.* New York: Humana Press; 2013:29–40.

*The author wrote an earlier version of this chapter that appeared in Domen RE. Ethical Issues in Transfusion Medicine and Cellular Therapies. Bethesda, Maryland: AABB Press; 2015. AABB Press has kindly given the author permission to borrow freely from the earlier text.

CHAPTER 15

Risk-Based Decision Making in Transfusion Medicine

J. MILLS BARBEAU, MD, JD

INTRODUCTION

How do we make decisions? Physicians make a constellation of medical decisions every day. Shall we start antibiotics? Recommend transferring the patient to hospice? Some healthcare decisions are more financially complex. Should we allocate funds to purchase a new MRI machine? Open a labor and delivery ward?

All decision making is fundamentally about change—deciding whether a change is indicated, and if so, choosing the best option among all others. Of course, change by its nature involves risk. Thus, for better or worse, all decisions are about change, and all change is accompanied by risk.

Risk-based decision making is the process of systematically assessing all of the risks that will accompany a contemplated change, in an effort to optimize one's decision. In our daily lives, we employ this process intuitively. We carry algorithms in our minds that guide us, such as when to start antibiotics, which drugs to choose, and when to discontinue or change the antimicrobial coverage. For higher-order decision making at the level of policy formulation, however, it is advisable to be more explicit and comprehensive in one's assessment of the risks that accompany a decision, and more systematic in the analysis of the options.

Formal risk-based decision making is used in a variety of contexts, both inside and outside of healthcare, and the process must inevitably be tailored to fit the subject matter.[1] The general principles of risk-based decision making remain similar, however, whether one is addressing environmental concerns, economic regulation, science funding, or healthcare policy. In all cases, the framework must not only provide a comprehensive technical analysis, but also include public and individual values within the decision framework.[2] The best available scientific judgment must be balanced against public risk perception and risk tolerance.[3] Fortunately, in the field of transfusion medicine, the process of risk-based decision making is already remarkably well defined, so we will begin by discussing how formal risk-based decision making is carried out.

THE PROCESS OF RISK-BASED DECISION MAKING IN TRANSFUSION MEDICINE

In the year 2011, risk-based decision making was not an entirely novel concept, particularly in government and industry. In transfusion medicine, however, 2011 was a watershed for risk-based decision making. In October of 2011, the proceedings of an international consensus conference on "Risk-Based Decision Making for Blood Safety" was published.[4] Hosted in Toronto by the Canadian Blood Services and Héma-Quebéc, the program included collaborators from France, Germany, UK, USA, Canada, Australia, and the Netherlands, primarily consisting of experts from academia, blood services, and governmental organizations. Blood services included the Alliance of Blood Operators, which is an international group comprised of Canadian Blood Services, America's Blood Centers, Australian Red Cross Blood Service, the European Blood Alliance, and the National Health Service Blood & Transplant (UK), as well as AABB, the American Red Cross, Blood Systems, Inc., and Héma-Quebéc.

Graham Sher of Canadian Blood Services provided the opening remarks. He began by stating:

> blood safety decision making has become increasingly complex and is not well served by traditional decision-making paradigms. An effective framework for risk-based decision making is needed, and there are diverse considerations implicated in the design of such a framework, including *scientific, medical, ethical, legal, regulatory, economic, and public policy perspectives.*

(Italics added.) He noted that blood safety decision-making was "increasingly complex, inconsistent, difficult to explain, and not obviously risk-based." He called for the development of a decision-making process that "addresses as much the science of blood safety as the ethics, social values, economics, public expectations, and historic context." The consensus statement generated by the conference was published in Vox Sanguinis the same year.[5]

Risk Management in Transfusion Medicine. https://doi.org/10.1016/B978-0-323-54837-3.00015-8

The consensus statement emphasized that the guiding blood safety paradigm has been to reduce risk to the lowest possible level, with negligible concern for cost. This was unsustainable, as perfect safety is unachievable. The costs and benefits of action—or inaction—must be ascertained using scientific evidence. Opportunity costs, meaning potential advantages that could be achieved if resources are deployed in other areas, must be considered in the cost-benefit analysis. Quality improvement must be an essential component of risk management, with an emphasis on product quality and unified standards. Risk management should be proactive, and risk-based decision making, as developed in other sectors of society, should be the standard. All stakeholders must be engaged in risk management decision making. Importantly, the ethical principles of autonomy, beneficence, and justice must guide the decision-making process. A very useful brochure published online by the Alliance of Blood Operators on April 2, 2015 provides an excellent guide to the risk-based decision-making process.[6]

The principles of risk-based decision making set forth in the 2011 "Risk-Based Decision Making for Blood Safety" consensus statement have stood the test of time. As healthcare costs rise and the demand for cost-saving measures increase, emerging infections continue to pose ever-increasing threats to the blood supply. Commentators continue to remind readers that the best way to manage costs and improve quality is through the disciplined use of risk-based decision making.[7-9]

On the first day of the consensus conference, Graham Sher's opening salvo announced that an effective framework for risk-based decision making is needed, and the design of the framework must include *scientific, medical, ethical, legal, regulatory, economic, and public policy perspectives*. Immediately thereafter he added *social values* and *historic context*. What might such a framework look like? How do the listed elements fit together? Why these elements and not others? Let us begin by listing the "perspectives" from which we are being asked to evaluate blood safety decisions.

> A risk-based framework for blood safety decision making incorporates the following perspectives:
>
> - Medical
> - Economic
> - Legal
> - Ethical
> - Regulatory
> - Public Policy
> - Historic
> - Social values

When healthcare decision makers consciously seek a broad range of perspectives, the process tends to look like this:

- Medical
- Economic

  - Legal
  - Ethical
  - Regulatory
  - Public Policy
  - Historic
  - Social values

Very often, when deciding whether to make healthcare expenditures, one hears an appeal to the cost-benefit ratio. If the cost-benefit ratio is favorable, then the cost is justified. Risk-based decision making is intended to raise the analysis to a level at which healthcare expenditures become sustainable. To achieve that goal, the items in the right-hand column need to be granted parity with those on the left. I propose to do so with a brief discussion of public policy.

I have proposed elsewhere a theory of public policy in which public policy and regulatory rulemaking are generated out of the daily workings of law, social values, history, and ethics, as shown below.

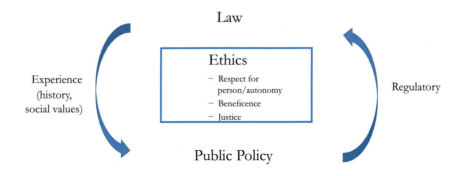

The process begins in the law, and there is no better place to start than with Justice Oliver Windell Holmes, Jr.

Why Law?

"A page of history is worth a volume of logic."
– Oliver Windell Holmes, Jr.

"The life of the law has not been logic; it has been experience."
– Oliver Windell Holmes, Jr.

Justice Oliver Wendell Holmes, from https://en.wikipedia.org/wiki/Oliver_Wendell_Holmes_Jr.

In a well-ordered civil society, people generally know the rules of behavior in a given social or commercial context. Sometimes in the course of daily life, however, an individual may engage in activities that another finds objectionable. Imagine that it is early in the Industrial Revolution, and one party builds a factory on a river immediately upstream from a prosperous farm. The farmer needs fresh water for her farm, but the industrialist needs to consume the water and discharge the effluent. The farmer believes her rights to fresh water have been violated, but if the industrialist is ordered to stop polluting, he will believe his rights have been violated.

There is a first time for every type of conflict, and if the parties cannot resolve the problem–and they are sufficiently motivated–they end up in court. In common law jurisdictions such as the United States and Great Britain, the courts seek precedent from earlier cases to guide them, and with the help of juries as fact-finders, courts do their best to craft a fair outcome in light of prior precedents. If the facts are distinguishable from all prior cases, or if prior precedents would unintentionally produce anomalous results as applied to the present case, parties can distinguish their case and appeal to justice. The common law is thus a learning legal system, based on experience, history, and the social values of the culture in which it evolved.

As a maturing body of case law develops in a given area of activity, various themes begin to appear, as solutions to particular types of conflicts are proven reliable. If the corpus of successful resolutions becomes robust, it may be possible to achieve great efficiencies by codifying the rules of conduct in that sphere of activity. In the United States, this is commonly achieved by a Congressional act authorizing regulatory rulemaking in that field. As regulatory activity in that sphere of activity continues to mature, so might formal and informal regulatory rulemaking.

A key point to recognize is that the ethical principles of autonomy, beneficence, and justice are at all times the glue that holds the process together. In the courtroom, in Congress, and in regulatory rulemaking, the desired outcomes are directed toward autonomy (self-determination), beneficence (care for others), and justice (distributive justice, a fair allocation of resources, responsibilities, and rights).

In the United States, the processes outlined above describe virtually everything that we refer to as public policy. Of course, once the wheel starts spinning, it is difficult to see where the process of public policy begins or ends. We continue to learn from experience, study history, have recourse to the courts, pass statutes, promulgate regulations, and moor our public policy activities to the three ethical pillars. It is instructive to start with the courts, however, because all new sources of conflict—cases of first impression—do, in fact, start in the courts. This may be public policy's creation myth, but it is one with considerable explanatory power.

We have examined the elements of risk-based decision making. Now, it is time to apply risk-based decision making to an actual case—indeed, a very interesting case–so that we may judge its utility for ourselves.

THE HOLY GRAIL

In late December, as the 2015 New Year was approaching, the Food & Drug Administration (FDA) surprised the United States' blood banking and transfusion medicine community by announcing the approval of a blood system[10] for inactivating infectious pathogens in plasma[11] and in platelets collected by apheresis (i.e., single-donor platelets).[12] Indeed, the newly approved blood system was capable of inactivating a remarkably large variety of infectious organisms. The system works by exposing the organisms to a photochemical process based on amotosalen, which is a psoralen compound. Psoralens possesses the inherent characteristic of intercalating into deoxyribonucleic acid (DNA) or ribonucleic acid (RNA). Once in place, amotosalen can be activated by exposure to ultraviolet A (UV-A) light, causing the amotosalen to cross-link the DNA or RNA pyramidine bases, rendering the organism incapable of replicating:

| 1 | Intercalates into Regions of DNA and RNA | 2 | Crosslinks upon UVA Illumination | 3 | Blocks Replication, Transcription and Translation |

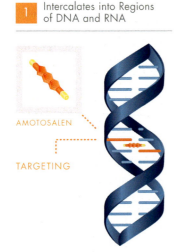

AMOTOSALEN

TARGETING

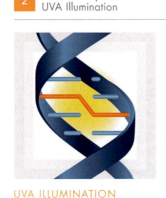

UVA ILLUMINATION

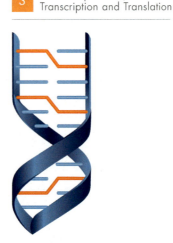

Psoralens possess a constellation of characteristics that suit them to the task of pathogen inactivation. Their reactivity with nucleic acid pyrimidine bases is highly specific, but since pyrimidines are universal, the psoralens are able to target a wide variety of infectious organisms, as long as their nucleic acids are accessible to the chemical. Amotosalen binds pathogen and lymphocyte nucleic acids equally well. Therefore, amotosalen not only cross-links the nucleic acids of infectious agents, preventing them from replicating, but also cross-links nucleic acids of lymphocytes in the donor's blood ("passenger" white cells), preventing the foreign lymphocytes from mounting an immune response against the recipient. In other words, amotosalen can protect against transfusion-associated graft-versus-host disease.

Psoralens interact with nucleic acids at a high frequency even at very low concentrations of reactants, effectively finding DNA and RNA among biologic molecules. They merely intercolate, however. They do not actually cross-link the nucleic acids unless they are activated by UV-A light. Therefore, psoralens have the dual attributes of covering a broad spectrum of targets (almost any organism with DNA or RNA), and they can be turned on and off like a light.[13] Psoralen activation is performed extracorporeally, and after the pathogen inactivation process is complete, a wash step is performed prior to transfusion. If any amotosalen remains in the plasma or platelets when they are transfused, it seems unlikely that the amotosalen would be exposed to UV-A light in the patient's bloodstream:

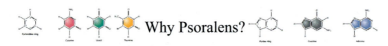

Why Psoralens?

- Reactivity with nucleic acid *pyrimidine bases* is highly specific
- Psoralens have no *sequence* specificity
  - Not selective for specific organisms: Binds pathogen and lymphocyte nucleic acids
- Interaction with nucleic acid occurs with high frequency at low concentrations of reactants
  - The psoralen hones in on DNA/RNA among biologic molecules
- Psoralen-nucleic acid crosslinking occurs only in UVA light
  - Broad spectrum, but turned on and off by light

One cannot help but be struck by the elegance of the new amotosalen-based pathogen inactivation system. However, certain questions needed to be raised. The processing steps in pathogen reduction lead to reduced potency of blood components. Could that reduction in potency lead to more deaths than it prevents?[14] Does the pathogen inactivation process neutralize every single pathogen that is present? If not, microbes may still be able to proliferate inside the patient. The FDA had to set a standard, and it settled upon a requirement that the extent of pathogen inactivation must be at least a 4 log reduction of infectivity. "Infectivity" is defined as the ability to replicate, which could be determined, for example, by PCR. If the burden of pathogens is high, might the unit of blood still sometimes be infective?

Another concern might be the class of drugs used for pathogen inactivation. Psoralen compounds are an important source of chemotherapy agents precisely because they are capable of cross-linking cancer DNA. Psoralens are associated with carcinogenesis. How likely might it be that blood recipients might develop various forms of cancer? If somehow pathogen inactivation could cause sporadic cancers, what kind of epidemiological surveillance would be able to detect that effect? Should we transfuse children with pathogen-inactivated blood?

How much will pathogen inactivation cost—and are there better uses for the money? Perhaps the impact would be greater if we spent resources on surveillance, domestically or in countries where emerging infectious diseases are endemic. Perhaps an investment in foreign public health initiatives would protect the US blood supply more effectively than adding amotosalen to donor blood in the United States.[15]

RISK-BASED DECISION MAKING CASE STUDY: PATHOGEN INACTIVATION

Within weeks of the FDA's announcement that it had approved a system for inactivating pathogens in plasma and apheresis platelets, AABB organized a symposium in Bethesda, Maryland, on implementation of pathogen-reduced blood components, which was held April 27–28, 2015. A chief goal of the symposium was to frame a risk-based decision-making approach to evaluating the risks and opportunities presented by the new technology, and to formulate a plan for filling gaps in the knowledge needed for decision making. The symposium included leaders in blood banking and transfusion medicine, representatives from FDA, Centers for Disease Control and Prevention (CDC), and industry, scientists and statisticians, and representatives from Canadian and European blood centers with experience implementing pathogen inactivation in clinical practice.

Very much in the spirit of risk-based decision making, the first speaker, Harvey Klein, MD, gave a talk entitled "Pathogen Inactivation: Rationale and Some History." And indeed, history plays a very important role in our thinking about transfusion-transmitted infectious diseases, particularly in light of the Acquired Immunodeficiency Syndrome (AIDS) epidemic. Throughout the symposium, AIDS, ethics, law, and societal preferences took their place beside scientific, medical, and economic considerations. An overview of the AABB symposium will provide an excellent illustration of risk-based decision making at work.

To illuminate the relevant historic background and resulting societal preferences, HIV is an appropriate place to start. HIV's entry into the blood supply in the 1980s led to an attitude toward transfusion-transmitted infectious diseases that has been characterized as the "safe blood paradox." Blood has never been safer—but it is never safe enough. This attitude is pervasive on an international scope, as seen in lead sentences of scientific articles, such as Kitchen et al. in the United Kingdom: "The safety of allogeneic blood and blood products in relation to infectious risk is paramount, even though absolute safety is an ideal that clearly cannot be attained,"[16] and Velthove et al. in the Netherlands: "The viral safety of plasma-derived medicinal products is of paramount importance."[17]

Canada, in response to HIV's entry into the blood supply, convened the Krever Commission, which issued a landmark report on "the tainted blood scandal of the 1980s".[18] The Commission collected evidence and held hearings beginning in 1993, issuing a final report in 1997. As a result of the Commission's findings, Canada restructured its national blood system and adopted a precautionary approach to blood safety. In formulating Canada's restructured blood system, the Krever Commission articulated the new Principles of the Master Agreement as follows:

1. Voluntary donations should be maintained.
2. National self-sufficiency … should be encouraged.
3. Adequacy and security of supply … should be encouraged.
4. Safety of all blood … should be paramount.
5. Gratuity of all blood … should be maintained.
6. A cost-effective and cost-efficient blood supply program … should be encouraged.
7. A national blood supply program should be maintained.[18]

Note that, among all of the principles of Canada's new Master Agreement, only the safety of blood on line 4 is singled out as being paramount, whereas cost-effectiveness and cost-efficiency on line 6 are only to be encouraged. When asked about "the conflict between safety on the one hand and cost-efficiency and cost-effectiveness on the other," one official, Mr. Desch, responded:

Safety should be paramount. Now, does that mean it should override everything else? My understanding of "paramount" is that is what it should be, the one and foremost. However, when you have a policy down below of cost effective and cost efficient, you may start to run into some inconsistences or some difficulties in balancing those two ... principles.

We thus recognize at the outset that, in applying risk-based decision making, decisions regarding implementation of pathogen inactivation will have to take into account an inherent conflict between a risk-benefit versus a zero-tolerance approach.

Michael Busch's iconic[19] graph depicts the time-line of the arrival of HIV in the United States, the virus' entry into the blood supply, and the effectiveness of early interventions to protect the blood supply:

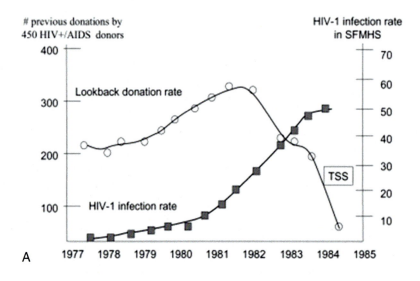

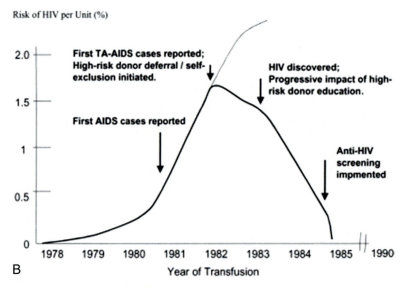

As one can see from the Busch graph, the first AIDS cases in the United States were identified in 1980–81. In 1982, it was proven that AIDS could be transmitted by transfusion. In 1983, the HIV virus was identified. During this time period, epidemiologic strategies established the existence of high-risk groups consisting of male homosexuals, IV drug abusers and their sexual partners, and—as users of Factor VIII concentrate–hemophiliacs. The increasing awareness that there were high-risk donor groups, that HIV was virus, and that the virus was transmissible by blood transfusion was sufficient in itself to begin to reduce the prevalence of HIV in the blood supply. Donor education and increasing awareness of HIV's transmissibility through blood transfusions led to donor self-exclusion, which drove HIV risk per unit of blood almost to the far-right edge of Busch's graph.

The ability to test donor blood for HIV was achieved in 1985. As one can see on Busch's graph, anti-HIV screening of donor blood using ELISA testing accounted for the post-1985 decrease at the extreme far right end of the tail. For more than 30 years, the United States has concentrated on driving the post-1985 transmission rates ever downward, most recently by universal screening using nucleic acid testing ("NAT testing"). It should be noted that this approach is a zero-tolerance approach—it is not a risk-benefit approach, but rather zero tolerance. During the 6-year period from 2002 to 08, there was not a single reported case of transfusion-transmitted HIV infection in the United States.[20] By way of comparison, during the 4-year period from 2005 to 2010, FDA reported 307 transfusion-related fatalities (~61/year) from all causes.[21] From a risk-benefit point of view, there may be other risks than HIV that could lay claim to our healthcare resources. Transfusion-related acute lung injury (TRALI), for example, went from being the highest source of transfusion-associated mortality to being relatively low-risk, simply due to implementation of proper interventions. In absolute numbers, more lives may be saved by targeting the lowest-cost interventions, yet we recognize that transmitting even a few cases of HIV each year through blood transfusions is not tolerable from a societal perspective, so universal nucleic acid testing (NAT) testing continues.

Today, the rate at which newly recognized emerging pathogens threaten the blood supply seems to be accelerating. For every such pathogen, a new blood test may need to be developed, approved by FDA, and implemented. By the time the first pathogen reduction technology was approved by the FDA, the biggest concern in the transfusion community was whether we can afford to hammer down to zero every infectious risk that threatens to enter the blood supply.

The idea of a single, one-size-fits-all approach that will eliminate virtually all infectious pathogens is enormously appealing. Pathogen reduction technology appears to provide that capability. Because the technology depends on cross-linking DNA or RNA, it can affect nearly all pathogens. The list of pathogens that are not reliably inactivated is short, including organisms such as nonenveloped viruses (Hepatitis A, Hepatitis B, Parvovirus B19, and Poliovirus), prions, and some spore-forming bacteria such as Bacillus cereus. So far, the recent emerging pathogens, such as Ebola and Zika viruses, appear to be susceptible to pathogen reduction.

It must be noted that the two FDA-approved pathogen reduction systems are only cleared for use in plasma and apheresis platelets. There are some technical hurdles to cross before pathogen inactivation can be approved for use on red blood cells, which is ultimately where the largest impact would be felt. Meanwhile, there are other companies developing analogous technology that may improve the inactivation process even further.

If we choose to move toward implementing a pathogen reduction technology that promises to render the blood supply safe from almost all infectious agents, will that technology replace NAT testing and other currently mandated screening? Here is where we may be the most burdened by history. Given our historic zero tolerance approach to infectious disease transmission in blood transfusions, will societal and historic pressures tolerate our abandoning current (and anticipated) testing for HIV, Hepatitis B and C, syphilis, West Nile virus, Zika, and other emerging pathogens?

At the AABB symposium on implementing pathogen inactivation, the economics experts reported that pathogen reduction could be affordable only if the present pathogen-specific testing is discontinued. In other words, to make pathogen reduction technology economically feasible, at least some of our current testing must be eliminated.[22-24] Here we feel most acutely the burden of history. Societal preferences are informed not only by our history of HIV in the blood supply, but also by our current experience with emerging infections, eagerly covered by the news and social media. We have thus identified an important knowledge gap that must be filled before our risk-based decision making can go forward: What is the level of societal tolerance for removing current testing and replacing it with pathogen reduction technology?

At this point, we have begun to glean how risk-based decision making is playing out in the context of pathogen reduction technology. We have touched on medical, scientific, and economic considerations, examined the historic context, and identified the need to better assess societal preferences. With the FDA, we have touched on regulatory policy, although we will have a few more observations regarding regulatory and public policy considerations at the end of our analysis. This leaves us with the legal evaluation as the only element of risk-based decision making that we have not yet addressed.

It may not seem immediately apparent how a legal analysis could contribute much to a decision whether to adopt pathogen reduction technology. Indeed, when I was asked to speak on the legal aspects of pathogen reduction at the AABB symposium, I was not certain how much one could expect to offer. Nevertheless, the point of risk-based decision making is to work systematically through a framework that is designed to ensure that all important risks are identified and considered in the decision process. In this case, adhering to the principles of risk-based decision making and taking a close look at legal considerations turned out to reveal some surprises.

We examined fundamental legal concepts in Chapter 10, and now we have an opportunity to apply them. The reader may recall the elements of a case for negligence:

Law Suit for Negligence

<u>Elements of a negligence claim</u>:

- Duty (duty of care)
- Breach
- Causation
  - Proximate cause
- Harm

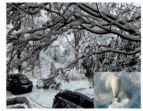

To be liable for negligence, one must first owe a duty of care toward the injured party. In the case of medical negligence (medical malpractice), the duty of care is established when the parties enter into a doctor-patient relationship. Once the duty is established, the plaintiff must prove that the physician breached the duty of care by failing to provide the level of care that an ordinary physician would have provided, and the failure to deliver that level of care caused actual harm to the patient.

Accordingly, the first element in a negligence case is proving that the defendant owed a duty to the plaintiff. A home owner owes a duty to pedestrians to keep sidewalks clear and free of ice. However, if a polar bear were to slip and fall, its lawsuit would fail, since the home owner does not owe a duty of care toward polar bears. Similarly, a physician does not owe a duty of care to someone unless that person is her patient.

Once a medical duty of care is established, the next step in a medical malpractice case is to determine whether the duty of care was breached. This requires a determination of whether the care lived up to the "standard of care" in medical practice. Here things get tricky. If a patient is injured by a pathogen that would have been inactivated by psoralen-treated blood, what standard of care would the treating physician be held to? What would be the standard of care for protecting blood recipients from infectious diseases? Is there a duty to eliminate infectious risks at all costs, i.e., zero tolerance? Or must treating physicians maximize the cost-benefit profile for blood, spending resources judiciously to maximize benefits for the greatest number of patients?

At this point, it may be useful to recall the three ethical pillars of autonomy, beneficence, and justice. Autonomy (patient choice) suggests that we should at least be certain to include patient preferences and social values into our risk-based decision making in the first place, since it would be impracticable for blood suppliers to offer a dual supply and allow each patient to choose whether to use the pathogen-reduced product. Beneficence and justice get to the standard of care issue. Beneficence is the treating physician's cardinal principle: The physician has a fiduciary duty to the patient, putting the patient's interests above other concerns. Justice, on the other hand, is more oriented to shepherding resources, maximizing overall benefit, and equitable sharing of rights and responsibilities. With a moment's reflection, one sees that a physician's standard of care is based on beneficence, which is individual-oriented, whereas public health is based on justice, which is community-oriented. As shown below, the same three ethical principles apply to both the doctor-patient and the public health roles, but the standard of care for evaluating pathogen reduction technology that would apply in the doctor-patient and public health contexts is likely to be different. An individual physician would be expected to provide the safest available option for her patient, whereas a public health official would be expected to provide options that maximize benefits for all:

Ethical Principles & Duty of Care

Relationship to Patient	Ethical Duty	Standard of Care For Evaluating PR
Doctor-Patient	Respect for autonomy **Beneficence** Justice	Choice/informed consent Maximize patient safety Clinical best practices
Public Health (FDA, AABB)	Respect for autonomy Beneficence **Justice**	Choice/informed consent Maximize risk-benefit Maximize cost-benefit

Armed with this legal review, we can make use of an important lawsuit, *William Snyder v. American Association of Blood Banks*.[25] The plaintiff, William Snyder, tragically contracted HIV in 1984 from a transfusion received during open-heart surgery. HIV-specific ELISA testing was not available until 1985. At the time of Mr. Snyder's surgery, donor screening questionnaires were in place, and the transfusion medicine community was debating whether to adopt a surrogate test, Hepatitis B core antibody, that correlated with HIV risk. The American Red Cross and AABB did not recommend the surrogate test. Their concerns included the impact on the blood supply, the cost and lack of specificity of the screening test, and what at the time appeared to be a low transmissibility of HIV by blood transfusion.

Snyder alleged that AABB was negligent for failing to recommend surrogate testing and screening, specifically claiming that AABB had a duty to recommend Hepatitis B core testing. Snyder won the case, and the judgment against AABB was affirmed on appeal.

One may well have misgivings about this judgment. First, the initial step in a negligence case is to prove that the defendant owed a duty to the plaintiff. AABB is a private, tax exempt, not-for-profit professional association. Why would AABB have a duty to Snyder to make any kind of recommendation on any subject? Snyder seems to be a polar bear! As it turns out, he was not. It is generally true that professional organizations do not owe a duty to promulgate recommendations. A professional association for swimming pool installers does not owe anyone a duty to promulgate guidelines for safe pool dimensions.[26–28] However, the appellate court was persuaded by the argument that AABB had placed itself in a position of authority and responsibility by establishing a near-monopoly on inspecting,

certifying, and issuing standards governing blood banking and transfusion medicine. According to the court, AABB had so much control over blood practices, and thus control over blood providers, that AABB had made itself almost governmental in its authority. Therefore, AABB had a duty to Mr. Snyder to promulgate regulations on HIV testing.

If the court was correct in finding that AABB owed a *duty* to Snyder to promulgate recommendations, the next step should have been to determine what the *standard of care* is for issuing recommendations, and whether AABB breached that standard. It seems quite possible that AABB could have protected itself considerably simply by improving its documentation regarding the reasoning for declining to recommend Hepatitis B surrogate testing. After all, the correlation between Hepatitis B status and HIV status was uncertain, and universal implementation of Hepatitis B core antibody testing would have been very expensive. Significantly, it was clear by 1984 that an enzyme-linked immunosorbent assay (ELISA) test specific for HIV would soon be approved.

Indeed, in July 1984, FDA's Blood Products Advisory Committee's Hepatitis B Core Antibody Testing Study Group reported its conclusions regarding the Hepatitis B core antibody test. The group consisted of 11 members, representing the FDA, plasma fractionators, AABB, and other important blood-industry associations. A majority of the group rejected the Hepatitis B core test, believing it would result in rejection of too many healthy donors, it was not sufficiently specific, and it cost too much. They also believed that self-screening was working effectively. A minority countered that the Hepatitis B core test would exclude a significant percentage of high-risk donors, which would have saved lives.[29]

If AABB was obligated, by virtue of its leadership role in transfusion practices, to promulgate recommendations regarding HIV testing, its standard of care should have been a "public health" standard (risk-benefit and cost-benefit rather than zero-tolerance). AABB appears to have done precisely that. Given the circumstances as they existed in 1984, AABB should not have been considered negligent in declining to recommend Hepatitis B testing. The record demonstrates that AABB performed an assessment of the strategies available at the time, in light of the science as known at that time, and it came to a rational conclusion regarding the utility of Hepatitis B surrogate testing.

The lesson to be learned today is that AABB should document its risk-based analysis regarding pathogen reduction technology. A holistic examination of the advantages, disadvantages, and remaining uncertainties regarding pathogen inactivation technology is already well under way. The industry standard for decision making in the field of transfusion medicine is risk-based decision making, so AABB has largely satisfied its standard of care by supporting the ongoing analysis of the technology. The evaluation is still ongoing, but plasma and single-donor platelets are now on the market, and fact-gathering in gap areas continues to go forward, with the expectation that pathogen reduction technology will eventually be available for red blood cells. AABB appears to be meeting the standard of care for policy-formulation in this field, although it has not issued formal recommendations.

Our legal considerations regarding pathogen reduction technology lead us to one last byway: Strict liability law. In Chapter 10, we addressed strict liability for harm caused by blood products. Strict product liability is a legal concept that originated in manufacturing. Product liability is "strict" because an injured plaintiff can recover for injuries without having to prove that the manufacturer was negligent. As we saw in Chapter 10, when infectious diseases like hepatitis entered the blood supply, patients began to sue hospitals and blood banks under a theory of strict liability. The blood provider may not have been negligent, but any patient who received "tainted blood" could sue under strict liability for injuries or death caused by the blood.

To protect the blood banking industry from ruin, states across the country passed so-called "blood shield" laws to protect blood providers from being sued under strict liability. The laws invariably declared that blood is not a product, and providing blood to patients is a medical service, not a sale. This legal history is quite important in the context of pathogen reduction technology. The chemicals that bind RNA and DNA in pathogen inactivation technology are not blood or blood products. They are chemicals that are added to blood. Therefore, physicians, hospitals, and blood banks may be strictly liable for any and all harm that is caused by pathogen reduction technology.

This discussion of legal aspects of pathogen reduction technology completes our review of risk-based decision making as it has applied to pathogen reduction. Appropriately, we will end with some comments about public policy. We began the chapter with a discussion of how public policy is compounded out of law, ethics, history, societal preferences, and regulatory initiatives. At precisely the time that AABB's Symposium on Implementation of Pathogen-Reduced Blood Components was being organized, the New England Journal of Medicine published a perspective piece by Edward Snyder, Susan Stramer, and Richard Benjamin, entitled "The Safety of the Blood Supply–Time to Raise the Bar."[30] All three authors were in attendance at the AABB symposium.

Snyder et al. begin their article with a discussion of the historic approach to blood pathogens, noting that the field has relied on a reactive approach, implementing screening tests in response to each new pathogen that is identified, an expensive approach that is not sustainable. They urge FDA to mandate a proactive approach by requiring universal blood treatment with approved pathogen reduction technologies. They note that new pathogens continue to emerge, including Ebola, dengue, chikunkunya, hepatitis E, pandemic influenza, and SARs viruses, and they argue that adoption of pathogen reduction technology could allow the elimination of at least some screening costs.

The authors urge the federal government to mandate universal pathogen reduction, driving adoption by supporting a reimbursement schema that recognizes the costs that will be avoided by a proactive strategy. By asking the federal government to mandate universal pathogen reduction, the authors are providing a way to protect blood providers from legal liability for unanticipated harms, while also shifting the responsibility away from blood providers to pay for the technology. The suggestion that adoption of pathogen reduction technology could allow "certain screening tests, along with their costs" to be eliminated, is a clear call to shift away from a zero-tolerance paradigm to a cost-benefit approach.

One may agree or disagree with the authors' call to action, but it is a remarkable piece of advocacy, and a clear call for a new public policy approach to protecting patients from infectious, blood-borne pathogens. As such, it is a compelling illustration of how a risk-based approach to public health problems can lead to more comprehensive and more nuanced decision making, and ultimately to better policy formulation.

REFERENCES

1. Walker D, ed. *Principles of Risk-based Decision Making*. Rockville: Government Institutes; 2001.
2. Bohnenblust H, Slovic P. Integrating technical analysis and public values in risk-based decision making. *Reliab Eng System Saf*. 1998;59:151–159.
3. Pidgeon N. Risk assessment, risk values and the social science programme: why do we need risk perception research? *Reliab Eng System Saf*. 1998;59:5–15.
4. Bennett JL, Blajchman MA, Delage G, Devine D. Proceedings of a consensus conference: risk-based decision making for blood safety. *Transfus Med Rev*. 2011;25(4):267–292.
5. Stein J, Besley J, Brook C, et al. Risk-based decision-making for blood safety: preliminary report of a consensus conference. *Vox Sang*. 2011;101:277–281.
6. Alliance of Blood Operators. *Risk-based Decision-making Framework for Blood Safety*, v1.1 ; April 2, 2015. https://allianceofbloodoperators.org/media/115522/rbdm-framework-2-april-2015-v11-for-website.pdf.
7. Devine DV. Implementation of pathogen inactivation technology: how to make the best decisions? *Transfusion*. 2017;57:1109–1111.
8. Custer B, Janssen MP. Health economics and outcomes methods in risk-based decision-making for blood safety. *Transfusion*. 2015;55:2039–2047.
9. Bennett JL. Making good policy decisions: a discipline we cannot afford to ignore. *Transfusion*. 2015;55:2775–2777.
10. Cerus Corporation's Intercept Blood System.
11. *FDA Announcement*. December 16, 2014.
12. *FDA Announcement*. December 19, 2014.
13. Wollowitz S. *Semin Hematol*. 2001;38(suppl 11):4–11.
14. Hess JR, Pagano MB, Barbeau JM, Johannson PI. Will pathogen reduction of blood components harm more people than it helps in developed countries? *Transfusion*. 2016;56:1236–1241.
15. Indeed, such a program may have positive externalities: improving public health in poorer countries could pay for itself, potentially generating an economic boon on a global scale.
16. Kitchen AD, Barbara AJ. Current information on the infectious risks of allogenic blood transfusion. *Transfus Altern Transfus Med*. 2008;10:102–111.
17. Velthove KJ, Over J, Abbink K, Janssen MP. Viral safety of human plasma-derived medicinal products: impact of regulation requirements. *Transfus Med Rev*. 2013;27:179–183.
18. Krever H. *Final Report: Commission of Inquiry on the Blood System in Canada*. Ottawa: The Commission; 1997:1012–1014. Part 4.
19. Busch MP. Transfusion-transmitted viral infections: building bridges to transfusion medicine to reduce risks and understand epidemiology and pathogenesis. *Transfusion*. 2006;46(9):1624–1640.
20. *Morbidity and Mortality Weekly Report (MMWR)*. 2010;59(41):1335–1339.
21. *Fatalities Reported to FDA Following Blood Collection, Transfusion: Annual Summary for Fiscal Year*. 2010. http://mnperfsoc.org/images/2010_FDA_Blood_TX_Collection_Fatalities.pdf.
22. Custer B, Agapova M, Martinez RH. The cost-effectiveness of pathogen reduction technology as assessed using a multiple risk reduction model. *Transfusion*. 2010;50:2461–2473.
23. Ellingson KD, Sapiano MRP, Haass KA, et al. Cost projections for implementation of safety interventions to prevent transfusion-transmitted Zika virus infection in the United States. *Transfusion*. 2017;57:16251633.
24. McCullough J, Goldfinger D, Gorlin J, et al. Cost implications of implementation of pathogen-inactivated platelets. *Transfusion*. 2015;55:2312–1241.
25. Snyder v. American Association of Blood Banks. 676 A. 2d 1036 144 N.J. 1996;269.
26. Meyers v. *Donnataci, 220 N.J. Super. 73, 531 A.2d 398 (Law Div; 1987)*.
27. Beasock v. *Dioguardi Enterprises, Inc., 130 Misc. 2d 25, 494 N.Y.S.2d 974 (Sup. Ct. Monroe Co. 1985)*.
28. Howard v. *Poseidon pools, Inc., 133 Misc. 2d 50, 506 N.Y.S.2d 523 (Sup. Ct. Allegheny Co. 1986)*.
29. Snyder, supra.
30. Snyder EL, Stramer SL, Benjamin RJ. The safety of the blood supply – time to raise the bar. *N Engl J Med*. 2015;372:20–23.

Index

Note: Page numbers followed by "f" indicate figures, "t" indicate tables.

Printed in the United States
By Bookmasters